Young Onset Dementia Reconsidered

Young Onset Dementia Reconsidered

A Solution-Focused Approach

Jan R. Oyebode and George Rook (eds.)

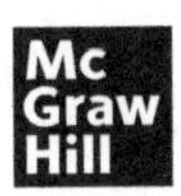

Open University Press

Open University Press
McGraw Hill
Unit 4
Foundation Park
Roxborough Way
Maidenhead
SL6 3UD

email: emea_uk_ireland@mheducation.com
world wide web: www.mheducation.co.uk

Executive Editor: Sam Crowe
Editorial Assistant: Hannah Jones
Content Product Manager: Graham Jones
Cover Design: Adam Renvoize
Cover Art: Gail Gregory
Logo Design: Julia Heron

A catalogue record of this book is available from the British Library

ISBN-13: 9780335252497
ISBN-10: 0335252494
eISBN-13: 9780335252503

Typeset by Transforma Pvt. Ltd., Chennai, India

Praise Page

progress and changes since, the book keeps its promise to reconsider what have learnt so far and how research outcomes are best applied in practice.

The editors have assembled contributions from a wide range of inspiring experts, thoroughly covering the specialist themes arising in YOD. My greatest joy in perusing this book though are the contributions from people living with YOD who bring alive the academic and research outputs with their insights and lived experience. This is what makes the book so readable and relatable, not only for professionals and students, but also for people affected by YOD and the general public."

Reinhard Guss, Consultant Clinical Psychologist,
Clinical Neuropsychologist;
Former Chair and Dementia Lead of Faculty of Psychology
of Older People in the British Psychological Society;
Former Convenor of European Standing Committee on Geropsychology
and Founding Member of the Young Dementia Network.

Contents

List of figures, tables and boxes

About the editors

George Rook worked as an accountant, an English teacher and a secondary school business manager. At the age of 62 he was diagnosed with Alzheimer's and vascular dementia. Since then he has established the Shropshire and Telford Dementia Action Alliance and chairs the Dementia Steering Group for his locality. He has chaired the 3 Nations Dementia Working Group. He is also a member of the National Audit of Dementia and Memory Service National Accreditation Project teams. George takes part in research as a co-researcher, and was one of the Dementia Enquirers with Innovations in Dementia, developing guidance for the role of people living with dementia in research. George also blogs about living as well as you can with dementia.

Jan R. Oyebode is Professor of Dementia Care at the University of Bradford, UK. She previously worked as a clinical psychologist in the National Health Service, which is where she became interested in how to better support people living with young onset dementia and their families. She has researched the personal and family impact of young onset dementia and frontotemporal dementia and led the post-diagnostic workstream of the Angela Project. She is currently principal investigator on an NIHR-funded project, DYNAMIC, on improving social care for people with young onset dementia and their family members, and is deputy director of the NIHR Policy Research Unit for Dementia and Neurodegeneration led by the University of Exeter. She leads the Research and Evidence workstream of the UK Young Dementia Network.

About the contributors

Rachel Allen is a PhD candidate at the Alzheimer Scotland Centre for Policy and Practice, University of the West of Scotland. Her research explores young onset dementia and career development, with a focus on women's experiences.

Christian Bakker is programme leader of the young onset dementia research programme at Radboud University Medical Center, Nijmegen. He also works as a healthcare psychologist with people with young onset dementia. His research is aimed at improving post-diagnostic care and support for people living with young onset dementia and their families.

Natasha (Tash) Bayes is a Researcher in the Faculty of Health, Education and Society at the University of Northampton. Tash has a particular interest in qualitative research as she enjoys talking to people to explore their expertise, views and insights, and the privilege of hearing their unique experiences through this rollercoaster journey we call life.

Janet Carter is Associate Professor, Division of Psychiatry, Faculty of Brain Sciences at University College London and Consultant in Old Age Psychiatry at North East London NHS Foundation Trust. She leads a specialist young onset dementia clinical service and led the Angela Project, the largest UK study of young onset dementia to date.

Laura Cole is a Senior Lecturer and Course Lead for MSc Dementia Studies at the Geller Institute of Ageing and Memory, University of West London. She is a psychologist and co-lead for the DEfIN-YD project (Development of a Young Onset Dementia Research Network).

Seb Crutch is Professor of Neuropsychology and a clinical psychologist at the Dementia Research Centre, University College London, and has been the clinical lead for Rare Dementia Support (RDS) since its inception in 2016, leading the expansion from large support groups to more intimate small-group and one-to-one services.

Suzannah (Sue) Evans is an Occupational Therapy Lecturer Practitioner, working in North Wales for Betsi Cadwaladr University Health Board and Wrexham University. She worked as the cognitive rehabilitation (CR) therapist and the trainer for other CR therapists in the clinical trials of GREAT cognitive rehabilitation, and enjoys supporting people with dementia achieve their goals.

Mel Hall is a Senior Lecturer in Childhood and Education at Manchester Metropolitan University. She is a sociologist with interests in families, health and narrative methods. Mel was the research associate on the Alzheimer's Society funded study, '*The perceptions and experiences of children and young people who have a parent with dementia*' (2014–17).

Jacqueline Hussey is a Memory Clinic Consultant in Wokingham, Berkshire. Jacqui has a long-term interest and passion to provide age-appropriate support for individuals living with young onset dementia and their families, and is one of the co-founders of the award-winning charity Younger People with Dementia CIO.

Torhild Holthe, PhD, worked as a clinical occupational therapist, specialising in older adults' health. She was a researcher and lecturer at the Norwegian National Centre for Ageing and Health and project leader for 'Young onset dementia and assistive technology project', part of the Norwegian Dementia Plan 2015, funded by the Norwegian Health Directorate.

Aud Johannessen is Professor Emerita at the University of South-Eastern Norway, Tönsberg. She is also working as a Senior Researcher at The Norwegian National Centre for Ageing and Health, a public competence and research environment. At the Centre she became interested in how to better support people living with young onset dementia and their families.

Laura Lebec is a Post-Doctoral Research Fellow in the Alzheimer Scotland Centre for Policy and Practice at the University of the West of Scotland. Her background is in the third sector, and she is currently working on a research project improving support for people in employment with dementia.

Calum Macdonald is a barrister specialising in financial services regulation and a Visiting Lecturer at the University of Law. His mother, Anne Macdonald, lived with posterior cortical atrophy and was Vice-Chair of the Scottish Dementia Working Group.

Clare Mason is Assistant Professor at the Centre for Applied Dementia Studies, University of Bradford and is lead volunteer at Pathways, a young onset dementia support group. Clare has worked with people living with dementia since leaving school and started the first service for people living with young onset dementia in Bradford, whilst working for Social Services.

Andrea M. Mayrhofer is a Senior Research Associate at Newcastle University. Her research focuses on post-diagnostic support for people affected by younger onset dementia.

Mary O'Malley is a Senior Research Fellow at the University of Worcester. Her research interests focus on improving the quality of life for people living with dementia. Mary has a particular interest in improving diagnosis and support for younger people living with dementia. She is passionate about public and patient involvement, co-research and disseminating research to the public.

Jacqueline Parkes is Professor of Applied Mental Health at the University of Northampton. She is the founder and co-lead of the University's Dementia Research and Innovation Centre. Jackie is a mental health nurse who continues to work with people affected by dementia in the community.

Jackie Pool, DipCoT, Dementia Care Champion, QCS Ltd, is an occupational therapist specialist in dementia with over 40 years of experience in supporting people to live well with dementia by using reabling approaches. She has worked as a clinical practitioner, educator, researcher, public speaker and published author across the NHS and social care sectors

Louise Ritchie is Reader in Dementia Research at the University of the West of Scotland. Her research aims to enhance the quality of life for individuals affected by dementia with a particular focus on working with dementia.

Pamela Roach is an Assistant Professor in Family Medicine at the University of Calgary, Canada and citizen of the Métis Nation of Alberta. She has worked with families living with young onset dementia in both Canada and the UK to improve approaches to dementia care and quality of life.

Pat Sikes is Professor Emeritus in Qualitative Inquiry at the University of Sheffield. Pat's interests are around qualitative – especially narrative and auto/biographical – approaches to research, research ethics and social justice. Her family's experiences, after her husband was diagnosed with dementia, led Pat to seek funding from the Alzheimer's Society to study the perceptions and experiences of children and young people with a parent with dementia.

Vasileios Stamou is an Honorary Visiting Researcher at the University of Bradford. He previously worked as a researcher on the Angela Project, which is where he became passionate about improving services and support for younger people with dementia and their families.

Kirsten Thorsen is a geronto-psychologist, a Senior Researcher and Professor Emerita. She has studied ageing as narrated by life histories, and loneliness over time in the longitudinal NorLag study. Young onset dementia and needs for support has been a theme in later studies. She has been affiliated to NOVA (Norwegian Social Research), the University of Tromsö and the Norwegian National Centre for Ageing and Health.

Marjolein de Vugt is Professor and Director of the Alzheimer Center Limburg at Maastricht UMC+ in The Netherlands. She is an expert in psychosocial research in dementia, with a specific interest in young onset dementia. As a healthcare psychologist at the Memory Clinic, she intertwines her clinical insights with research, focusing on developing impactful psychosocial interventions.

Jennifer Walker is a Haudenosaunee member of the Six Nations of the Grand River and a health services researcher. She is an Associate Professor at McMaster University in the Department of Health Research Methods, Evidence, & Impact. Dr Walker runs an active research community-engaged research programme in ageing and dementia.

Nikki Zimmermann is the Direct Support Lead for Rare Dementia Support, leading an experienced specialist team providing one-to-one, small and large group support incorporating education and empowerment for people affected by a rare dementia. Nikki has many years' experience supporting people and families living with young onset dementia within the community and cognitive neurology clinics, as well as her own personal family experience.

Lived experience

The experiences of people living with young onset dementia and of family members run throughout this book. As an editor, George Rook has been fully involved and has also contributed two chapters (2 and 18). Three online discussions with people living with young onset dementia were held on the topics of each section before chapter authors wrote their material. All chapter authors were invited to come and listen in. Chapter 2 gives an account of these discussions. All who took part gave permission for anonymous quotation of their words. Many other chapters include words spoken by people living with young onset dementia or supporting someone with young onset dementia. These are greatly enriching to the content. In some places (especially Chapter 16), people have given their explicit written consent to be named – something that is their right to do. Most other quotations have been made anonymous with individuals being given pseudonyms (that is, names that are not their own). At all times, the publishers have ensured that we, the editors and chapter authors, have explicit permission to include these anonymised quotations.

The Reconsidering Dementia Series

The dementia field has developed rapidly in its scope and practice over the past 25 years. Many thousands of people are newly diagnosed each year. Worldwide, the trend is that people are being diagnosed at much earlier stages. In addition, families and friends increasingly provide support to those affected by dementia over a prolonged period. Many people, both those diagnosed with dementia and those who support them, have an appetite to understand their condition. Care professionals and civic society also need an in-depth and nuanced understanding of how to support people living with dementia within their communities over the long term. The *Reconsidering Dementia* book series sets out to address this need. It takes its inspiration from the late Professor Tom Kitwood's seminal text *Dementia Reconsidered* published in 1997, which, at the time, revolutionised how dementia care was conceptualised.

The book series is jointly commissioned and edited by Professor Dawn Brooker MBE and by Dr Keith Oliver. Dawn has been active in the field of dementia care since the 1980s as a clinician and an academic. She draws on her experience and international networks to bring together a series of books on the most pertinent issues in the field. Keith is one of the foremost international advocates for those living with dementia. He also brings an insightful perspective of his own and others' experience of what it means to live with dementia gained since his diagnosis of Alzheimer's disease in 2010.

Dawn and Keith have been professional colleagues for many years. They worked together on the second edition of Kitwood's book entitled *Dementia Reconsidered, Revisited: The Person Still Comes First.* This 2019 publication was a reprint of the original text by Tom Kitwood alongside contemporary commentaries for each chapter written by current experts. Many topics in the field of dementia care, however, were simply unheard of in Kitwood's lifetime. When Open University Press approached Dawn and Keith with the idea of developing a book series dedicated to dementia, they were very pleased to accept. The subsequent titles in this series are cutting-edge scholarly texts that challenge and engage readers to think deeply. They draw on theoretical understandings, contemporary research and experience to critically reflect on their topic in great depth.

This does not mean, however, that they are not applicable to improving the care and support of those affected by dementia. As well as the scholarly text, all books have a 'So what?' thread that unpacks what this means for people living with dementia, their families, people working in dementia care, policy-makers, professionals, community activists and so on. Too many books either focus on an academic audience OR a practitioner audience OR a student audience OR a lived experience audience. In this series, the aim is to try to address these perspectives in the round. The *Reconsidering Dementia* book series brings together the perspectives of professional practice, scholarship and the lived experience as they pertain to the key topics in the field of dementia studies. All the books aim to help us to think afresh, to reconsider our standpoint and to ultimately improve the experience of those affected by dementia for years to come.

Preface

The traditional stereotype of dementia is that it affects older people who are in the post-retirement stage of life. Although it is true that dementia prevalence increases considerably in older age groups, it has always been the case that there are a significant number of people who live with dementia in earlier life stages. Indeed, Auguste D, who was the patient that Alois Alzheimer first described as demonstrating the symptoms of the disease process that was named after him, was only aged 51. At the time that Tom Kitwood wrote *Dementia Reconsidered*, however, young onset dementia was not a term that was used at all. If people were under the age of 65, they were considered to have pre-senile dementia. The term senile was then taken to be synonymous with dementia.

It is now widely recognised that dementia is not simply just part of the ageing process. However, despite the fact that the numbers of people with young onset dementia are significant, there are still huge barriers to diagnosis and post-diagnostic support for people who present with symptoms of dementia under the age of 65. People with young onset dementia and their families still experience challenges at every stage of the dementia journey.

It is timely then that we have a book that reconsiders the concept of young onset dementia for the twenty-first century. Jan Oyebode and George Rook have brought together an impressive number of contributors, including many from the Angela Research Project team. This project generated a rich source of evidence to improve diagnosis and post-diagnostic support for people and families living with young onset dementia. In this book the authors draw on this evidence to help readers understand the particular importance of autonomy, identity and relationships to those living with young onset dementia. They show us how this applies to the differential diagnosis and the diagnostic process. They consider how best to support people with technology, cognitive rehabilitation. and financial and legal advice. The book also covers how people living with young onset dementia can engage in research and planning services. Employment, leisure activity, and relationships with life partners, children and wider family and friends and peers living with dementia are also covered in depth.

Everyone working in the dementia care field also owes an enormous debt of gratitude to those living with young onset dementia who have given huge amounts of time and energy to advocate for people living with dementia now and into the future. Without these direct voices of the lived experience, the world would be a poorer place. When people speak from lived experience, it changes the hearts and minds of professionals and those with the power to shape services and prioritise funding. Many of the early pioneers of direct dementia advocacy were diagnosed with dementia before the age of 65.

Many have not lived to see changes in their lifetime but it is their vision that will inform the future shape of the response to dementia.

We hope that this book will help our readers share this vision of what good looks like for those living with young onset dementia.

Series Editors: Dawn Brooker and Keith Oliver

Additional thoughts from Keith Oliver

Whilst young onset dementia remains in the realm of rarer dementias, and those of us who live with it are often considered rarities and even viewed with doubt and suspicion. In reading this book, you will be made aware of how different young onset is from old onset dementia but also that there are similarities. This ground-breaking book informs and guides readers with insight and wisdom in order to reconsider their views on dementia, particularly how dementia affects younger people with a diagnosis.

When Dawn Brooker and I first spoke about subjects we felt should be included in this book series, an area I felt worthy of inclusion was young onset dementia. This was partly because it is very relevant to my life having been diagnosed with it aged 55, and secondly recognising that whilst some literature exists it is worthy of a reconsidered view. The next consideration was who to ask to write this book and immediately I could think of no one better than Professor Jan Oyebode, who I have had the utmost respect for since meeting her nine years ago. I was delighted when she accepted and told me she would be co-editing the book with my friend George Rook. Turning to the eminent writing team, I have known many of them through my involvement with the Young Dementia Network, whose advisory board I served on from its formation to 2022 when due to my dementia I stood down, and with the Angela Project, which I was also very much involved with.

I applaud the solution-focused approach, which runs consistently throughout this book, and this focus recognises the many challenges people affected by young onset dementia face alongside realistically centring upon both the person and positive possibilities rather than the problem. What is now required is that the good practice we see spreads further and is able to have a greater impact in helping more people.

Since being diagnosed with young onset dementia, many labels have been attached to me – patient, service user, sufferer, living with dementia, expert by experience. Now as I approach my seventieth year, it is interesting to be regarded forever as a youngster which brings Peter Pan to mind, though sadly for the past four years I have not flown anywhere!

Many people with a diagnosis of, or caring for someone with, young onset dementia carry a beacon of hope – this book will help the beacon shine more brightly as together we reconsider the way forward for us all.

Acknowledgements

First and foremost, we would like to thank those members of the DEEP Network living with young onset dementia who gave their time to the three online discussions held to help chapter authors and ourselves as editors to hear their views on the book's themes of autonomy, identity and connection. *Young Onset Dementia Reconsidered* is better for their input.

We would also like to express our appreciation to everyone living with young onset dementia, or supporting someone living with young onset dementia, who has been quoted in our book, either anonymously or credited. Your words convey your experiences far more richly than our own ever can.

We would like to acknowledge all who were part of the Angela Project team: Jan's colleagues, Dr Jenny LaFontaine and Dr Vasileios Stamou from the Centre for Applied Dementia Studies at the University of Bradford; Dr Janet Carter, the principal investigator, Professor Jacqueline Parkes and Dr Mary O'Malley; and the experts-by-experience, including Jane Twigg and Dr Keith Oliver.

We would like to thank and acknowledge all the chapter authors who put precious time into their contributions and responded graciously to our demands.

Administrative support from Rachel Niblock and Mozalfa Ilyas made all the difference at those moments that mattered.

Finally, huge appreciation from Jan to Wendy Mitchell and Keith Oliver for being sources of inspiration and motivation. Wendy is much missed but has contributed so much to thinking about young onset dementia. If Keith had not approached Jan to suggest that she might tackle producing this book, it would not have happened, and if Wendy had not suggested George to be co-editor, this book would have been much the poorer.

Acronyms and abbreviations

AD	Alzheimer's disease
ADAD	Autosomal dominant Alzheimer's disease
ADL	Activities of daily living
ADRT	Advance directive to refuse treatment
BAME	Black, Asian and Minority Ethnic
BGSI	Bangor goal-setting interview
bvFTD	Behavioural variant frontotemporal dementia
CADASIL	Cerebral autosomal dominant arteriopathy with subcortical infarcts and leukoencephalopathy
CHC	Continuing health care
CJD	Creutzfeldt-Jakob disease
CPR	Cardiopulmonary resuscitation
CSF	Cerebrospinal Fluid
CST	Cognitive stimulation therapy
CR	Cognitive rehabilitation
CT	Computerised tomography
DEEP	Dementia Engagement and Empowerment Project
DNACPR	Do not attempt CPR
DOLS	Deprivation of Liberty Safeguards
DVLA	Driver and Vehicle Licensing Agency
ECG	Electrocardiogram
FAD	Familial Alzheimer's disease
FCA	Financial Conduct Authority
fFTD	Familial frontotemporal dementia
FTD	Frontotemporal dementia
FTD-MND	Frontotemporal dementia with motor neurone disease
GPS	Global positioning system
GREAT-CR	Goal-oriented cognitive rehabilitation
IMCA	Independent Mental Capacity Advocate
LBD	Lewy body dementia
LPA	Logopenic aphasia
LPA	Lasting Power of Attorney
lvPPA	Logopenic variant of primary progressive aphasia
MMSE	Mini Mental State Examination
MRI	Magnetic resonance imaging
nfvPPA	Non-fluent/agrammatic variant of primary progressive aphasia
NHS	National Health Service
NICE	National Institute for Health and Care Excellence
PCA	Posterior cortical atrophy

PIP	Personal Independence Payment
PNFA	Progressive non-fluent aphasia
PPA	Primary progressive aphasia
QoL	Quality of life
RCT	Randomised controlled trial
SD	Semantic dementia
SMART	Smart, Measurable, Achievable, Realistic, Timely
SPECT	Single-photon emission computed tomography
svPPA	Semantic variant of primary progressive aphasia
TRCC	Truth and Reconciliation Commission of Canada
VaD	Vascular dementia
WHO	World Health Organisation
YOAD	Young onset Alzheimer's disease
YOD	Young onset dementia

1 Introduction and overview

Jan Oyebode

Overview

This chapter provides an introduction and overview of *Young Onset Dementia Reconsidered*. The aim is for the book to take a holistic, solution-focused approach, showing what can be done to live as well as possible with young onset dementia. The chapter gives a brief introduction to young onset dementia and its impact, highlighting the lack of age-appropriate and condition-appropriate support. It summarises findings from a major UK-based research study: 'The Angela Project: Improving Diagnosis and Post-Diagnostic Support for People with Young Onset Dementia and their Supporters'. This established the key needs that helpful services and support meet for people with young onset dementia and their families. This set of needs is introduced as the underpinning framework for the three-part structure of the book:

- to maintain or regain autonomy or control over life (as much as is possible);
- to have opportunities to express individual identity; and
- to have meaningful connections with family, friends and wider society.

The chapters in each section have been written by leading researchers and subject experts who summarise research evidence and best practice in ways of living and types of support that are helpful for people living with young onset dementia and their families. The topics covered by each are introduced.

Introduction

Being diagnosed with any serious, progressive, terminal condition in your forties, fifties or early sixties can be devastating: you are in the thick of life, expecting to have at least 20 years of reasonable health ahead and anticipating a fulfilling life after retirement from work. A diagnosis of young onset dementia is especially unnerving because dementia is commonly portrayed as affecting the very old and involving complete disorientation, confusion and loss of self (Gerritsen et al., 2018). Not surprisingly, dementia is the second most feared illness, after cancer (Watson et al., 2023). To receive a diagnosis of dementia at any age can be frightening but to be diagnosed in middle age, when you may be caring for children or young people, supporting elderly parents, working, still paying your mortgage and building up your pension, is a huge blow. In this book, we look at the impact of young onset dementia on the lives of those diagnosed and their families. We examine what we know about how living with young onset dementia affects independence, personal identity and relationships with others. Beyond considering impact, the book aims to be positive and solution-focused, concentrating on research evidence and best practice in ways of living and types of support that are helpful for people living with young onset dementia and their families.

So why reconsider young onset dementia? Dementia is defined as young onset when symptoms manifest before the age of 65 years (van de Veen et al., 2022). There are two important reasons why it requires special consideration: these are the time of life at which it occurs and the wide range of diagnoses that differ from those found in late onset dementia. Regarding range of diagnoses, while most types of dementia can occur both under and over 65 years, the constellation of diagnoses and the way dementia presents is different at younger ages. This, along with its rarity, poses issues for awareness and education of the public and of health and social care professionals, who need different knowledge and skills to diagnose and provide support. In relation to time of life, being younger makes a huge difference to dementia's impact on the person, their way of life, identity, relationships, family and friendships, finances and future. 'Pre-senile' dementia was first identified more than 100 years ago but there was little concerted attention paid to understanding its impact or the associated support needs until the last 20 years or so. However, a significant body of knowledge has been building up over recent years around its distinctive nature and needs, making this a good time to reconsider young onset dementia so that age-appropriate support can be offered.

The sub-title, *A Solution-Focused Approach*, captures the book's emphasis on what is possible rather than focusing only on problems. Our inspiration for this comes from high-profile examples of those with young onset dementia themselves, who have blazed a trail showing that a diagnosis of young onset dementia need not signal the start of despair and, indeed, may open new satisfying chapters of life. Tom Kitwood revolutionised the way we think of dementia, giving us a person-centred understanding that helped to break down barriers between people with and without dementia. His work helps us understand important aspects of relating to and supporting those who are living with dementia. We hope this book engenders the same degree of empathy and optimism concerning young onset dementia. We wish to ensure positive knowledge about young onset dementia is passed on, so it can be harnessed to improve the lives of those diagnosed.

Overall, this book is:

- Holistic, including emphasis on aspects such as financial well-being, co-production of services, and meaningful physical and creative activity, that take it beyond the more usual health-dominated approach.

- Solution-focused, going beyond deficits and lack of service provision, to look at what can help and what can be done to ensure people with young onset dementia and their families are better supported to live as well as possible.

Who is *Young Onset Dementia Reconsidered* for?

This book aims to be of value to policy-makers to help them to take age into account and provide equitable, non-discriminatory services for people living with dementia. It will also serve a need for service commissioners, for example in Integrated Care Boards in England, who need facts and figures to understand why it is vital that they have age-appropriate dementia services. The information across the range of chapters will arm health and social care practitioners in the statutory, voluntary and community sectors, with useful information that will give them confidence to be able to understand and support those affected. It will also be of value to staff in training for health or social care roles, and students and their teachers. There is often little time in the curriculum for dementia, let alone young onset dementia, so the information provided here will be a useful resource to draw on.

This is primarily an evidence-based text. The chapter authors have summarised the findings of authoritative well-designed research studies, including qualitative studies that give voice to people living with young onset dementia or supporting those with young onset dementia. The text should inspire dementia researchers to turn to this under-researched but impactful area. It will enable those planning projects to base their proposals on a firm foundation and will direct researchers to areas where more knowledge is required. Research commissioners as well as researchers will see that there are major research gaps on some important issues.

Last but not least, *Young Onset Dementia Reconsidered* will be an empowering source of information for those with young onset dementia and their families. Most people living with young onset dementia receive poor support due to health and social care professionals lacking knowledge about the condition and about what can be done to support people with a diagnosis. People with young onset dementia are often discharged from services after diagnosis and left to fend for themselves. In this book, anyone with a diagnosis, family and friends will be able to find out about the latest evidence in relation to a wide range of facets of life that are affected by living with young onset dementia.

In the remainder of this chapter, we:

- Provide a brief introduction to key issues that will be covered in greater depth later in the book: the nature of young onset dementia, the impact of receiving a diagnosis, and the lack of age-appropriate and condition-appropriate support.
- Summarise the key findings of the Angela Project, a major study that explored what sort of services and support people with young onset

dementia and their families find helpful in living with dementia, which informed the structure of this book.

- Provide an overview of the structure and scope of the book.

From pre-senile to young onset dementia

The significance of age to dementia was recognised from the first days of modern classifications of mental illness. The psychiatrist Emil Kraepelin, in the early 1900s, distinguished between senile and pre-senile dementia (Hippius and Neundörfer, 2003). For a long time, dementia had been recognised across a wide range of societies as a condition associated with old age but it was its occurrence at a younger age in Auguste Deter that captured the attention of Kraepelin's pupil, Alois Alzheimer. Auguste was admitted, aged 51 years, to the institution where Alzheimer worked. He described her symptoms in detail and studied her brain after her death. In her brain, he distinguished the plaques and tangles that are now recognised as typical brain changes of the disease that became named after him. Around the same period, Ludwig Binswanger, a Swiss psychiatrist and neurologist, described early onset vascular dementia, which Alois Alzheimer named Binswanger's disease (Yang et al., 2016). These early distinctions between pre-senile and senile dementia left a major legacy on the conceptualisation of dementia which lasted into the 2000s.

Nowadays, it is recognised that young onset dementia is not in itself medically distinct from late onset dementia. The eminent neurologist Martin Rossor referred in an influential article to the age cut-off of 65 years like this: 'This cutoff point is indicative of a sociological partition in terms of employment and retirement age, but this age has no specific biological significance and there is a range of disease features across this arbitrary divide' (Rossor et al., 2010: 793). But although there is no categorical diagnostic reason to separate young and late onset dementia, it is still helpful, from the point of view of services and support, to distinguish between them. Initiatives to establish age-appropriate services stretches back at least 30 years. I worked in dementia services in the 1980s and 1990s and was aware that when I met younger people with dementia, I needed to think differently and draw on different knowledge. I was Head of Older Adult Psychology Services in my area in the 1990s when we set up a specialist team known as the Working Age Dementia Service to provide age-appropriate expertise and support. Around the same time, a small number of equivalent teams were established across the UK, and the Clive Project (precursor to Young Dementia UK, now part of Dementia UK), a charity to serve people living with young onset dementia, was established.

Sadly, the EU Equality Framework Directive (2000), the UK Equalities Act (2010) and austerity combined to cut short this nascent growth. Where I worked it became considered discriminatory to have a young onset dementia service. Our Working Age Dementia Service was rebadged as the Rare Dementia Service and initial assessment once more became the province of 'all-age' dementia services. The social worker who was an integral part of the team was withdrawn into the local authority base and the Citizen's Advice worker post, which had provided invaluable information on finances and legalities, was cut.

This retrenchment has started to be reversed again recently. Two key landmarks within this in the UK have been the establishment of the Young Dementia Network in 2016 and the outcomes of the Angela Research Project (see more on page 8). The former has brought together people living with young onset dementia and their families, professionals and academics into an active working alliance to try and improve the lives of those with young onset dementia. The latter has produced a wide range of research evidence that can be used by the Young Dementia Network and others to influence provision. This includes evidence that specialist young onset dementia services are superior on a number of quality indicators to all-age dementia services (Stamou et al., 2021a).

Along the way, there has, of course, been a change in terminology. With the term 'senile' becoming pejorative, dementia in younger people became referred to by other terms, such as early onset dementia, working-age dementia, younger people with dementia and young-onset or young onset dementia. Researchers in the Netherlands invited a panel of 44 leading clinicians and researchers to suggest and select their preferred terms (Van de Veen et al., 2022). They reached consensus on young-onset dementia as the preferred term and this, and young onset dementia, are now increasingly used in research and health service contexts and are used throughout this book.

This brief dip into the historical context provides the backdrop for our reconsideration of young onset dementia.

The nature of young onset dementia

Dementia is defined as being of young onset when symptoms occur under the age of 65 years (Van de Veen et al., 2022). As mentioned above, the age divide is somewhat arbitrary but serves as a rough marker to distinguish between phases of middle age and later life. Of all people living with dementia, 7.5% of cases of dementia are thought to be of young onset (Carter et al., 2022) and there are estimated to be 70,800 people with young onset dementia currently living in England (Carter et al., 2022). The overall incidence is calculated at 11 per 100,000 people-years and this rises steeply with age (Hendriks et al., 2021). Numbers affected are more than those living with some other better-known conditions; for example, the numbers with young onset dementia are 14 times more than the number living with motor neurone disease.

Young onset dementia, like late onset, is an umbrella term encompassing a range of specific types. The spectrum of young onset dementia diagnoses is wider than in late onset but exact figures for the different sub-types are hard to find. Hendriks et al. (2021) found incidence was highest for Alzheimer's disease at 9.8 per 100,000 people-years; followed by vascular dementia at 4 per 100,000 and frontotemporal dementia at 1.1 per 100,000. Despite the highest proportion having Alzheimer's disease, overall, young onset dementias are not as heavily dominated by Alzheimer's disease as late onset. It is estimated that 15% of all young onset dementias are of rarer types (see Chapter 3 for detail of these).

O'Malley et al. (2019: 1) draw attention to the fact that as well as considering the more common types of dementia, clinicians also need to consider 'autoimmune, inflammatory, late-onset metabolic and hereditary/familial causes'.

Given this wide range of diagnoses, the first signs of young onset dementia may be very different from the progressive memory loss commonly seen in late onset Alzheimer's disease. Early signs for people with frontotemporal dementias, for example, could include difficulty with planning ahead, trouble inhibiting impulses (e.g. to swear, to eat sweet foods or to act on sexual thoughts), loss of empathy or language difficulties (Gorno-Tempini et al., 2011; Greaves and Rohrer, 2019). Even the way Alzheimer's disease presents is often different from its presentation in old age, as it is more frequently associated with visual problems connected with damage to the posterior lobe at the back of the brain. There is much more information on this in Chapters 3 and 4.

The range of symptoms makes it hard for those developing dementia to recognise that this may be the case. Also, the GP and diagnosing clinician need to be aware of how the different types of dementia present. With young onset dementia being quite uncommon and with it presenting differently from late onset dementia, the 'red flags' that might usually lead a GP to suspect dementia are often not present and the alternative symptoms can be mistaken for other physical or mental health problems (Vieira et al., 2013). This means that diagnosis is often delayed. One study found that the waiting time from approaching a GP to getting a diagnosis was over 4 years, compared with a period of 2 years for people with late onset dementia (van Vliet et al., 2012). It is therefore vitally important that those in primary care and in dementia assessment services have accurate information and awareness of young onset dementia.

The impact of being diagnosed with young onset dementia

Young onset dementia brings a wide range of problems related to its various sub-types, as well as a host of issues related to life stage. In terms of sub-types and their associated challenges, people with posterior cortical atrophy, for example, are likely to experience difficulty in processing information about what they see and where things are, so they may have trouble finding objects or judging distances (Crutch et al., 2012). People with frontotemporal dementias can have problems using language, finding words, planning ahead or inhibiting impulses (Gorno-Tempini et al., 2011; Greaves and Rohrer, 2019). These varying symptom profiles cause various difficulties in employment and in negotiating everyday life and social relationships. In addition, more cases of young onset dementia than late onset dementia have a genetic component, which means they are more likely to be passed down through the generations; those diagnosed and their families may have to consider these implications too.

In late onset dementia, the person affected has usually already retired from work, has adjusted to living on a pension, has probably started to adjust to living with age-related changes in cognition, sensory functioning and physical health, and their children (if any) are adults. By contrast, for those with young onset dementia, middle age is a time when most people are at their busiest and most productive, whether in a career or in home life. The development of a disease that impairs brain function therefore brings huge disruption. It usually results in a person facing premature termination of their employment and career, and not knowing where to turn to find renewed purpose.

The condition not only affects the individual but also impacts on the whole family. In late onset dementia, many households consist of two retired people supporting each other or a single person supported by grown-up children. In young onset dementia, many of those affected live with a partner or spouse who is likely to be working, who may have to reduce or leave employment, impacting further on family finances. In addition, there may be children or young people who are still at home or reliant on their parents, whose lives are affected (Hall and Sikes, 2017). People diagnosed may find themselves shunned by long-term friends who do not understand the idea of young onset dementia or who are afraid of the changes they see. One experimental study found students held significantly more negative attitudes when a person with dementia was described as younger as opposed to older. The students were more likely to think of the young person as dangerous and expressed being less willing to offer them help (Werner et al., 2020). Not only this, but the progressive nature of the disease means the person and their family have to continually adjust and face an uncertain future. Overall, young onset dementia poses severe existential challenges to a person's sense of who they are.

Support for people with young onset dementia

In the UK, about 80% of people with young onset dementia receive ongoing health and social care from dementia services that deal with all age groups (Stamou et al., 2021a). Services are typically geared up to those who are in their late seventies or eighties, who have different generational experiences and a different pace of life from those in their fifties and early sixties. Against this backdrop, health and social care staff are usually unfamiliar with the issues of young onset dementia. They may not often see people with the different subtypes of dementia that are more common at earlier ages, so they do not know how to assess, where to refer on to, or how to help people overcome changes in cognition and behaviour. They may not have easy access to speech and language therapists, family therapists, specialist neuropsychology or occupational therapy services. They are unlikely to know how to provide employment advice, to know the rules around benefits for people of working age, or to know how to access services for children and young people.

As young onset dementia is relatively rare, there tend not to be dedicated community services for younger people to provide opportunities for peer support or age-appropriate activities in the local area. Activities and social groups for people with dementia of all ages are usually experienced as age-inappropriate by those with young onset dementia due to the age differences.

Such groups are usually catering for a majority of people of an older generation whose attitudes, expectations, hobbies, likes and dislikes generally differ from those born, not in the 1940s or 1950s but in the 1960s and later.

Overall, current ongoing age-appropriate support for people diagnosed with young onset dementia is patchy in that good services are available only in some places. In many areas there is no specialist young onset service with the appropriate knowledge and skills to signpost people or provide them with support.

The Angela Project

The Angela Project was a three-year research study (2016–19) funded by the Alzheimer's Society aimed at generating evidence to improve diagnosis and post-diagnostic support for people living with young onset dementia and their families. With permission from her family, the project was named after Angela, who experienced symptoms from the age of 48 years but waited 3 years to get a diagnosis. This important research study led to a number of significant findings and related publications and it is the foundation on which the structure and content of *Young Onset Dementia Reconsidered* is built. The project had invaluable input from people living with young onset dementia (Oliver et al., 2020; Parkes et al., 2022) who shaped the questions and the way they were addressed. The key findings are described below finishing with the aspect that underpins this book. All the academic papers and outputs can be easily accessed in full through the Young Dementia Network website (https://www.youngdementianetwork.org/research-evidence/the-angela-project/).

The Angela Project work on diagnosis led to recommended 'minimum' and 'gold' standards for conducting assessment and diagnosis of young onset dementia (O'Malley et al., 2020). These were developed with an international panel of 23 international clinical experts. The minimum standard comprises 15 items that all panel members regarded as 'absolutely essential' or 'very important' to follow when assessing someone for possible young onset dementia. The gold standard adds another 33 standards that over 80% of the experts agreed were 'absolutely essential' or 'very important'. The work on diagnosis also included consultation with 36 people living with dementia and family supporters on best practice for conducting and communicating diagnosis (O'Malley et al., 2021). This work and its outcomes are described in depth in Chapter 2.

A survey of post-diagnostic services showed how important specialist young onset dementia services are (Stamou et al., 2021a). Only one in five people with young onset dementia received ongoing support from a specialist young onset dementia service, yet specialist services were superior on a range of counts. People with young onset dementia who were in contact with young onset services were more likely to have a follow-up appointment within 6 weeks of diagnosis, experience care continuity, have a care plan and be more satisfied with the support they were receiving. Interviews were conducted with managers of services and commissioners to understand what helps to set up and sustain specialist young onset dementia services. Seven aspects were identified as essential: 'having knowledgeable, committed local champions; involvement of people living with young onset dementia and family supporters; initial delivery within existing resources; partnership working within and between sectors; having a reflective, supportive organizational culture; gathering evidence of impact; and having wider support and guidance' (Oyebode et al., 2023: 1).

The survey showed the crucial role family members play in providing support, which contrasted with low levels of service use and cost. Over half of those with young onset dementia had a family member who spent more than 5 hours a day helping or 'supervising'. Almost half of these family members also estimated spending 15 hours or more per week more on household tasks now than they had before the diagnosis. The equivalent cost of family support was £8000 per family per 3 months, contrasting with the median costs of community-based health and social care, which were just £400. This pattern holds true for people with late onset dementia too but is exaggerated in those with young onset dementia with family care being at a higher level and services being at a lower level. Only one in five respondents had contact with a dementia-related charitable body (e.g. Alzheimer's Society, Dementia UK), implying that people with young onset dementia either did not know about the support available or did not want to take advantage of it. The high levels of family support raise the question of how people who live alone or do not have such supportive relationships manage.

A key focus of the Angela Project was to find out what services or support people with young onset dementia considered helpful and why. The survey showed eight aspects of services were valued (Stamou et al., 2021b).

- specialist advice and information on young onset dementia;
- signposting to age-appropriate services;
- interventions to maintain physical and mental health;
- opportunities for social participation;
- opportunities to have a voice;
- enablement of independence while managing risk;
- enablement of financial stability; and
- support interventions for family relationships.

These valued attributes are wide-ranging and indicate the breadth of service required for young onset dementia.

Through further analysis of the survey and additional in-depth interviews (Stamou et al., 2022), the project considered what it was about the services that were organised and delivered made them helpful. The findings emphasised the importance of three tiers of delivery – the individual staff level, service level, and the level of the wider network of services:

- At the level of the person, person-centredness was the key quality. It was found to be vital for health and social care staff to take a collaborative, positive attitude, to be flexible, to provide in-person support and to provide user-friendly information.

- At the service level, a good fit between a person's needs and what was available in the service was crucial. To be helpful, services needed to be age-appropriate, to be able to meet the needs of symptoms associated with rarer dementias and to provide for the whole family.
- At the level of the wider organisation, service systems were helpful when there was specialist young onset dementia provision, integration across services, and stability and consistency over time.

Having looked at what services or support needs to be provided and how, the researchers then considered *why* it was that services provided in these ways were experienced as helpful. This involved identifying the needs that positive services met (Stamou et al., 2023). This led to 16 themes that we clustered into groups to form three high-level, over-arching themes.

The first theme, 'maintaining autonomy', was about the importance people living with young onset dementia placed on maintaining their independence. Services that helped people with young onset dementia to be in control were those that offered empowering information and advice about young onset dementia; supported activities of daily living as needed; were appropriately tailored for someone of middle age; and gave the person a voice in what was provided, so that the individual had a sense of agency rather than feeling like a bystander in their own care.

The second theme, 'being myself', captured the emphasis placed by those living with young onset dementia on maintaining their own identity and way of life. Support that helped people to regain a positive outlook and re-establish either a sense of continuity or a 'new normal' were central. This might be, for example, by supporting someone to maintain or return to longstanding interests and hobbies, or by supporting and encouraging them to develop new activities and talents. Meaningful occupation – that is, having something to do that suits the individual – was core to this. To be well enough to pursue meaningful activities, it was vital to maintain cognitive, emotional and physical health as well as possible, and services that assisted across these areas were highly valued.

The third important theme was 'togetherness'. People with young onset dementia valued support that helped them to maintain those relationships that were important to them, including, where needed, having family-centred interventions to enable close relationships to continue, as well as being able to access support for all family members. People also found it helpful to establish new peer support relationships where they could share experiences and feel they were in the company of others who understood. In addition, those with young onset dementia wanted to continue to contribute to society and appreciated opportunities to do so.

The content and structure of *Young Onset Dementia Reconsidered*

Young Onset Dementia Reconsidered has been structured around these three overarching themes and their sub-themes. We have changed the labels of the overarching themes slightly to: 'maintaining autonomy', 'retaining identity' and 'being connected'. Each section of the book centres on one of the overarching themes and the chapters within each section reflect the sub-themes.

The first section, 'Maintaining Autonomy', has six chapters. A major turning point in living with young onset dementia is being given a diagnosis. Two chapters are focused on this aspect. The first of these introduces a number of rare dementias. This chapter concludes with a call to action for people to have diagnosis-centred as well as person-centred care. This can be understood through reference to Tom Kitwood's well-known equation that dementia = neurological impairment + biography + personality + health + social psychology. The chapter authors suggest that in young onset dementia, it is important to pay specific attention to the nature of the neurological impairment as well as considering the person's health, life story, personality and relationships. The second is centred around findings from the diagnosis work stream of the Angela Project, mentioned above. The work involved a consensus study which gathered the views of people living with young onset dementia on how a diagnosis of young onset dementia can be given in a sensitive way that is empowering.

Three core chapters in this section then consider particular ways to maintain independence. One looks at how to maintain autonomy through the use of technology; the next looks at using cognitive rehabilitation techniques (these are evidence-based strategies) to overcome or get around cognitive impairment; and the third addresses the legal and financial implications of being diagnosed, outlining how people can use their rights to maintain control over their own lives.

Finally, in this section, is a chapter on how important it is for those living with young onset dementia to be involved as partners in service planning to ensure that services are age-appropriate and provide what is needed.

The second section, 'Retaining Identity', has six chapters that look at ways to maintain and support identity for people living with young onset dementia as well as for partners who are family carers.

The first chapter in this section is focused on culturally safe dementia care. This considers the position of people from Indigenous communities in Canada, where Indigenous people are a minority in their own country and have experienced both historical and current prejudice and discrimination. The chapter highlights the importance of understanding cultural context in order to provide safe, trustworthy, strengths-based support. Many of the issues raised have relevant parallels for supporting those from minoritised ethnic communities in the UK and other countries.

The subsequent three chapters address issues around the roles of work, hobbies and activities, and research involvement, in maintaining individual identity. The first describes experiences in relation to employment and the support required to enable a positive employment outcome. The second considers the benefits of taking part in meaningful social, creative and sporting activities and how these can be offered in a personalised way to suit people living with young onset dementia. The third looks at the sense of purpose and satisfaction many people with young onset dementia have found from getting involved in dementia research. It draws on the author's experiences of running the Dementia Experts for Involvement-Young Dementia (DEfIN-YD) Project as a model for how to foster genuine involvement.

Dementia is by definition a progressive condition, and the next chapter in this section tackles the issue of changes of identity as cognitive impairment and its consequences become more pronounced. Drawing on research which followed people living with young onset dementia over a 7-year period, it shows the benefits for identity of living in an accepting, considerate and supportive environment.

The impact of young onset dementia on family members who become 'primary carers' is addressed in the final chapter of this section. The vast majority of support for those with young onset dementia is provided by spouses or partners, of the opposite or same sex, and this is the area which is most researched. This chapter therefore focuses on summarising the impact on spouse/partner carers and looks at evidence-based approaches that can alleviate stress and promote the well-being of this group.

The third section of the book includes three chapters on the theme of 'Being Connected'. The first picks up on the impact on families and outlines challenges to family relationships that arise in the context of young onset dementia. It summarises the ways that continuing family-centred care from specialist teams can be significant in helping families to overcome these difficulties and it calls for action to make such services more widely available. It is followed by a chapter specifically focused on the impact of young onset dementia on children and young people, acknowledging how hard it is to have a parent with young onset dementia but placing the emphasis on some of the aspects that can generate hope or inspiration for others. This chapter also makes suggestions for the types of support needed by children and young people, highlighting the value of connections with each other. The third chapter concentrates on peer relationships, drawing on the author's experience of running a young onset dementia support group and showing the benefits of peer support in providing a sense of understanding that reduces isolation.

Finally, George has summarised the content in a short final chapter.

Involvement of people living with young onset dementia in the production of this book

I put forward the initial proposal for *Young Onset Dementia Reconsidered* as a result of direct encouragement from Keith Oliver, so effectively the idea came from someone living with young onset dementia. During the process of the proposal being agreed, Dawn Brooker and Keith (series editors) encouraged me to approach a person living with young onset dementia to be a co-editor. This resulted in George joining me and we have been working as a team of two.

George suggested early on that before inviting chapter authors we should meet people living with young onset dementia to find out what they thought should be in the book. We held three online sessions and received inspiration, facts and anecdotes that this book reflects. The following chapter summarises these discussions. A big thank you to those who took part.

As co-editors, we read each chapter as it came in and discussed each online. I made notes and suggestions to feedback to authors on the basis of these discussions. Our emphasis has been on the evidence base from published research that draws on experiences of those living with young onset dementia. We have placed emphasis on clarity rather than simplicity, avoiding duplication and trying to ensure scientific or medical jargon does not interfere with understanding or readability.

We hope that this book will be easily readable by health and care professionals, researchers and lay readers alike. For those who seek deeper understanding, our authors have provided comprehensive references for readers to follow.

References

Carter, J., Jackson, M., Gleisner, Z., et al. (2022) Prevalence of all cause young onset dementia and time lived with dementia: analysis of primary care health records, *Journal of Dementia Care*, 30 (3): 1–5.

Crutch, S.J., Lehmann, M., Schott, J.M., et al. (2012) Posterior cortical atrophy, *Lancet Neurology*, 11 (2): 170–78.

Gerritsen, D.L., Oyebode, J. and Gove, D. (2018) Ethical implications of the perception and portrayal of dementia, *Dementia*, 17 (5): 596–608.

Gorno-Tempini, M.L., Hillis, A.E., Weintraub, S., et al. (2011) Classification of primary progressive aphasia and its variants, *Neurology*, 76 (11): 1006–14.

Greaves, C.V. and Rohrer, J.D. (2019) An update on genetic frontotemporal dementia, *Journal of Neurology*, 266 (8): 2075–86.

Hall, M. and Sikes, P. (2017) 'It would be easier if she'd died': young people with parents with dementia articulating inadmissible stories, *Qualitative Health Research*, 27 (8): 1203–14.

Hendriks, S., Peetoom, K., Bakker, C., et al. (2021) Global prevalence of young-onset dementia: a systematic review and meta-analysis, *JAMA Neurology*, 78 (9): 1080–90.

Hippius, H. and Neundörfer, G. (2003) The discovery of Alzheimer's disease, *Dialogues in Clinical Neuroscience*, 5 (1): 101–8.

Oliver, K., O'Malley, M., Parkes, J., et al. (2020) Living with young onset dementia and actively shaping dementia research – The Angela Project, *Dementia*, 19 (1): 41–48.

O'Malley, M., Parkes, J., Stamou, V., et al. (2019) Young-onset dementia: scoping review of key pointers to diagnostic accuracy, *BJPsych Open*, 5 (3): e48. Available at: https://doi.org/10.1192/bjo.2019.36.

O'Malley, M., Parkes, J., Stamou, V., et al. (2020) International consensus on quality indicators for comprehensive assessment of dementia in young adults using a modified e-Delphi approach, *International Journal of Geriatric Psychiatry*, 35 (11): 1309–21.

O'Malley, M., Parkes, J., Campbell, J. et al. (2021) Receiving a diagnosis of young onset dementia: evidence-based statements to inform best practice, *Dementia*, 20 (5): 1745–71.

Oyebode, J.R., La Fontaine, J., Stamou, V., et al. (2023) Establishing and sustaining high-quality services for people with young onset dementia: the perspective of senior service providers and commissioners, *International Psychogeriatrics*. Available at: https://doi.org/10.1017/S1041610223000443.

Parkes, J., O'Malley, M., Stamou, V., et al. (2022) Lessons learnt from delivering the public and patient involvement forums within a younger onset dementia project. *Dementia*, 21 (7): 2103–16.

Rossor, M.N., Fox, N.C., Mummery, C.J., et al. (2010) The diagnosis of young-onset dementia, *Lancet Neurology*, 9 (8): 793–806.

Stamou, V., La Fontaine, J., Gage, H., et al. (2021a) Services for people with young onset dementia: The 'Angela' Project national UK survey of service use and satisfaction, *International Journal of Geriatric Psychiatry*, 36 (3): 411–22.

Stamou, V., La Fontaine, J., O'Malley, M., et al. (2021b) The nature of positive post-diagnostic support as experienced by people with young onset dementia, *Aging and Mental Health*, 25 (6): 1125–33.

Stamou, V., La Fontaine, J., O'Malley, M., et al. (2022) Helpful post-diagnostic services for young onset dementia: findings and recommendations from the Angela Project, *Health and Social Care in the Community*, 30 (1): 142–53.

Stamou, V., Oyebode, J., La Fontaine, J., et al. (2023) Good practice in needs-based post-diagnostic support for people with young onset dementia: findings from the Angela Project, *Ageing and Society*. Available at: https://doi.org/10.1017/S0144686X22001362.

van de Veen, D., Bakker, C., Peetoom, K., et al. (2022) Provisional consensus on the nomenclature and operational definition of dementia at a young age, a Delphi study, *International Journal of Geriatric Psychiatry*, 37: 3. Available at: https://doi.org/10.1002/gps.5691.

van Vliet, D., De Vugt, M.E., Bakker, C., et al. (2012) Time to diagnosis in young-onset dementia as compared with late-onset dementia, *Psychological Medicine*, 43 (2): 423–32.

Vieira, R.T., Caixeta, L., Machado, S., et al. (2013) Epidemiology of early-onset dementia: a review of the literature, *Clinical Practice and Epidemiology in Mental Health*, 9 (1): 88–95.

Watson, R., Sanson-Fisher, R., Bryant, J., et al. (2023) Dementia is the second most feared condition among Australian health service consumers: results of a cross-sectional survey, *BMC Public Health*, 23: 876. Available at: https://doi.org/10.1186/s12889-023-15772-y.

Werner, P., Raviv-Turgeman, L. and Corrigan, P.W. (2020) The influence of the age of dementia onset on college students' stigmatic attributions towards a person with dementia, *BMC Geriatrics*, 20: 104. Available at: https://doi.org/10.1186/s12877-020-1505-4.

Yang, H.D., Lee, S.B. and Young, L.D. (2016) History of Alzheimer's disease, *Dementia and Neurocognitive Disorders*, 15 (4): 115–21.

2 What people living with young onset dementia told us

George Rook

At the outset of working on this book, we wanted to hear from people living with young onset dementia to ensure that we dealt with issues that are important to them, and that their voices were reflected in the book.

We organised three webinars over Zoom in which six people with young onset dementia took part, alongside several chapter authors. The webinars were recorded, with consent, and participants agreed that their contributions could be quoted anonymously. We would like to thank Rachel Niblock, who worked within the DEEP Network (for Innovations in Dementia) for her work in making these webinars happen.

Each webinar explored one of three themes: Control, Connections and Identity. These themes were identified in the Angela Project, in which Jan (my co-editor) was involved. The Project found that services and support experienced as helpful most often met one of these three key needs. The three themes form the basis for the structure of our book (see Chapter 1 for more on this).

Control

The first discussion was attended by three people living with young onset dementia, whom we identify as P1–P3, and three chapter authors (A1–A3). G is George, who also facilitated these discussions, and J is Jan, my co-editor.

There is a perception that living with dementia at any age brings with it a loss of control over one's life. A person becomes incapable of making decisions and living independently, whether as part of a family group or alone. Our contributors felt differently. They were enjoying their lives, meeting new friends, doing things that they found worthwhile. *'It has changed how our lives are going, but in a very good way'* (P3).

They really enjoyed going out and about to talk to people about dementia, to lots of different groups. *'It's eye opening ... people have asked questions like "can you go out on your own?", and I say "yes I can". Educators we call ourselves'* (P3). P2 enjoyed meeting people he otherwise would not have met. *'With my dementia I feel I am having a wonderful time and feel I am helping people with dementia.'*

P1 was involved in a range of projects: '[it's] *good to know you are being listened to and your opinion is being taken seriously*'.

> *For me the main thing about maintaining control is that people don't presume what I need or want, but that I am asked. The thing I find frustrating is when others, probably with the best of intentions, feel they know what I need or what is best for me without asking me. For me, that is keeping control. I may not be able to do things as freely or easily as before, but involve me … don't make decisions about me without me. (P1)*

P2 said: '*When I was diagnosed I took it very hard, was down for about twelve months. But when I accepted it I came flying back. Now I say it's the best thing that ever happened to me.*'

P3, formerly a doctor, said: '*it was difficult when I started telling people about my illness … people couldn't believe it*'. After the COVID-19 pandemic,

> *I got to a point when I had told my close family and a few of my very close friends. But when everything started opening up I thought I just have to tell people. What am I doing not telling people! And I had a great time because it makes you so much freer. (P3)*

G summarised that having control over when to tell people about the diagnosis was an important part of retaining control.

Everyone spoke of feeling really down for a while after their diagnosis. P1 said she told people about her diagnosis as a way of taking control: '*I honestly felt my life was over. I felt this was very much the beginning of the end and I couldn't see a way out. It was only though finding peer support that I got back.*' P1 also said that she had made friends she never would otherwise have met, and had been doing things that she would not have been doing without dementia: '*It's not the best thing to be diagnosed with dementia, but now I live the best I can*' (P1).

J asked what should have been done differently to have a better experience of diagnosis. P1 replied:

> *I had a good consultant. But I was told to 'put my affairs in order', then handed a bag of bumph … I wasn't given any hope leaving that room. Once the consultant said the word 'dementia', all of a sudden I felt I would be sitting in a corner unable to do anything. That really threw me … Like P2, I thought I was going to die and would be at the end stage within a few weeks. (P1)*

But P1 said she was put in touch with a dementia navigator who gave her some hope.

G was told soon after diagnosis: '*Don't take risks, don't get tired, and put your affairs in order.*' But, he went on:

> *For me, Zoom during COVID and afterwards has been not quite my life but not far short. It's got me into research and has found me loads of friends whom*

I really know well now. We used to meet only once or twice a year at confer-ences, but then it became every week. It's fantastic. (G)

G referred to the way some people, including professionals, are sceptical of 'all this nonsense about having a new life! He commented: *'Well I'm not saying it's good to have dementia but it does give you a new life, because by definition one thing comes to a slow grinding end, and another starts … it's like rebirth.'*

The discussion moved on to technology as a way of helping to keep control. P1 said:

The technology I use to help me keep control is Alexa. I set timers on her con-stantly and I name them. So if I put something in the oven I will say 'set oven timer for … or set washing timer', etc. When Alexa goes off I know what I need to do. It's helped me a lot because I don't have anyone else to help. (P1)

P3 also used Alexa for cooking timers. She liked to cook but found it hard to do the measures, so she has a device that speaks to you as you are putting the ingredients into a bowl. It counts for you as you measure. P3 also said she would like the chance to speak to people who invent and design things so she can explain what they need.

P2 said he used to read two or three books a week, but now cannot recall where he is in the book or what is happening.

Another aspect of being in control related to employment. P2 stated:

Employment laws absolutely annoy me. When you're given a diagnosis of dementia, the companies instantly fall behind the Health and Safety rules to suit them. You become unemployable because you have been diagnosed with dementia.

Once you have a diagnosis, insurance companies don't want to know you. And employers try to avoid paying you out. We need a statement or law so that insurance companies and employers understand this is a terminal illness and we don't have to beg to be paid what we are entitled to.

My truck licence was taken away from me on the day of my diagnosis. They told me not to worry! (P2)

Finance was identified as a massive issue for those with a diagnosis. P1 said: *'I personally don't have any control over my own finances, and that is my per-sonal choice.'* She had stopped working as an interpreter before her diagnosis. The mortgage was paid off and her husband was still working, so they could manage. She thought it must be horrendous for younger people with family at home and mortgages to pay.

G described transport and driving as big issues. He cannot get a bus from where he lives and taxis are very expensive and hard to book. G and P1 both took control over their own safety on the road, restricting themselves to day-time driving. They do not drive at night any longer because of the difficulties with bright lights and orientation.

G summarised that losing financial control and a driving licence are two very impactful things to happen to anyone in terms of losing control over their lives.

What about continuing to make decisions as a means of retaining control? P1 said she was still involved in decisions and could stand up for herself. G said he insists on being part of decisions on things he regards as important for him, but has realised that some things really are no longer important and is happy to defer.

P2's partner, as part of planning ahead, had a wet room installed. P2 was happy to go along with this decision but he found the noise and disruption of construction very disturbing. He used to go out for hours to get away from the noise.

Family gatherings can present difficulties for people living with dementia, regardless of age. G finds it hard to deal with the noise and disruption of routines, like taking medications or having wake-up time with a mug of tea. The only practical way to take control is to withdraw from the company, but this can make one feel guilty.

P2 didn't see any guilt in this. He said he gets dragged to family gatherings but cannot wait to get back home. '*If we choose to do something we can prepare and know what's going to happen, but if people descend on us we cannot always choose, so that's the big difference.*'

One of our authors then asked how we learned to use Alexa. P1 said her husband got a device with a screen and uploaded recipes for her to read on the screen. She said setting the alarms was very easy. P2 had a niece who recommended Alexa and set up his favourite music.

P3 said she no longer used devices; she sees them but can't really use them. She asks her husband or daughter to do it for her. She finds it very frustrating and sometimes wants to throw the things away.

G ended by saying he believes that at diagnosis, every person should be provided with a computer tablet of some sort and trained to use it. '*It would give everyone a whole new world.*' Others strongly agreed.

Connections

Our second webinar was attended by four people living with young onset dementia (P1, P3–5), a former carer (P2) who had looked after their daughter with young onset dementia, and two chapter authors (A1 and A2). The facilitator also lived with young onset dementia, and again is referred to as G.

P1 was diagnosed with early onset dementia aged 53 and lives alone. His most important connections are with family and with the support networks he is involved with in the wider community. He is very active in peer support and activism networks which helps connect him to peers. The membership of his group is intergenerational.

P3 had found it hard to connect with others who had had a similar diagnosis, but now, largely as a result of the COVID-19 pandemic, Zoom was having a dramatic effect, widening his circle of friends and peers. Conversely, for those who could not use Zoom (or an equivalent), COVID-19 had had a dramatic negative effect, breaking connections with others and restricting opportunities to connect with new people.

G commented that using technology, such as Zoom, was very much a *'use it or lose it'* situation. It was important not to stop doing things for any reason as you might not be able to re-learn what you forget after a few weeks or months.

For P4 peer support was very important, *'but you have to choose the most appropriate group for yourself'*. Both P2 and P3 found that people stopped visiting after a diagnosis, probably due to stigma and lack of understanding of the disease. P3 now has a new set of friends, as well as his own close family.

G equated establishing or connecting with peer support with having *'a new family'*. He said he wanted to be with the right people who listen.

P4 said: *'With peers you don't have to explain about things like keeping up with conversations. They understand and allow a free flow of discussion.'* Others agreed that conversation can go all over the place, often with little logic, just connections in someone's mind but this isn't a problem when you are with peers.

P1 feels comfortable when with peers because *'they are like me. There is mutual understanding.'* He added that the reaction is different when you encounter people you don't know. P1 wears the disability sunflower lanyard when going shopping but gets second looks from people because there is no obvious, visible disability.

P5, who lives in Europe, is still a member of a choir, a samba band and other groups, and uses their diagnosis to educate people around them about dementia.

We then moved on to connections with neighbourhoods.

P3 used to take the bus and just go to Costa and watch the world go by, but recent cuts in services had made this much more difficult. And losing this frequent connection had adversely affected his mental and cognitive health.

P2 said their daughter had been connected to objects. *'For example, she had an old handbag and a stuffed toy that became important to her.'* These things were taken away by staff when she moved into a care home because they were 'unhygienic'. G said he felt connected to some trees and plants (e.g. the primroses beginning to flower), especially where he often walked.

G next asked about the effect or impact of working in the dementia world, as in activism.

P4 had found this *'very important'*. Activism had given them *'a third profession and a purpose'*. G said he found his work tended to go in cycles of activity, which could get tiring, *'but it involves my brain'*. P3 looked forward to *'retiring from activism. It can get too busy. There's not enough time to relax.'*

P1 had lost connection with his work colleagues, and lost some confidence playing the trombone, but continued to pick it up to play on his own.

P2's daughter used to be a nurse and after moving into a care home would go round taking people's pulses. *'But nobody helped her to find a substitute for nursing.'* The daughter *'had a dog but dogs were not allowed into the care home'*. And the daughter was not allowed to go out.

G commented that *'Things are taken away but not given back.'* P2 said that *'care takes away control'*, and P1 said he was fearful of losing being normal to the demands and opinions of the care staff.

P4 was frustrated that *'people turn activities or hobbies into therapies, pet therapy, art therapy, etc.'*. P5 spoke about still studying music and playing tennis. They had appeared on the television programme 'The restaurant that makes mistakes', and through this became a celebrity.

Speaking of the Dementia Friendly Communities initiative, P4 said they tried to be part of their local dementia-friendly community, but they had to elbow their way in because people were patronising and wanted to exclude people living with dementia. *'Dementia-friendly often means customer-friendly.'*

A1 asked if 'therapies' are often developed for family members rather than the person with dementia. P3 said he had attended some Alzheimer's Scotland activities but felt he was 'treated like a kid'.

Identity

This webinar was joined by five people living with young onset dementia, and the former carer of one. They are referred to as P1–P6, with P3 being the former carer. Three chapter authors attended (A1–A3) and were invited to ask questions at the end.

G started the discussion by asking, *'How does dementia affect the sense of who you are?'*

P1 felt their identity had changed as a result of being pushed out of work, until they got involved in DEEP, in research and in painting. *'I never made it to retirement; I was forced out of work. Identity is so linked to occupation. People say "Hi, what do you do?" It's a conversation stopper if you have no occupation to talk about.'*

For P2, a healthcare professional for 20 years, *'identity was a big theme at work. At 53 I was not performing well enough at work, and I was assessed and forced to retire … there are so many assumptions about who you are when you have the label "dementia".'*

P1 said, *'Isn't identity about doing things for yourself, not others doing them?'* And that 3–6 months post-diagnosis, there's often a loss of self for people who are diagnosed. P1 wondered whether it is the same for carers? P3, a former carer, explained that their identity *had* changed as a result of providing care.

P4 said they had lost their self, purpose and worth after diagnosis: *'It took me a while to find a new self.'* And P5 commented on what identity means to them: *'The first thing is our name. Hobbies, interests, character, likes and dislikes, faith … it's linked with dignity … people need to be respected and valued.'*

P1 noted that *'identity has a strong link with relationships. Some people go into diagnosis as man and wife and come out as patient and carer'*. One of P1's family members referred to them having *'so-called dementia'* because it was so early in their life. P6 said they would be furious if that was said to them: '*How many times can you keep on educating and telling people about dementia?*'

P2 missed the camaraderie of work; their self-esteem plummeted after retirement. They felt like 'Billy No Mates', and became anxious about joining groups.

G summarised the discussion as follows: '*We have spoken about identity being linked to self-worth, being valued and respected, reciprocal relationships, positive relationships ... you often lose people who imagine that they can't relate to you anymore.*'

P5 spoke about the way you dress. If you wear traditional South Asian dress, it affects how people perceive you, and '*tarnishes* [your] *identity.*'

> *We're all different, we all bleed, we have different languages ... but people don't always accept you for who you are. The biggest factor is trust, knowing each other. I trust G so I'm comfortable to talk here. But it can be very hard when English is your second language.* (P5)

P1 felt that their identity was tied to peer support and dementia activism, '*especially as I live alone; otherwise I would turn inwards and turn my face to the wall. It's about you in your community and your environment. Does identity depend on inner strength?*'

P2 revealed having been told that, '*You don't dress (or look) like you've got dementia.*' The others agreed that this can be '*very, very annoying*', and reveals just how little such people know about dementia. And the participants agreed that identity was an emotional topic. P1 and P2 both said they choose carefully the company they keep in order to feel comfortable and confident.

P5 emphasised that '*we need to be connected socially*'. COVID might have forced physical distancing, but not social distancing over Zoom.

A1 shared that her own mum had dementia. '*She was a very strict person. When she got dementia, she lost control and she hugged and kissed. It was a gift. We had to re-learn how to relate to her.*'

G commented: '*Personality is what others see; identity is what I feel.*' While P2 said that '*it's confusing. It's a semantic thing, but I know I've changed ... but I don't know which part.*'

Speaking as a sociologist, A2 said that '*we see ourselves through reflections of society. We all have deep down identity and we have to hang onto that.*' A3 said that much of what we had said reflected psychological theories. She also asked, when we spoke of work whether we meant paid work only? P1 felt that work was paid employment, while P2 felt that giving a talk about dementia felt like work.

G ended the session by saying that taking part in activism, talks and so on gradually gets into your system and becomes a part of your identity.

Key points

The key issues and concerns raised during the webinars, which we address in this book, are as follows

Control

1. A diagnosis of dementia does not of itself reduce a person's being in control of their life.
2. Life after diagnosis can be very different and very positive, likened to having a 'new life'.
3. Feeling in control depends upon being included in decision-making, however trivial or important.
4. People around you can assume they know what is best for you, and may slip into not including you in discussions and decisions.
5. People with a diagnosis of dementia (at any age) have to preserve their inner strength and identity in order to maintain their control over their lives.
6. Nothing about me without me!
7. Part of having control is deciding when to share your diagnosis with others, with whom and when.
8. People usually feel very low in the months following diagnosis. The consensus was that gaining peer support is the best way out of this, and leads to a much more positive attitude to living with dementia.
9. Technology enables people to retain control in their lives by helping them to continue to be independent of others, particularly using reminders when cooking, or for medications.
10. Specifically for young onset dementia, the ramifications of diagnosis for employment generally mean the end to paid work. Experience suggested that employers use health and safety and any other regulations they can to terminate your employment. They do not generally seek to understand dementia or the law relating to disability.
11. Our contributors had perhaps been lucky in not finding themselves in dire financial circumstances after diagnosis, due to partners continuing to work and mortgages being paid off, but the impact of suddenly ceasing to be employed can be shattering, contributing to the sense of loss and low mood after diagnosis.
12. Family and other gatherings present difficulties for people with dementia, such as noise, disrupted routines and general 'disorder'. People said they felt guilty about not taking part or enjoying family occasions, but they had to withdraw to escape the dementia-related challenges.

Connection

1. Support networks in the community are important to all our participants, with an emphasis on peer support. Peers understand dementia and do not question, they just 'get it'.
2. Participants did acknowledge, however, that it is important to find a peer group that suits you, as not all of them did initially. Once they did so, they said it was like having a 'new family'.

3. Connection through activism and campaigning was very important too, and provided added meaning to people's lives.
4. During COVID-19, the use of Zoom in particular increased connection for many, since meetings were frequent and regular, and some found opportunities (e.g. research) that might not otherwise have presented themselves.
5. Neighbourhood connections are valuable. Our contributors found being out in their community, whether simply taking a walk or sitting in a coffee shop watching the world go by, really valuable. One person noted that when local bus services were reduced, it made it much more difficult to get into town and as a result his mental and cognitive wellbeing were affected.
6. Transport is an issue for most people in maintaining connection. Many lose their driving licence, rely on a reduced bus service – that is, if there is one! – and find taxis both expensive and difficult to arrange.
7. One person with young onset dementia had been moved to a care home, only to have their dog taken away and to be prevented from going out. There was a general fear of going into a care setting and losing control and connection, and having to go along with staff decisions and opinions.
8. There was agreement that dementia-friendly communities generally mean 'customer-friendly' communities, and have little impact on people's daily experiences.
9. Finally, there was also anxiety about ordinary, enjoyable activities becoming 'therapised'.

Identity

1. It is no surprise that identity was associated with one's job. And for people with young onset dementia this is especially relevant. Retirement is one thing, but being forced out of a job that (at least partly) defines one's identity was found to be particularly difficult.
2. However, participants said that becoming involved in activism and campaigning gave them back their identity – indeed, a new and enjoyable identity.
3. Being able to speak freely in peer groups also endorsed people's identity and feelings of self-esteem.
4. Identity was defined by some as doing things for yourself, not what others want you to do.
5. When you have dementia, people make assumptions about you, which undermines your identity. It is important to maintain inner strength to ignore this, and indeed to educate people. Everyone said they had become an educator since diagnosis.
6. Identity is linked to self-worth, being valued and respected, reciprocal relationships and positive relationships.
7. Personality is what others see; identity is what I feel.

Part 1

Maintaining Autonomy

The analysis of responses to the Angela Project found that people living with young onset dementia find services and support helpful when they contribute to them keeping as much control over their life as possible, for as long as possible. This could be through:

- having access to high quality empowering health care, including a sensitively conducted assessment that results in an accurate diagnosis of the type of dementia;
- accessing new technologies and therapies that support and promote independence;
- taking action to manage the financial and legal implications of the diagnosis and future care;
- having a voice in the sort of services that are provided.

The chapters in Part 1 reflect these themes.

Different diagnoses, different people, different needs

Nikki Zimmermann and Sebastian Crutch

Overview

This chapter explores different forms of dementia, and the value that understanding the nature of the condition may bring for the young person living with dementia, their families and friends, and the health and social care professionals working with them. The first part of the chapter explains what we mean by rare dementias and examines three specific forms: frontotemporal dementia, primary progressive aphasia and posterior cortical atrophy. This section contains some technical information about the brain and underlying diseases. It also tries to capture the 'essence' of these conditions, which is most often revealed by individuals' and families' stories about the changes they have experienced. The second part of the chapter concerns the practical and emotional impact of these conditions, and describes some of the ways information, advice and support can be tailored to the individual. Overall, we argue that 'rare' dementias are in fact not that rare (though they are often not recognised or diagnosed) but also that they offer precious insights into the challenges that anyone with any dementia may experience as their condition progresses.

Keywords

Frontotemporal dementia, primary progressive aphasia, posterior cortical atrophy, symptoms, syndromes, practical and emotional support.

Learning points

Enable readers to:

- make distinctions between different forms of dementia, and feel more confident to ask 'Dementia? What type?';
- be able to explain or give a few examples of why understanding both the person and their type of dementia can be helpful when supporting someone with their needs;

- recognise that the experiences of people with 'rare', non-memory-led dementias may reveal something of what people with 'common' dementias may experience as their condition progresses;
- help address the problem of slow and inadequate diagnosis by considering, or encouraging others to consider, the underlying cause of someone's dementia.

Introduction

Awareness of dementia has increased markedly in recent years but the breadth of that understanding is often not matched by depth, with ideas persisting that dementia only affects older people and memory and is the same thing as Alzheimer's disease. Alzheimer's disease is the most common cause of dementia but there are many other diseases that can lead to dementia. These conditions are rarer, can occur at a younger age, and can cause symptoms that are not memory-related. These include difficulties with visual perception, language and communication, movement and behavioural changes.

'Rare dementia' is a term of convenience that refers to forms of dementia which are:

- atypical;
- young onset (with symptoms emerging before the age of 65 years); and/or
- inherited.

It is most easily defined as dementias other than typical late onset Alzheimer's disease, vascular dementia or mixed dementia, the forms of dementia with which most people are familiar. However, despite the term 'rare dementia', the conditions are likely not that rare, and may account for approximately 15% of all dementias – around 147,300 of the estimated 982,000 living with any dementia in the UK (Alzheimer's Research UK, 2024). See Figure 3.1 for an illustration of the main types of dementia and the percentage of cases each accounts for. Conditions falling under the rare dementia umbrella include:

- frontotemporal dementia (FTD);
- primary progressive aphasia (PPA);
- posterior cortical atrophy (PCA);
- Lewy body dementia (LBD);
- young-onset Alzheimer's disease (YOAD).

Two inherited conditions are also covered in this chapter:

- familial frontotemporal dementia (fFTD);
- familial Alzheimer's disease (FAD).

Figure 3.1 Pie chart illustrating the different types of dementia and approximately how common they are.

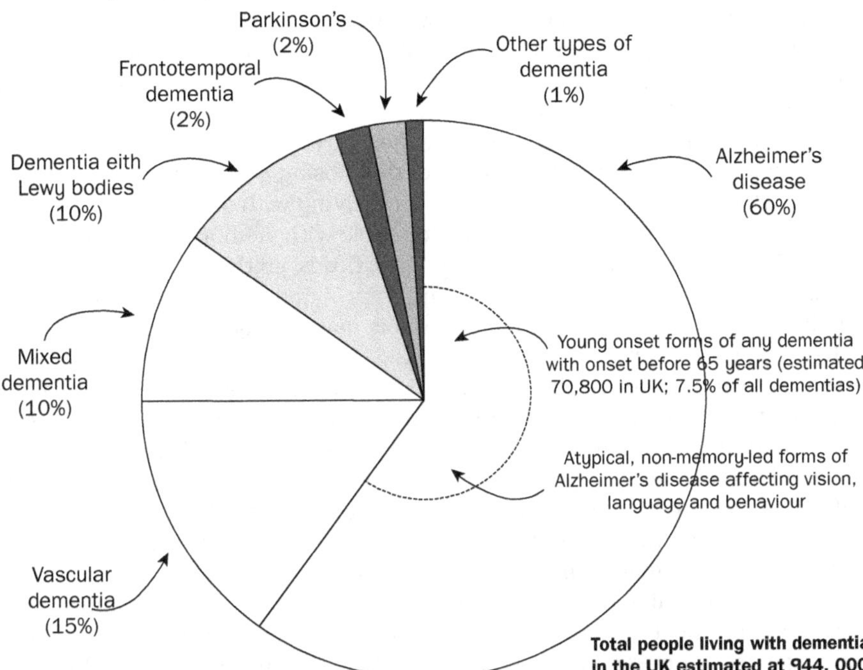

Key: The rare dementias are shown by the various shaded segments. People with young onset dementia are placed at the centre. An additional concentric circle with dotted lines in the Alzheimer's disease segment illustrates atypical forms of Alzheimer's disease. This is placed near the centre because rare dementias are more common but not exclusively seen in younger people.

Adapted from a figure created by Alzheimer's Research UK (2024).

Making a specific diagnosis of these atypical and young onset conditions is critical for planning a trajectory for people living with the condition and their families that ensures there is a fit-for-purpose holistic care plan in place.

Due to the symptoms differing from what is perceived as typical for dementia and occurring at a young age, symptoms are frequently initially mistaken as resulting from menopause, stress, mid-life crisis or relationship problems. Around 30% of people living with a rare dementia initially receive an incorrect diagnosis, and there is a widespread lack of understanding and a shortage of dedicated resources to support those affected. A Memory Assessment Service audit (Royal College of Psychiatrists, 2021) found that 13.3% of dementia diagnoses were other than Alzheimer's disease, vascular dementia or mixed; however, a specific diagnosis was only coded for 42% of those individuals, with the majority listed as 'unspecified dementia'. This highlights the difficulty and delays many experience in getting the correct diagnosis.

Primary care data are equally discouraging about the number of people receiving the specific diagnosis they require. The UK Government began in June 2023 to collect data on just four sub-types of dementia: Alzheimer's disease, vascular dementia, mixed and 'other'. The resulting reports show that the proportion of 'other dementia types' recorded in different locations across England varied between 16% and 66%. This highlights a lack of precision and consistency in diagnosing even common dementias let alone their rarer cousins. (See Chapter X for further detail about the general process of diagnosing young onset dementia.)

Most resources produced to support people living with dementia are targeted at the most affected group, who are older people with memory problems caused by Alzheimer's disease. People in their forties, fifties, sixties and sometimes earlier may have few memory problems but a varying subset of other symptoms and challenges. In some cases, a diagnosis is made of 'young onset dementia', the limitations of which need to be recognised. Age is significant but young onset dementia does not specify the disease, so cannot help the individual or family fully understand their symptoms, or fully anticipate the likely impacts and needs.

The diagnosis of a rare type of dementia can bring with it a set of unique and complex challenges. With such conditions proportionately more likely to develop in individuals at a younger age, this raises additional challenges relating to individual and family responsibilities and transitions, for example, work, medical retirement planning, financial commitments (such as for mortgage and rent), childcare and care transitions, along with challenges to the specific symptoms related to the type of dementia. Many of these age-related challenges are addressed in later chapters. As noted in Chapter X, following a diagnosis, many people find that existing health, social and voluntary services do not cater adequately for their individual needs. In particular, individuals may find that established dementia support groups are not particularly relevant to their situations, owing to different ages, interests and life situations as well as them having different symptoms.

Before describing a few of the rare dementias and their impact upon individual and family lives in more detail, it is worth noting that 'rare' also means precious. The experiences of those living with rare dementias frequently shed light on under-recognised symptoms that may develop later in those with 'common' dementias – which are by their nature progressive – at a point at which memory, communication and other issues may limit others' awareness of such challenges. So, we argue that understanding something about different diagnoses and the impact they may have for different people and their different needs may aid not only those living with or caring for or about someone with one of these conditions, but anyone, with any dementia at any age.

Rare types of dementia

Although there are over a hundred types of dementia, we will focus on three with prominent non-memory-based symptoms: frontotemporal dementia (FTD), primary progressive aphasia (PPA) and posterior cortical atrophy (PCA).

This selection is partly due to their frequency – for example, as we shall see, posterior cortical atrophy is the most common type of 'atypical Alzheimer's disease' – and partly to illustrate the huge contrast in symptoms and challenges when degeneration preferentially affects the very front (FTD), side (PPA) or back (PCA) of the brain.

There are many reasons for seeking the correct diagnosis, but clinically, it is particularly important when it comes to prescribing medications. It is worth noting that frontotemporal dementia and Alzheimer's disease result from changes in the brain that are not only in different locations but are also due to disturbance of different brain proteins building up in an abnormal way in and around brain cells (Dubois et al., 2014; Convery et al., 2019). This is why medications may benefit one condition but not another. At present, there is licensed medication to treat symptoms of Alzheimer's disease. The four currently licensed medications are described in brief on the National Health Service website (2023). Three of them (including Donepezil) are acetylcholinesterase inhibitors, which work by supporting messages between brain cells to get through. Although they can have a modest benefit, there is no evidence that they are helpful in diseases with a pathology of frontotemporal dementia, and in some cases they have been shown to increase anxiety and agitation.

In the new era of disease-modifying therapies (these are medications that can actually slow the course of disease progression, not just treat the symptoms) that we are moving towards, the potential for disease-specific treatments may also motivate greater precision in the diagnostic process in some settings.

The outside layer of the brain, the 'cortex', has four lobes: frontal, temporal, occipital and parietal. Figure 3.2 shows that different lobes are affected in different dementias:

- the left-hand panel shows that the frontal and temporal lobes are affected in frontotemporal dementia;
- the middle panel shows that the temporal lobe is affected in primary progressive aphasia; and
- the right-hand panel shows that the occipital and parietal lobes are most affected in posterior cortical atrophy.

Figure 3.2 Illustrations of the brain regions primarily affected in frontotemporal dementia.

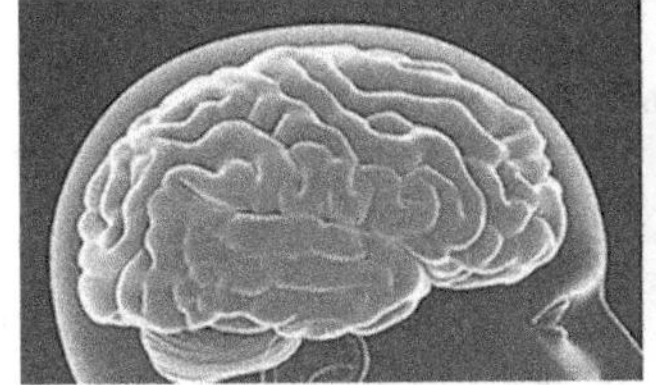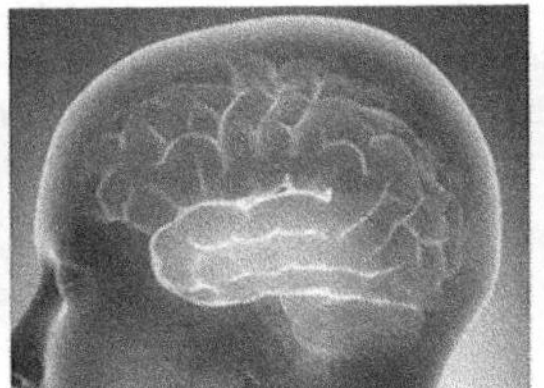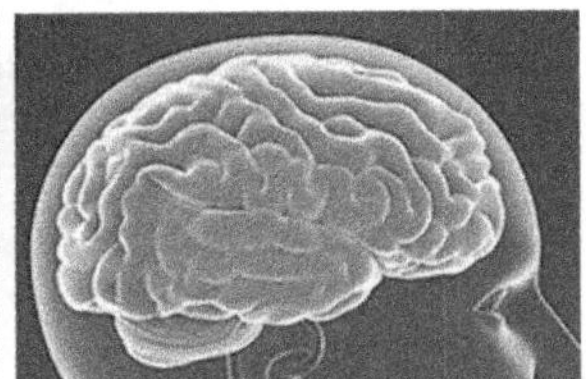

Frontotemporal dementia

Frontotemporal dementia (FTD) is a group of dementias mainly affecting the frontal and temporal lobes of the brain (Figure 3.2). These areas of the brain are involved in particular in regulating personality and behaviour, and enabling communication and speech. Frontotemporal dementia is subdivided into two types:

1. Behavioural variant FTD (bvFTD), mainly affecting behaviour and personality.
2. Primary progressive aphasia (PPA), a group of dementias mainly causing a loss of speech and language abilities. These include:
   o progressive non-fluent aphasia (PNFA) and
   o semantic dementia (SD).

Frontotemporal dementia is caused by the loss of brain cells caused by an abnormal build-up of certain proteins (i.e. Tau, TDP-43 and FUS) in the front of the brain. The processes that lead to the loss of these brain cells are varied and not well understood. In around 30–40% of cases, a person with FTD may have a family history of the condition in which a parent or sibling has been affected. In these cases, the cause of FTD is likely to be genetic.

In a small number of people, FTD overlaps with one of a number of diseases that affect movement of the body such as motor neurone disease, progressive supranuclear palsy and cortico-basal syndrome (see Table 3.1). The symptoms of these diseases can be more physical and can occur alongside FTD, with initial diagnosis sometimes reflecting the order in which cognitive or motor symptoms emerge.

Primary progressive aphasia

Primary progressive aphasia (PPA) refers to a group of dementias that affect speech and language (see Figure 3.2). There are three common types, of which two were listed above as sub-types of FTD; the third is logopenic aphasia, which shares underlying pathology with Alzheimer's disease.

Table 3.1 Common overlaps between types of frontotemporal dementia and diseases that affect movement

	Frontotemporal dementia			
Overlaps	Behavioural variant FTD	Familial FTD	Progressive non-fluent aphasia	Semantic dementia
Progressive supranuclear palsy	X	X	X	
Cortico-basal syndrome	X			
Motor neurone disease	X	X		

Progressive non-fluent aphasia

Progressive non-fluent aphasia (PNFA), also known as the non-fluent/agrammatic variant of PPA (nfvPPA), can affect a person's ability to use speech, to form sentences that make sense, or to use grammar appropriately. For instance, somebody with PNFA might have problems producing the words that they want to say. Their speech might sound very slow or physically difficult, or they may get the order of words in a sentence mixed up. Difficulties with word order and sentences can be present in writing as well as speech. By contrast, comprehension of others' speech is relatively well preserved.

Semantic dementia

Semantic dementia (SD), also known as the semantic variant of PPA (svPPA), affects a person's 'semantic memory', which is the store of knowledge that we gain throughout our lives – our memory for facts rather than events. This includes, for example, knowledge about who people are, what objects are and what words mean. If you said to somebody with semantic dementia, 'Please pass me the scissors', they might reply, 'Scissors? What are scissors?' – although this might only happen with less common items in the early stages. The speech of people with semantic dementia can be quite fluent, but they may start to use more general words, such as 'thingy', as their access to precise words in their vocabulary declines. The loss of understanding of words and objects can differ greatly between people and in the early stages can be quite subject-specific (see Julia's story).

Julie's story of living with semantic dementia

Julie was an A-grade student who graduated from Oxford University with a first class honours degree before pursuing a career in law. Julie excelled at her job and was promoted to a partner in her law firm before the age of 30. As well as juggling a successful and demanding career, Julie and her husband had three children. With a busy family life and many community and social commitments, including charity trustee and school governor roles, Julie decided to step back from work in her forties. Pre-COVID Julie felt she had menopausal problems causing brain fog. Feeling this was quite normal and with no concerns from her GP, she thought these difficulties would pass.

During COVID, Julie and her husband spent a lot more time together, and the specific issues Julie was experiencing became more apparent. On walks in the countryside, she could not distinguish between the different farmyard animals. Her husband would point to a sheep and she suddenly had no concept of the name of the animal.

Later, Julie started to struggle to identify well-known films, which frustrated and concerned her as she had been an avid cinema-goer from an early age.

She also had no recognition of the faces of famous actors, drawing a blank with names she would have known such as Dame Judi Dench or Brad Pitt. When asked if she had enjoyed films that she would have seen even in her earlier years such as *Grease*, *Pretty Woman* and *Dirty Dancing*, she had no idea if they were famous or what they were about.

Julie was diagnosed with semantic dementia at the age of 55. Speaking with Julie, she seems very articulate and coherent, and can hold a basic conversation very well. She admits to struggling in the company of ex-colleagues and loses track in more intellectual conversations, making her feel inferior and having a severe impact on her mental well-being.

Logopenic aphasia

Logopenic aphasia (LPA) is also known as the logopenic variant of PPA (lvPPA). Somebody with LPA might have difficulties with searching for the right word to say, although their ability to physically produce speech is not affected. These word-finding difficulties can lead to long pauses in conversations. People with LPA can also get parts of words muddled up, such as saying 'aminal' instead of 'animal'. Whereas progressive non-fluent aphasia and semantic dementia are types of frontotemporal dementia, LPA, by contrast, is usually caused by the same proteins in the brain that cause Alzheimer's disease. It is often referred to as an unusual ('atypical') form of Alzheimer's disease.

Given the contrasting benefits and negative consequences of prescribing acetylcholinesterase inhibitor medications to people with Alzheimer's disease and frontotemporal dementia mentioned above, the primary progressive aphasias are a prime example where it is important that a diagnosis of not only the syndrome but also the likely underlying disease is in place before prescribing medication.

These different levels of explanation and the fact that some dementias have a general name and specific sub-types, has given rise to a confusing variety of diagnostic terms. The relationship between different dementia clinical diagnoses, syndrome clusters and underlying diseases is described in Figure 3.3.

Posterior cortical atrophy

The most common atypical presentation of Alzheimer's disease is posterior cortical atrophy (PCA). As the name suggests, posterior (= 'back') cortical (= 'of the brain') atrophy (= 'shrinkage') is caused by the progressive loss of brain cells in the parietal and occipital lobes (see Figure 3.2). This results in a profound loss of the ability to see what and where things are, as the brain fails to interpret information about shape, movement, texture and colour. This is very much a 'brainsight' rather than an eyesight problem; episodic memory (i.e. memory for events) and insight are relatively well preserved. Typical early

Figure 3.3 Diagram describing the relationships between diseases that cause dementia and the syndromes (collections of symptoms) they give rise to.

Underlying diseases (and proteins)

Alzheimer's disease (amyloid plaques + tau tangles)

Frontotemporal lobar degeneration (tau/ TDP-43/ FUS)

Clinical diagnoses

Alzheimer's disease (AD) or Young Onset Alzheimer's disease (YOAD)

Posterior cortical atrophy

Logopenic aphasia

Behavioural/dysexecutive AD

Frontotemporal dementia (FTD)

Behavioural variant FTD

Semantic dementia

Progressive nonfluent aphasia

Primary progressive aphasia

Directly inherited form (and responsible genes)

familial Alzheimer's disease (APP/PSEN1/2)

familial FTD (C9orf72/ MAPT/ GRN)

The figure shows the relationship between: diseases (thick solid lines), general or overarching clinical diagnoses (dotted lines), specific diagnosis or sub-types (thin solid lines). (1) Sub-types that come under Alzheimer's disease or young onset Alzheimer's disease; (2) sub-types of frontotemporal dementia; (3) sub-types of primary progressive aphasia.

Adapted from an unpublished figure created by Dr Chris Hardy.

symptoms include difficulty with complex spatial tasks such as judging distances or clipping wing mirrors when driving and parking, orienting clothes correctly when getting dressed, and getting lost on a page when reading.

Posterior cortical atrophy also affects a range of other abilities supported by the back of the brain. These include difficulties with calculation and spelling, as well as spatial judgements in other sensory modalities such as hearing or feeling where things are. Alzheimer's disease is by far the most common disease underlying the syndrome of PCA, accounting for more than 90% of cases, although PCA can also have other causes, including Lewy body dementia, cortico-basal degeneration and, rarely, Prion disease.

Posterior cortical atrophy is commonly a young onset condition with an average age at onset of 58 years, but can occur in much older and much younger people (see Kate's story).

Kate's story of living with posterior cortical atrophy

Kate was a lively young woman in her late twenties. After graduating from university, she worked in London and New York briefly before returning to her home town to be near her family. She had a good job, lots of friends and an active social life. Friends had reported Kate had always been a worrier, being overly cautious and doing slightly odd things, like taking photos of her plugs in her bedroom to ensure she had switched her electrics off before she left the house. She had struggled with dyslexia at school and was often described as 'easily distracted' but always generally happy. Kate started to have high anxiety and complain of visual problems. She was losing the ability to read. Even following basic instructions resulted in severe panic attacks. Her parents suspected a mental health problem. After a referral from the GP, a brain scan was arranged for a suspected brain tumour. However, the scan revealed shrinkage at the back of the brain, and possible PCA. Kate was 29 years old.

Through seeking specialist support and navigation to a specialist cognitive neurology clinic, further investigations were carried out to exclude Creutzfeldt-Jakob disease (CJD) and a brain tumour. The experienced neurologist gave a probable diagnosis of PCA, but also referred on to an international expert on the condition. After further assessments and imaging, this expert confirmed the diagnosis. Kate was the youngest person they had known to be diagnosed with PCA. This referral pathway demonstrates the vital importance of expertise and willingness to refer on, when assessing people with unusual symptoms occurring outside the age range expected for dementia.

The support needed for Kate has been difficult to obtain as she does not fit the remit of most services or the characteristics of most people with the condition. Specialist support has provided help for the family to plan for the future, to adapt the house and their social environment. This has included transforming a room downstairs into a bedroom with ensuite bathroom for Kate. The bedroom has been decorated with contrasting colours to help with visual problems of identifying furniture and spaces. Wardrobe doors have been removed to enable easy access to clothes. Shelves in the wardrobes have been painted in different colours to help Kate identify where different articles of clothes are kept. Voice-activated 'Alexa' and speakers were added to the bedroom and various rooms of the house to help Kate with her independence and choose her favourite music. Motion sensor lighting is also used to help with night-time trips to the bathroom.

The diagnosis has had a huge impact on the lives of the whole family, physically, socially and psychologically. Two years later, Kate is living at home with paid carers helping, but family providing 24/7 care. Her mother is performing all personal care and dressing. Kate struggles walking outside unaided and the internal home environment is now completely adapted to meet her needs as she is easily confused. Continuous support is required as her needs change. Further help is now provided by the community mental health team who regularly visit to help with more pronounced psychological symptoms and the battle for continuing health care (CHC) funding. The CHC assessment criteria do not easily capture or reflect the needs of someone with very rare symptoms at a very young age.

Genetics

Through years of research, it has been discovered that the cause in some individuals of Alzheimer's disease and frontotemporal dementia is a genetic mutation. This means that in each family the disease is caused by a mutation in a single gene. A single copy of the mutated gene, inherited from one parent, will cause the disease. This is known as an *autosomal dominant pattern of inheritance*. Each child of an affected parent will have a 50/50 chance of inheriting the gene mutation and therefore developing the disease, which commonly develops at a similar age to when their parent developed it. This pattern of inheritance accounts for less than 1% of Alzheimer's disease cases overall but is much more common in frontotemporal dementia, since around 30–40% of people diagnosed have a family history of the condition and are likely to have a genetic cause. Those with a strong family history may be referred for genetic counselling in relation to possible genetic testing.

Familial Alzheimer's disease

Familial Alzheimer's disease (FAD) is the name of the inherited form of Alzheimer's disease, also sometimes referred to as autosomal dominant Alzheimer's disease (ADAD). Mutations in three genes are known to cause most cases of FAD. These are the presenilin 1 (PSEN1), presenilin 2 (PSEN2) and amyloid precursor protein (APP) genes, with mutations in PSEN1 being the most common.

Unlike typical Alzheimer's disease (the non-inherited form), which usually occurs in people in their seventies or eighties, FAD usually occurs much earlier. People with FAD typically first develop symptoms before the age of 65, most commonly in their forties or fifties. However, this varies considerably between families. In some families, individuals may be as young as their early thirties when diagnosed. The initial symptoms of FAD are usually similar to those of typical Alzheimer's disease, primarily progressive memory loss, but there are might also be difficulties with communication and mobility, as well as behaviour changes.

Familial frontotemporal dementia

Familial frontotemporal dementia (fFTD) is the name of the inherited form of frontotemporal dementia (FTD). Three genes are responsible for the majority of cases of genetic FTD: progranulin, tau and C9orf72. At least six other genes can cause familial FTD, and more may be discovered. Table 3.2 shows the risk of inheritance of the different types of FTD and some of the related movement disorders.

Table 3.2 Risk of inheritance of frontotemporal dementia and related movement disorders

Type of dementia	Risk of inheritance (%)	No. inheriting the condition
Behavioural variant FTD	40–45%	c. 4 out of 10
Frontotemporal dementia with motor neurone disease	20–40%	2–4 out of 10
Progressive non-fluent aphasia	5–10%	510 out of 100
Cortico-basal syndrome	5%	5 out of 100
Semantic dementia and progressive supranuclear palsy	1%	1 out of 100

Practical and psychological support and well-being

Daily living activities can be hugely disrupted by a diagnosis of a rare dementia and this can also have grave repercussions for the psychological well-being of the person living with the disease and their caregivers. There are many examples where this occurs. For example, the young gentleman with primary progressive aphasia who was once an avid and adventurous cook, who is now totally reliant on his wife to do the food shopping because mixing up his words has had a real impact on his confidence. Even tasks that used to be simple, like ordering the morning coffee at the local café, now induce anxiety, having ordered a 'flat wife' rather than a 'flat white'. Although this can be viewed as humorous, it has also been stigmatising and it has impacted on the couple's relationship as this role has moved away from him.

Sad situations are also regularly faced by families impacted by behavioural variant frontotemporal dementia if disinhibition takes over, interfering with enjoyment of social situations. Examples include family weddings when the affected person makes inappropriate remarks to female family members, or inappropriate jokes made at funerals. Families frequently describe how such events slowly cause the invitations to dry up and the caregivers to feel ostracised and isolated. There are practical ramifications too, for if the person with bvFTD can no longer be asked to go to the shop for bread and milk without the fear of them making suggestive remarks to the female shopkeeper, that becomes another task for the caregivers' to-do list.

The challenges faced by younger people diagnosed with posterior cortical atrophy may be focused much more on practical everyday tasks, but nonetheless have their psychological consequences. For example, common practical impacts of having the condition include always putting jackets on inside out, knocking clear glasses off the table at a restaurant, and struggling to distinguish between sinks and urinals in pubic bathrooms. Having to rely constantly on someone else for help with what are perceived as basic tasks can rob people of their sense of independence and identity.

It is important that the person is seen by an experienced clinician, preferably a cognitive neurologist or a psychiatrist experienced in the field of rare disorders. It is also paramount that the practical and social impacts are fully supported along with psychological needs. Younger people with a diagnosis are often at the heart of many social situations with a variety of responsibilities due to the place and time within their lives. Many are still working and carry professional responsibility and accountability. Many, with young families, are playing a pivotal role in their schools and communities, and may have both upward and downward caring (that is, from the generation above as well as the generation below) and other responsibilities. Many people at this age are also very active with social engagements, sports and other events. Their place in society at this time in their lives often differs greatly to those who are older.

The vulnerabilities and risks associated with a diagnosis of a rare dementia can have a devastating impact on all of these personal, family, professional and community connections, with of course significant emotional, practical and financial impacts that will endure. These are addressed in depth in the following chapters.

Many people living with a rare dementia are very conscious of the terminology used around their condition. Receiving and accepting a diagnosis is never easy. Through the experience of small groups we have facilitated over the years, we have learnt that people feel they live alongside the diagnosis. Whilst not wishing to be labelled as 'suffering', many find it hard to describe themselves as 'living well', often instead stating they are 'living as well as they can'. Despite this rejection of banal positivity, many people with a diagnosis live their best lives and try to be as positive as possible.

Sharing experience reveals powerful stories of people adapting, creating strategies, joining peer support groups, living by routines and changing their ways of coping periodically to meet their evolving and increasing needs. Despite all the challenges, many also demonstrate a profound ability to live with hope, sharing experiences, tips and encouragements with their peers, and joining research programmes through the altruistic desire to enable chances, hopes, interventions and treatments for future generations. (See Chapters 11 and 16 for more on these themes.)

If people have insight into their disease and the symptoms this presents, then through acceptance and understanding many find strategies and solutions to maintain a purposeful life. However, many people living with frontotemporal dementia have a lack of insight due to the damage in the frontal lobe of the brain. The frontal lobe is responsible for behaviour regulation, self-monitoring and the moral coding that underpins knowing what is and is not acceptable. It is hard in this situation to find solutions because the person concerned is unaware that there is anything wrong or different. Often it becomes the responsibility of the family and friends to find ways to adapt their own responses and behaviours to anticipate, navigate and negotiate problematic situations. Whilst challenging, such adaptations are frequently aided by:

- a clear and collective understanding of why certain behaviours occur;
- how those behaviours can be attributed to the disease, not the person; and
- sharing symptom-impact-solution lists of what others have done in similar situations.

An example of a symptom-impact-solution list is:

- A symptom is that the person with frontotemporal dementia has become drawn to sweet foods and every day insists on going to the sweet shop.
- The impact is that their spouse becomes worked up and angry every day.
- The solution found is that instead of getting angry that the person is insistent on going to the sweet shop every morning on the way to the park, the couple have a large breakfast with sweet tasting fruit before going out; the spouse changes their route so they do not go so near the sweet shop; the spouse takes a small bag of sweets as a later 'reward'.

Sometimes we have to accept that obsessions are part of the disease and the focus of obsessions changes over time. Sometimes an understandable sense of hopelessness and annoyance at an obsession can be reduced by hearing from others about similar obsessions that did not last for too long.

The often-used phrase *'when you have met one person with dementia, you have met one person with dementia'* is true for anyone with any dementia but perhaps especially true in relation to individuals with frontotemporal dementia, which can affect people so differently, as illustrated by the quote below:

> *The emotional support I receive is such a lifesaver. My husband has FTD and sometimes life is so hard and I am so fed up. I REALLY need family to 'get' it … it's not THAT hard surely – after eleven years! HE is not making a choice, the ghastly illness is. Trouble is, it is SO good at disguise that our adult children cannot see past Dad who he has always been, and Dad who he is FORCED to be now. Thank goodness I have this emotional support.* (Individual with fronto-temporal dementia)

In other types of rare dementias, such as posterior cortical atrophy and progressive primary aphasia, people are often very insightful and hypervigilant about their symptoms and the impacts these have on their and others' everyday lives. This awareness, which again runs contrary to prevailing stereotypes about people with dementia, can have significant consequences for someone's changing sense of identity, purpose and loss. Preserved insight may also be connected to changes in mood and anxiety, although the psychology and psychiatry of these conditions and other forms of young onset dementia remain relatively poorly understood.

Each different type of dementia typically has an associated group of professionals who have the relevant skills and expertise. However, it is worth noting that the rarity of a diagnosis means some professionals themselves require support in adapting relevant techniques and approaches they use more commonly with people with 'typical' dementia, stroke or other conditions. This support may be provided by cognitive neurologists, via onward referral or discussion of complex or unusual presentations. Cognitive neurologists not only regularly see people with certain symptoms in their clinics but also often spend a significant amount of time in clinical research studies bolstering their understanding of these diseases. Specialist cognitive clinics often have access to specific equipment to provide complex investigations, such as different types of brain scans and lumbar punctures, which Memory Assessment Services may not have access to.

Many people living with progressive primary aphasia reach out to speech and language therapists to instil their knowledge and guide them through a whole host of communications strategies to boost their confidence. Pictures, storyboards, script writing and keyring tags are among the aids and strategies used to help fill in the gaps in conversation and enable people to continue their roles in society, whilst approaches such as communication partner training can often support relationships and friendships.

Many people living with or caring for someone with posterior cortical atrophy find the advice of occupational therapists and local sensory teams very helpful, and also themselves may find creative solutions such as using high contrasting tableware, putting colour tags into clothing to show which way round to wear them, brightly coloured stickers to draw attention to light switches, and adaptations to bathroom furniture and lighting to aid independence. One person who felt well supported by her team commented:

> *Through support I found that finding solutions and creating habits was one of the best skills I could possibly give myself if I were to continue living a life that gave me a level of quality, boosted my self-esteem and the ability to tackle the never ending maze of challenges.* (Individual with posterior cortical atrophy)

In the case of families with directly inherited dementias, specialist psychological and counselling support is often needed. This is to help family members make decisions around specific issues, such as genetic testing and whether or how to have children, and to address the wider implications for individuals and families. The complexity of the situation gives rise to a large number of issues that are rarely addressed in standard dementia practice, including rumination on risk, disclosure of genetic risk to children, and gene-non-carrier survivor guilt. Ideally, support is tailored to individuals' evolving needs, as they move from caring for family members and being at risk to potentially becoming affected themselves.

Activities of daily living and social needs

Everyone living with dementia and their families will have struggles at some point with activities of daily living (ADLs). It is important that these are assessed appropriately so adaptations and support can be put in place to allow people to enjoy fulfilled lives. The remaining chapters in the first part of this book address a number of approaches to help people maintain independence.

The type of care needs to be individually catered to the person living with dementia or a family carer. In the UK, Social Needs Assessments or Carers' Assessments should be carried out by the local authorities. There is no charge for a care needs assessment and everyone is entitled to one regardless of income, savings or level of need. A social care professional will usually do a home visit or online assessment interview to find out how someone is managing everyday tasks. The person will ask about:

- your health, and what you can and cannot do, or struggle to do;
- your cultural and religious background and support network;
- your current living arrangements;
- how you would like to be supported; and
- information about your needs from your carer, if you want them to be involved in your assessment.

The local council must do their best to help each person, and should consider what support is needed right now, and what might help in the future. As with much form-filling, there are a lot of generic areas to cover, in order to reveal any risks. The basic categories cover: nutrition, mobility, hygiene, personal care, dressing, safety at home, maintaining personal relations, being part of the community, and wellbeing and being safe from harm.

Problems arise due to the very wide range of conditions and disabilities these assessments need to cover. It is often perceived that the ideal candidate for such an assessment is a frail elderly lady with memory problems who may forget to eat and become malnourished, or eat food that is out of date and become ill; or who has mobility problems and may fall in the car park going to the supermarket; or who may dress unwisely for the season and wear a winter coat in summertime with risk of overheating. But there are quite different risks in many younger onset and rare dementias. For example, a younger person with frontotemporal dementia:

- Would typically not be frail and may be physically fit and with lots of energy. Therefore, they might not be perceived to have any problems relating to mobility. However, the compulsive behaviour associated with FTD often reduces people's ability to weigh up risk, leading to risks crossing roads or to excessive walking to the extent of becoming exhausted and getting lost, or in the home attempting unsafe DIY repairs, to name but a few.
- Would likely not forget to eat; quite the contrary, they would eat excessively and often be attracted to carbohydrate-rich or sugary foods putting them at risk of obesity. They may even steal to fulfil the compulsive need for sweet foods.
- Rather than dressing with excessive clothing, a common symptom of FTD is disinhibition, and the lack of understanding what is and is not appropriate in public, so in hot weather the risk might be of the person removing all items of clothing.

It is therefore imperative that advice is given to prepare for such social care and needs assessments, as those with rare dementia need to have their specific needs identified and support plans in place to meet these needs.

Diagnosis of different types

The key point about diagnosing most rare dementias is that the clinical history is key. The diagnosis rests primarily on clinical assessment, with other investigations, including neuropsychological, neuroimaging and biomarker support where appropriate. In that sense, with the right knowledge and experience, many rare dementia diagnoses are accessible, and not all require specialist equipment or laboratory processes. A guide to key questions, signs and symptoms for healthcare professionals can be accessed in table 1 of an article written by a team of clinical-academics from specialist cognitive clinical and research centres (Johnson et al., 2021).

Some generic cognitive assessment tools may not be suitable to diagnose non-memory-led dementias, as they are often based primarily on evaluation of episodic memory. Furthermore, some investigations, such as specific forms of brain imaging, lumbar puncture to gather cerebrospinal fluid and detailed neuropsychometric testing, may not be deliverable within some Memory Assessment Services, so are often better conducted via referral to a cognitive neurology clinic.

As noted in the introduction, the wide variation in rates of 'dementia unspecified' diagnoses across different services and areas in the UK strongly signals inconsistencies in the depth and appropriateness of assessment processes. This variation is reflected clearly in the accounts of people living with dementia and their families. Assessment and diagnosis in the case of a rare dementia may take several visits, and ongoing monitoring with follow-up appointments is necessary. The neurodegenerative nature of such conditions means it is important that those with a rare dementia are monitored periodically after diagnosis by specialists to review their changing needs. Sadly such services are not commissioned in all areas.

Conclusions

Whilst it may seem counterintuitive to finish rather than start a chapter about rare dementias with the practicalities of diagnosis, we placed the discussion at the end to make the point that expert diagnosis is vital for all, yet is not currently available or provided to all. The call to action really has to be for more people – both those living with dementia and professionals who are diagnosing and supporting those who do – to ask the question: 'Dementia? What type?' Without the appropriate diagnosis, too much time and too many opportunities to understand, adapt and receive support will continue to be wasted.

With the right diagnosis, people are much better equipped to anticipate, plan for and address their needs and the needs of those around them. People can reduce the sense of loneliness and dislocation that often accompanies a diagnosis by finding and meeting others in a similar situation. And professionals can tailor the care and support they offer to best meet the needs of those they serve.

The time of the naysayers who disparage the value of a diagnosis 'because there is no treatment' has passed – not just because we are entering a new era of disease-modifying therapies, but because of the overwhelming evidence that offering the right support at the right time delivers real benefits for individuals, families and care systems.

The arguments of those who exalt person-centredness above all are incomplete – to misquote William Osler, we need to 'ask not *just* what disease the person has, but *also* what person the disease has'. Tom Kitwood acknowledged neurological impairment as one influence on how a person is affected by dementia and as a factor that needs to be understood to provide person-centred care. However, having broadened thinking to be holistic, the importance of the nature of neurological impairment is sometimes overlooked or even dismissed as reflecting a narrow biomedical approach. In young onset dementia, knowing the nature of neurological impairment is vital. A growing collective acknowledgement and response to different diagnoses, not just different people, will help to identify and cater for different needs, ultimately benefiting anybody with any dementia.

So what does this mean in practice?

If you have had a diagnosis or have a family member or friend who has a diagnosis or maybe you have some suspicions or concerns

Do you know where to go and what questions to ask? Do you know you are entitled to a second opinion or to have further investigations to establish a specific diagnosis and that the GP or Memory Assessment Service can refer on for this? Having a correct and specific diagnosis is just the start, and post-diagnostic support is essential to understand and to live as well as possible.

If you are a clinician working in a Memory Assessment Service

Do you feel you have an awareness of the early signs of the different subtypes of Alzheimer's disease, frontotemporal dementia and related conditions? And do you and your team have the confidence to offer adequate advice and support to people and their families who have a suspected diagnosis of these sub-types? Familiarity with the distinctive early signs of these different types of dementia can minimize the likelihood of overlooking or misattributing symptoms to depression, anxiety and menopause.

The key factor in the majority of rare dementia diagnoses is listening to the clinical history and experiences of the people sat before you and evidencing this with the appropriate procedures. Those with dementia should not necessarily have to visit an academic specialist centre to gain an accurate diagnosis. The real question is whether you feel confident to make the diagnosis and whether you have access to the services for required extra investigations? If not, you should consider making an onward referral to a specialist centre.

If you work in a social care team

Is your knowledge extensive enough to be able to carry out symptom-relevant needs and care assessments for people living with atypical dementias and their families? It has been established that the 'one-size-fits-all' approach is no longer appropriate and people with atypical dementias will often have non-memory-based needs, which need to be met to enable them to live a fulfilled life.

References

Alzheimer's Research UK (2024) *Breakdown of dementia by disease type*, Dementia Statistics Hub. Available at: https://dementiastatistics.org/about-dementia/subtypes/ (accessed 20 May 2024).

Convery, R., Mead, S. and Rohrer, J.D. (2019) Review: Clinical, genetic and neuroimaging features of frontotemporal dementia, *Neuropathology and Applied Neurobiology*, 45 (1): 6–18.

Dubois, B., Feldman, H.H., Jacova, C., et al. (2014) Advancing research diagnostic criteria for Alzheimer's disease: the IWG-2 criteria, *Lancet Neurology*, 13 (6): 614–29.

Johnson, J.C.S., McWhirter, L., Hardy, C.J.D., et al. (2021) Suspecting dementia: canaries, chameleons and zebras, *Practical Neurology*, 21 (4): 300–12.

National Health Service (NHS) (2023) *What are the treatments for dementia?* Available at: https://www.nhs.uk/conditions/dementia/about-dementia/treatment/ (accessed 20 May 2024).

How sensitive delivery of diagnosis can be empowering

Mary O'Malley and Janet Carter

Overview

This chapter provides evidence-based information about how to deliver a diagnosis in a way that is both sensitive and empowering. It is centred around some key findings from the diagnostic workstream of the Angela Project. The chapter first considers why it is vital for the clinician, who tells the person with young onset dementia about their diagnosis, to have empathy. This is followed by an overview of the issues that make it challenging for clinicians to undertake assessment and diagnosis of young onset dementia and a summary of research into how well standards for good quality assessment and diagnosis are being met. The chapter then turns to the communication of the diagnosis, looking at why clinicians find this hard to do and at what those living with young onset dementia want from the process. Twenty-seven consensus statements from people living with young onset dementia and their supporters are presented with a view to spreading information about how to improve practice in disclosing to someone that they have young onset dementia.

Keywords

Sensitivity, empowerment, the Angela Project, diagnosis, functional statements, relational statements.

Learning points

- Receiving a diagnosis of young onset dementia can be experienced as destabilising and associated with shock, stigma and fear.
- Educating clinicians has potential to improve sensitivity and awareness about the impact of a diagnosis of young onset dementia.
- Being honest about uncertainty in diagnosis allows development of partnerships and shared decision-making that can improve engagement in services after diagnosis.

- Empowering individuals and families to understand their diagnosis is a reasonable expectation of all healthcare professionals, whether working in dementia services or in more general mental health, physical health or primary care settings.

Introduction

Empathy: the foundation for empowering delivery of a diagnosis of young onset dementia

Receiving a diagnosis of any type of young onset dementia has a profound impact on an individual's future. It is a life-changing diagnosis that may be experienced with feelings of shock, stigma, fear and destabilisation. On the other hand, it can also be experienced as empowering and enabling as it offers answers to uncertainty and a way forward (Wawrziczny et al., 2016; Rabanal et al., 2018).

A literature review conducted as part of the Angela project emphasised how unique the impact of receiving a diagnosis is to each family affected and how vital the role of the clinician is in communicating the diagnosis (O'Malley et al., 2019). When a diagnosis is made, the clinician needs to consider what information to give and how to communicate that information. In doing so, the clinician needs to bear in mind the potential impact on the individual and any family members. Empathy with the person and family is vital.

Doctors view diagnosis of dementia as a process, from pre-diagnostic counselling to support after diagnosis, as opposed to a single event or consultation (Hellström and Torres, 2013; Bailey et al., 2018). Delivering a diagnosis of dementia is a challenging process. It requires the clinician to balance the need to provide clear diagnostic information with being sensitive to the emotional experience of the person with dementia and their family.

A sensitive approach to delivery of the diagnosis involves discussion. This allows the person being diagnosed to 'have a voice' and ensures that their preferences, needs and values guide clinical decision-making. This in turn should result in care that feels respectful and responsive. When those making the diagnosis show sensitivity about the potential impact of diagnosis, this fosters an openness in the discussion. This empowers the person to feel more in control of the process and thus supports autonomy. This lays the foundation for the person being diagnosed and those providing the diagnosis to work together in partnership to plan for the future. The diagnostic complexity of young onset dementia means there is the need to remain open to review, and the diagnosing clinician may potentially modify his or her opinion over time as symptoms emerge and final diagnoses may change. The impact of this is better facilitated by strong partnerships and openness about uncertainty. Development of a trusting partnership between the clinical team and the person with young onset dementia can support the development of a positive outlook and make it more likely that the person receiving the diagnosis will engage with support services in the post-diagnostic stage.

Why is making the diagnosis of young onset dementia particularly challenging?

For many clinicians in general practice, adult psychiatry, general neurology and older adult memory services, the presenting symptoms of dementia in younger people may rarely be encountered. This makes it particularly challenging for these healthcare professionals to make a diagnosis. Dementia diagnosis is dominated by the view, derived from the numerical dominance of late onset Alzheimer's disease, that all dementia is associated with older age, day-to-day memory loss and decline in functioning. It may be rare for staff to be faced with a younger person with a different sort of presenting picture, so this situation demands a skill set that may not feel familiar.

As noted in Chapter 3, in young people, dementia often arises from rare causes and even frequent-cause dementia such as Alzheimer's disease may present with atypical symptoms such as visual problems, personality and behaviour change, and language problems. This can make diagnosis in younger individuals more challenging (Rossor et al., 2010; Rosness et al., 2016; Cations et al., 2021). Misdiagnosis may include psychiatric conditions such as depression and anxiety, and other neurological illnesses (Vieira et al., 2013; Tsoukra et al., 2022), which are common in this age group.

One in three people with young onset Alzheimer's disease presents with problems associated with posterior cortical atrophy (PCA). People with PCA experience problems with recognising objects and other visual changes (Crutch et al., 2012). Inherited forms of frontotemporal dementia (FTD) and Alzheimer's disease that run in families are also common and may present with neurological symptoms, such as repetitive involuntary movements, or with psychiatric symptoms, such as hallucinations or delusions (Greaves and Rohrer, 2019). People with behavioural variant frontotemporal dementia (bvFTD) may start to show lack of empathy or concern for others. In addition, some of the first signs might be social disinhibition, for example enthusiastically embracing someone they have only just met, or acting on aggressive or appetitive urges that would normally be repressed. For example, someone who has not usually used swearwords might swear in polite company or the person may over-eat sweet foods, for example, consuming several packets of biscuits in one sitting (Greaves and Rohrer, 2019). Changes in managing complex tasks may be identified by individuals becoming apathetic, repetitive or failing to plan ahead. Similarly, those with primary progressive aphasias are likely to experience various problems with language, such as retaining the meaning of words, producing or finding words (Gorno-Tempini et al., 2011).

How good is current assessment and diagnosis of young onset dementia?

A recent Australian study found that almost four in ten people who received a diagnosis of a young onset dementia at some point experienced a change in diagnosis, either from dementia to a different condition or vice versa (Tsoukra et al., 2022). On one hand, this demonstrates the complexity of making an accurate diagnosis, especially at an early stage; on the other, it raises questions about the quality of the diagnostic process. Several studies have evaluated the quality of the assessment and diagnosis of possible dementia in people aged 65 and younger. Most of these studies compared current practice against evidence-based guidelines for assessment and diagnosis (Salem et al., 2014; Konijnenberg et al., 2017). Such guidelines state that assessment, for people with suspected dementias of any age, should include as a minimum:

- history of cognitive symptoms;
- cognitive testing;
- psychiatric evaluation;
- physical examination including neurological examination;
- assessment of activities of daily living (ADLs);
- a set of blood tests; and
- an electrocardiogram (ECG) together with computerised tomography (CT) or magnetic resonance imaging (MRI) scans of the brain.

An acceptable assessment including all items of recommended basic diagnostic evaluation was performed in only 24% of younger people (Salem et al., 2014; Konijnenberg et al., 2017). This raises concern in terms of basic quality of assessment.

Even if fully followed, the investigations listed above are often insufficient to identify the complexity of presentation in young onset dementia. The Royal College of Psychiatrists (RCP) Memory Services National Accreditation Programme (Jethwa et al., 2022) includes three specific standards related to assessment of young onset dementia:

> The service has access to in-depth assessment of occupational functioning and neuropsychological assessment as required (e.g. for young onset dementia, complex or abnormal presentations).

> Specialist advice is taken when interpreting investigations/assessments/scans in people with complex needs, such as … those with young onset or rare dementias.

> The service can refer on to specialist services for rare or young onset dementia and/or complex care needs (e.g. regional/tertiary neurology/neuropsychiatry services …).

Further, most clinicians would recognize other crucial supplementary investigations may be needed, such as lumbar puncture for cerebrospinal fluid (CSF) analysis and genetic testing. Evidence suggests, however, that under-investigation is particularly common in non-specialist settings such as generic memory clinics that cover all age groups rather than specialising in young onset dementias (Eriksson et al., 2014).

As part of the Angela Project, the research team worked with international experts in the field of diagnosis of young onset dementia to develop a quality standard for assessment of the condition. The quality standard consisted of 31 different indicators that summarised expert opinions about how to make a comprehensive assessment (O'Malley et al., 2020). The project team undertook a benchmarking exercise of current UK practice across eight NHS memory services in England. They compared practice in these services against the quality standards. A thorough investigation of 402 patient records of individuals diagnosed with young onset dementia showed that there were gaps in practice, with most services meeting on average only 36% of these gold standard indicators (O'Malley et al., 2022). These findings confirmed earlier studies of the variations in clinical practice across sites and identified commonly missed items compared to expert consensus. The Angela Project focused on typical NHS mental health trusts and did not include people with young onset dementia diagnosed in neurology and specialist services. However, the study helped highlight gaps in current practice.

Over 20 years ago, Williams, Dearden and Cameron (2001) highlighted that most younger people with suspected dementia experienced chaotic pathways into care, with many seeing between two and five different specialist consultants before receiving a definitive diagnosis. Although this was many years ago, it appears from personal accounts that this is still a common experience. Care pathways for younger people with dementia differ significantly across the UK (Stamou et al., 2021). Influencing factors include whether:

- there are clinicians who have expert knowledge in young onset dementia;
- there is access to appropriate diagnostic teams (such as neurology, neuroradiology, speech and language therapy, clinical psychologists); and
- there are established young onset dementia support services in the area (Carter et al., 2017).

The RCP Memory Services National Accreditation Programme (Jethwa et al., 2022) now includes a standard related to the need for a local integrated care pathway for young onset dementia, so it remains to be seen whether this has a positive influence.

The Angela Project literature review (O'Malley et al., 2019) confirmed that under-recognition of and awareness about dementia in younger people, together with misattribution of symptoms, were major contributing factors to the much longer delays in receiving a diagnosis for younger adults compared to older adults. A study by Roach et al. (2013) additionally highlighted that clinicians and healthcare professionals doubted dementia as a cause of the symptoms, specifically because the person was young, looked physically healthy and was still working (Harris, 2004). Rohra (2016) reported that unnecessary delays arose from misdiagnosis of depression or burnout, indicating that psychiatric disorders are more immediately considered as a primary diagnosis. Despite evidence of day-to-day difficulties, getting professionals to listen to what was wrong proved difficult and concerns were often dismissed. This illustrates why it is crucial to raise awareness of young onset dementia among clinicians and the importance of its inclusion in clinical training.

Arguably, misdiagnoses resulting from insufficient or inadequate investigation of symptoms may be preventable by improving the knowledge and specialist training of general practitioners and dementia specialists involved in primary and secondary care. Enabling a timely diagnosis would protect people with young onset dementia from experiencing prolonged periods of uncertainty without understanding the underlying cause for their difficulties (van Vliet et al., 2012). Additionally, it could further prevent unnecessary service costs and speed up access to post-diagnostic care (Carter et al., 2017).

For young people, the consequence of the complex issues outlined above can mean a delay to referral due to under-recognition, under-investigation of key symptoms, misdiagnosis, and a long and daunting process to obtaining a definitive diagnosis (van Vliet et al., 2011; Draper et al., 2016; Millenaar et al., 2016). Providing individuals with an accurate diagnosis allows them and their families access to suitable treatments, support and research opportunities. Timely diagnosis and improved recognition have been rated by those with young onset dementia as the highest priority for service improvement (Armari et al., 2012).

Why is delivering the diagnosis of young onset dementia challenging for staff?

We have looked above at the complexity of diagnosis of young onset dementia itself but the process of giving the diagnosis is also challenging for clinicians. Studies show that clinicians may prevaricate in their explanations and avoid using necessary or appropriate medical language that the person and their family need in order to fully understand the diagnosis (Dhedhi et al., 2014; Dooley et al., 2015; Bailey et al., 2018). One study identified that communication training in memory services was inadequate in preparing doctors to deliver honest yet hopeful information about dementia diagnosis (Bailey et al., 2018). This was extra challenging when the person had difficulties with comprehension. The diagnostic feedback usually involves the individual and family members, and often friends and extended family. Balancing what can be discussed in front of disparate parties is also challenging for clinicians to gauge.

The journey to diagnosis – the younger person's perspective

Young people with dementia have spoken eloquently about the impact of diagnosis. Kate Swaffer, who is living with young onset dementia, has argued that an early diagnosis can be regarded as empowering, enabling and assisting the individual to remain independent for longer (Swaffer, 2016). Another key advocate for younger people living with dementia was Wendy Mitchell, who contributed greatly to research involvement for younger people with dementia, writing books and raising awareness of the importance of diagnosis. In an opinion piece for the *British Medical Journal* (Mitchell, 2019), Wendy emphasised the importance of 'hope' during and following diagnosis. She asked doctors to re-phrase how they deliver the diagnosis of dementia, suggesting that it is given like this:

> Yes, the diagnosis is that of dementia and not something anybody would wish to have. But think of it as the start of a different way of living; a way of adapting. I may not be able to offer any treatment, but I can offer help and there is still so much you can do, albeit differently and with support. (Mitchell, 2019)

The lived experience – evidence-based statements

One of the main aims of the Angela Project was to understand what mattered most to people living with young onset dementia and their family 'supporters' when receiving a diagnosis of young onset dementia. The direct voice of people and family living with young onset dementia is crucial to shaping good clinical practice in diagnosis. To find out what mattered most, the research team used a Delphi study to explore the real-world experience of young people and their families who had recently received a diagnosis. This method involves recruiting a panel of people who are invited to give their individual opinion in relation to an issue. The opinions are turned into statements and the panel members are asked to rate each one, saying whether they feel it is important or not. The average ratings are then fed back to the panel, along with any comments that were made. Over successive rounds of feedback, the aim is to find out which statements are very widely supported. These form a consensus opinion.

In this Delphi consensus study, 18 younger people with dementia and 18 'supporters' from across England were asked to rate individually what they felt was absolutely essential and very important to them when undergoing assessment for and feedback about a diagnosis of dementia (O'Malley et al., 2021). From initial open-ended questions, summary statements were refined and rated in two subsequent rounds to gain consensus on their views. Most of the panel agreed that 27 statements were absolutely essential or very important. These fell into two principal areas of concern:

- those connected with the relational aspects of assessment and diagnosis (i.e. aspects such as communication and inclusion, which were linked to the relationship between the person and their family members and the clinical team); and
- those related to the way the service systems function (i.e. aspects connected with the set-up and organisation of the assessment and diagnosis process).

The statements are shown in Boxes 4.1 and 4.2.

Box 4.1 lists the 11 statements related to relational factors about how the diagnosis was communicated and what is essential for a positive diagnostic experience.

Box 4.1: Relational aspects of the diagnostic process

1. **Private discussions:** Clinicians should offer opportunities for the person with dementia and their supporters to speak separately about any issue they wish to discuss.
2. **Reaction to diagnosis:** Remember that receiving the diagnosis is a lot to take in for the person with dementia and supporters.
3. **Explanation of assessments:** Clinicians should provide information about investigations (for example, on what the SPECT scanning was all about).
4. **Understanding all forms of dementia:** Clinicians should inform the person during the assessments about why certain tests are used, e.g. inclusion of visual tests to assess for posterior cortical atrophy.
5. **Being involved:** Being kept in the loop and feeling involved in the assessment.
6. **Meeting in person:** Communication with clinicians should ideally be in person.
7. **Avoid repetition:** Avoiding the same questions being asked by the separate clinicians where possible.
8. **Considerate use of language:** Clinicians should be compassionate, empathic and respectful and particularly sensitive when providing information about a diagnosis.
9. **Time to ask questions:** Give the person with dementia and their family enough opportunities to ask questions.
10. **Calm approach:** The clinician should be calm, approachable and easy to talk to.
11. **Using lay terms:** Clinicians should explain medical terms in a simplified manner.

Adapted from: O'Malley et al. (2021).

Box 4.2 lists the 16 statements related to how the memory service operated, which were viewed as absolutely essential or very important to people with young onset dementia and their supporters.

Box 4.2: Functional aspects of the diagnostic process

1. **Appointment:** Ensure there is enough notice between letters being issued and appointments.
2. **Convenience:** Make appointments convenient for working adults.
3. **Follow-up letter:** Provide the person with dementia and their supporters with a letter which details the diagnosis.

4. **Contact family supporters:** Healthcare professionals should contact family supporters if unable to get through to the person with dementia directly regarding appointments.
5. **Single point of contact:** Have an identified key person as a single point of contact throughout the whole diagnostic process.
6. **Quick referral**: The referral process from GP to first assessment needs to be shorter.
7. **Referrals to specialist services:** Referrals should ideally be made to specialist young onset dementia clinicians and services.
8. **Home visits:** Patients should be seen at home for assessments and post-diagnostic support where appropriate.
9. **Multidisciplinary team:** There should be a multidisciplinary team involved in diagnosis to provide appropriate support.
10. **Enhanced awareness of young onset dementia:** More awareness and training on rarer dementia types as well as the issues faced by young people with dementia in mental health trusts.
11. **Improved access to clinics:** Better access to sleep and anger clinics.
12. **Pleasant MRI experience:** The MRI experience should provide blankets, ear protectors to reduce noise and allow supporters to be in the room if the person being assessed so wishes.
13. **Results issued more quickly:** Results need to be given in the clinic more quickly.
14. **Shorter time to diagnosis:** The time taken to achieve a formal diagnosis needs to be shortened if possible.
15. **Recognition:** For the GP to identify dementia in younger people.
16. **Assessments:** Assessments should be conducted in a quiet and private room.

Adapted from: O'Malley et al. (2021).

Why are the statements important?

The statements on how to convey the diagnosis of young onset dementia are important to inform clinicians about what is important to those receiving the diagnosis. The statements represent the most essential elements of assessment and diagnosis for people who have experienced the process. Prime concerns were sensitivity in relaying the diagnosis, including what information was given, how it is communicated, and recognition of the potential impact on the individual and their family, and the need for an empathic approach.

Guidance from the British Psychological Society (Watts et al., 2018) provides advice for clinicians on how best to communicate a diagnosis of dementia, recommending that it be person-centred, considerate of individuals' expectations, preparedness and expressed wishes, and that consent be taken. Ensuring these principles are considered when diagnosing younger adults may be more challenging. For example, language variants, visuospatial variants and behavioural change are more common in younger people and understanding of the user perspective can be hard to gain. This might be overcome by avoiding delivering too much information at once, avoiding medical jargon, making explanations specific to an individual rather than generic, going at a slow pace and avoiding over-complicated explanations. Delivering information that is specific to the individual, and embedding information about the diagnosis within an explanation of findings from investigations, will make it more likely that the information will be recalled, understood and accepted.

Dementia Australia (2017) has published helpful guidance on better ways to communicate more generally with people with dementia, including recommendations to improve understanding, and seeking ways to encourage communication and expression when language and communication are significantly affected. These recommendations, which apply equally to those with young onset dementia, highlight the positives of treatment and new research, of being culturally and linguistically sensitive to those from diverse backgrounds, and of recognising that disclosure may be more appropriate over multiple visits.

Bill's experience of receiving his diagnosis

Bill (pseudonym) is a 61-year-old engineer and has recently been diagnosed with Alzheimer's disease after noticing changes in his ability at work and in concentration over the last year. His friends had also noticed he struggled to add up the scores at golf, and his wife thought he was more distant and less interested in going out and seeing family. After his initial visit to the GP his GP, he was referred to the local memory service team who invited Bill and his wife for an initial assessment to understand the changes they had both noticed. The memory service staff were reassuring and listened to their concerns. The staff explained that if Bill consented to proceed with further assessment, it was possible that a diagnosis of dementia could be the outcome.

Bill underwent detailed assessments with the multidisciplinary team who made him feel comfortable, explained the assessments and provided ample opportunity to answer any questions. The memory service team and clinicians took care to use lay terms when relaying the findings from the assessments to Bill and his family, and they were flexible in how they delivered results. Bill and his family chose to receive a follow-up visit in the comfort of their own home shortly after the feedback of the diagnosis when they had had a chance to take in the results. Bill and his wife were then provided with information about local post-diagnostic services they might be interested in exploring in future. Overall, Bill felt his journey to receiving a diagnosis was handled well. He was always kept informed of what was happening and now feels his diagnosis has given him an answer to the problems he had been experiencing.

Conclusions

This chapter has highlighted the importance of sensitivity in diagnosis of young onset dementia. It shows how recent research can provide new learning for clinicians and existing services about good practice. The style of communication, understanding of the impact of diagnosis and the clinicians' empathy can make a difference to personal experience and foster openness in discussion to support autonomy and partnership working. Combined, these factors can contribute to a positive outlook and promote engagement with services after diagnosis.

So what does this mean in practice?

For individuals and families

A new diagnosis is a lot to take in and each party may have different concerns that require private conversations.

For clinicians working in memory clinics

Remember that a sensitive empathic approach, giving time to individuals and families to discuss, absorb and learn about the diagnosis, can help support strong partnerships and shared decision-making for the future.

For organisers of memory services

Remember that convenient appointment times will be essential for working adults and a named contact can be helpful for organising this.

For clinic staff and healthcare professionals working in the field

Remember that new information and accessible resources about best practice are available via the Young Dementia Network.

References

Armari, E., Jarmolowicz, A. and Panegyres, P.K. (2012) The needs of patients with early onset dementia, *American Journal of Alzheimer's Disease and Other Dementias*, 28 (1): 42–46.

Bailey, C., Dooley, J. and McCabe, R. (2018) 'How do they want to know?' Doctors' perspectives on making and communicating a diagnosis of dementia, *Dementia*, 18 (7/8): 3004–22.

Carter, J.E., Oyebode, J.R. and Koopmans, R.T.C.M. (2017) Young-onset dementia and the need for specialist care: a national and international perspective, *Aging and Mental Health*, 22 (4): 468–73.

Cations, M., Loi, S.M., Draper, B., et al. (2021) A call to action for the improved identification, diagnosis, treatment and care of people with young onset dementia, *Australian and New Zealand Journal of Psychiatry*, 55 (9): 837–40.

Crutch, S.J., Lehmann, M., Schott, J.M., et al. (2012) Posterior cortical atrophy, *Lancet Neurology*, 11 (2): 170–78.

Dementia Australia (2017) *Assessment and diagnosis of dementia*. Available at: https://www.dementia.org.au/professionals/assessment-and-diagnosis-dementia.

Dhedhi, S.A., Swinglehurst, D. and Russell, J. (2014) 'Timely' diagnosis of dementia: what does it mean? A narrative analysis of GPs' accounts, *BMJ Open*, 4 (3): e004439. Available at: https://doi.org/10.1136/bmjopen-2013-004439.

Dooley, J., Bailey, C. and McCabe, R. (2015) Communication in healthcare interactions in dementia: a systematic review of observational studies, *International Psychogeriatrics*, 27 (8): 1277–1300.

Draper, B., Cations, M., White, F., et al. (2016) Time to diagnosis in young-onset dementia and its determinants: the INSPIRED study, *International Journal of Geriatric Psychiatry*, 31 (11): 1217–24.

Eriksson, H., Fereshtehnejad, S.M., Falahati, F., et al. (2014) Differences in routine clinical practice between early and late onset Alzheimer's disease: data from the Swedish Dementia Registry (SveDem), *Journal of Alzheimer's Disease*, 41 (2): 411–19.

Gorno-Tempini, M.L., Hillis, A.E., Weintraub, S., et al. (2011) Classification of primary progressive aphasia and its variants, *Neurology*, 76 (11): 1006–14.

Greaves, C.V. and Rohrer, J.D. (2019) An update on genetic frontotemporal dementia, *Journal of Neurology*, 266 (8): 2075–86.

Harris, P.B. (2004) The perspective of younger people with dementia: still an overlooked population, *Social Work in Mental Health*, 2 (4): 17–36.

Hellström, I. and Torres, S. (2013) A wish to know but not always tell – couples living with dementia talk about disclosure preferences, *Aging and Mental Health*, 17 (2): 157–67.

Jethwa, J., Fern, M., Abhayaratne, C., et al. (2022) *Quality Standards for Memory Services*, 8th edition. London: Royal College of Psychiatrists. Available at: https://www.rcpsych.ac.uk/docs/default-source/improving-care/ccqi/quality-networks/memory-clinics-msnap/msnap-7th-edition-standards-final.pdf?sfvrsn=b68c8fdb_0.

Konijnenberg, E., Fereshtehnejad, S.M., Ten K.M., et al. (2017) Early-onset dementia: frequency, diagnostic procedures, and quality indicators in three European tertiary referral centers, *Alzheimer Disease and Associated Disorders*, 31 (2): 146–51.

Millenaar, J.K., Bakker, C., Koopmans, R.T., et al. (2016) The care needs and experiences with the use of services of people with young-onset dementia and their caregivers: a systematic review, *International Journal of Geriatric Psychiatry*, 31 (12): 1261–76.

Mitchell, W. (2019) Wendy Mitchell: For those living with dementia, we need hope – research gives us that hope, *BMJ Opinion*, 1 August. Available at: https://blogs.bmj.com/bmj/2019/08/01/wendy-mitchell-for-those-living-with-dementia-we-need-hope-research-gives-us-that-hope/.

O'Malley, M., Carter, J., Stamou, V., et al. (2019) Receiving a diagnosis of young onset dementia: a scoping review of lived experiences, *Aging and Mental Health*, 25 (1): 1–12.

O'Malley, M., Parkes, J., Stamou, V., et al. (2020) International consensus on quality indicators for comprehensive assessment of dementia in young adults using a modified e-Delphi approach, *International Journal of Geriatric Psychiatry*, 35 (11): 1309–21.

O'Malley, M., Parkes, J., Campbell, J., et al. (2021) Receiving a diagnosis of young onset dementia: evidence-based statements to inform best practice, *Dementia*, 20 (5): 1745–71.

O'Malley, M., Parkes, J., Stamou, V., et al. (2022) Current UK clinical practice in diagnosing dementia in younger adults: compliance with quality indicators in electronic health records from mental health trusts, *Aging and Mental Health*, 26 (11): 1–10.

Rabanal, L.I., Chatwin, J., Walker, A., et al. (2018) Understanding the needs and experiences of people with young onset dementia: a qualitative study, *BMJ Open*, 8 (10): e021166. Available at: https://doi.org/10.1136/bmjopen-2017-021166.

Roach, P., Keady, J., Bee, P., et al. (2013) 'We can't keep going on like this': identifying story lines in young onset dementia, *Ageing and Society*, 34 (8): 1397–1426.

Rohra, H. (2016) *Dementia Activist: Fighting for Our Rights.* London: Jessica Kingsley.

Rosness, T.A., Engedal, K. and Chemali, Z. (2016) Frontotemporal dementia, *Journal of Geriatric Psychiatry and Neurology*, 29 (5): 271–80.

Rossor, M.N., Fox, N.C., Mummery, C.J., et al. (2010) The diagnosis of young-onset dementia, *Lancet Neurology*, 9 (8): 793–806.

Salem, L.C., Andersen, B.B., Nielsen, T.R., et al. (2014) Inadequate diagnostic evaluation in young patients registered with a diagnosis of dementia: a nationwide register-based study, *Dementia and Geriatric Cognitive Disorders Extra*, 4 (1): 31–44.

Stamou, V., La Fontaine, J., Gage, H., et al. (2021) Services for people with young onset dementia: The 'Angela' Project national UK survey of service use and satisfaction, *International Journal of Geriatric Psychiatry*, 36 (3): 411–22.

Swaffer, K. (2016) *What the Hell Happened to My Brain?* London: Jessica Kingsley.

Tsoukra, P., Velakoulis, D., Wibawa, P., et al. (2022) The diagnostic challenge of young-onset dementia syndromes and primary psychiatric diseases: results from a retrospective 20-year cross-sectional study, *Journal of Neuropsychiatry Clinical Neurosciences*, 34 (1): 44–52.

van Vliet, D., de Vugt, M.E., Bakker, C., et al. (2011) Caregivers' perspectives on the pre-diagnostic period in early onset dementia: a long and winding road, *International Psychogeriatrics*, 23 (9): 1393–1404.

van Vliet, D., De Vugt, M.E., Bakker, C., et al. (2012) Time to diagnosis in young-onset dementia as compared with late-onset dementia, *Psychological Medicine*, 43 (2): 423–32.

Vieira, R.T., Caixeta, L., Machado, S., et al. (2013) Epidemiology of early-onset dementia: a review of the literature, *Clinical Practice and Epidemiology in Mental Health*, 9 (1): 88–95.

Watts, S., McCabe, R. and Guss, R. (2018) *Communicating a diagnosis of dementia.* Leicester: The British Psychological Society. Available at: https://cms.bps.org.uk/sites/default/files/2022-10/Communicating%20a%20diagnosis%20of%20dementia.pdf.

Wawrziczny, E., Pasquier, F., Ducharme, F., et al. (2016) From 'needing to know' to 'needing not to know more': an interpretative phenomenological analysis of couples' experiences with early-onset Alzheimer's disease, *Scandinavian Journal of Caring Sciences*, 30 (4): 695–703.

Williams, T., Dearden, A.M. and Cameron, I.H. (2001) From pillar to post – a study of younger people with dementia, *Psychiatric Bulletin*, 25 (10): 384–87.

Resources

Two useful websites are:

https://www.dementia.org.au/information/for-health-professionals/clinical-resources/communicating-the-diagnosis

https://www.youngdementianetwork.org/research-evidence/the-angela-project/

5 How technology can help people living with young onset dementia

Torhild Holthe

Overview

A number of modern technologies have potential to support everyday life for people with young onset dementia. However, technology is not always properly adapted for use by people with young onset dementia. When considering the use of technology, therefore, it is vital to consider what tasks the person needs support with, and to pick a device or solution that can address their needs, wishes and preferences. The device needs to be easy to use and have potential to solve a problem that the person living with young onset dementia feels is important to their everyday life. If not, the device will never be accepted or used. All people are unique and thus a technology that works well for one person might not be usable for another. Bringing a technological device into the home often affects family members as well, so there is a need to discuss the pros and cons of the device for the whole household.

Keywords

Home-dwelling, digital technology, activities of daily living, coping, security, safety, independence.

Learning points

- receive reminders and keep appointments;
- keep track of time and know day from night;
- be located if they get lost;
- alert others in case of a fall;
- manage remotes, mobile phones, codes, and keys.

Introduction

Technology may have the capacity to help people maintain independence in the face of cognitive difficulties, such as impaired memory, impaired time orientation or impaired sense of direction. Technological development is rapid and new products and applications are frequently brought to the market. One of the recent trends is that stand-alone devices have become smaller and body-worn, so they can be carried around at all times (Holthe et al., 2022), opening up many new possible means of assistance.

It can be challenging for anyone to learn to use a new technological device, to judge whether it is useable, and to know if it will really provide the support that is needed. Incorporating the use of new technology in day-to-day life comes at a cost, as we have to adapt our habits, routines and roles to be able to use technologies (Kottorp et al., 2016). People vary in how much they already use technologies and how confident they are to adopt new ones. A person's motivation for trying and using a new device depends on how successful they think it will be. For those living with young onset dementia, these individual differences are relevant but also the process is likely to be made more difficult because of their cognitive impairments.

Despite this, the effort that is needed to embrace new technology can be worthwhile because, if we choose to do so, technology has potential to help people living with young onset dementia with many things, contributing to independent living. In doing so, it may also reduce the need for assistance and also reduce the concerns of friends and family. When there is moderate to severe cognitive impairment, it can be helpful for family members or other supporters to be involved with incorporating use of technologies into everyday life. Engaging friends and family could help people with young onset dementia who have more severe cognitive problems to benefit from technology. This chapter will summarise recent research about ways some people with dementia can successfully incorporate and benefit from technology in everyday living.

Research on technology with people with young onset dementia

Research on technology to maintain independent living specifically for people with young onset dementia is limited. A recent literature search looking at preferences for supportive services among persons with young onset dementia and their caregivers (Bannon et al., 2022), found only three research studies on assistive technology for everyday living. One finding was that both people with young onset dementia and their family carers strongly preferred age-specific resources and services adapted to the current stage of the disease. Examples were technologies that addressed practical support with day-to-day tasks, helped with social communication and/or enabled coping with self-care. However, the review did not provide any details about the specific technologies used (Bannon et al., 2022).

Research on technology use for people living with dementia, independent of age, is more common. It may very well be that age is of less relevance when it comes to technology use than it is for some other issues. One systematic literature review included 253 articles on technologies used by people living with dementia in general and their family caregivers (Fabricatore et al., 2020). The review found that the main reasons for using technology were to address cognitive impairments and enable activities of daily living. Key functions were:

- compensation for cognitive deficits, e.g. ensuring orientation to time and place, helping with sequencing of complex actions, such as preparing a snack or shaving (Lancioni et al., 2009, 2010), memory support and communication;
- modification of the environment to reduce risks and increase independence, such as a timer to monitor how long food is in the oven;
- cognitive training to reinforce brain functions, such as through playing computer games;
- monitoring of a person's safety or whereabouts where there is a particular risk, e.g. via global positioning system trackers, cameras, motion sensors, bed and fall sensors;
- carer support, including Telecare for a carer from a service provider to provide education and emotional support; and
- activity recognition, including sensor technology to monitor the behaviour of a person, such as if they are prone to get out of bed in the middle of night and leave the home, and calls for appropriate assistance.

The review suggested it was crucial that the technology provides cognitive support and is simple, reliable, intuitive and cognition-enhancing. In addition, size, portability, concealability and familiarity were reported as important factors for increasing user involvement. The relational elements required to obtain a dynamic interaction between human and technology must fit, so the person with dementia can trust the technology and feel in control of it (Lindqvist et al., 2013).

In order to have an impact on well-being, the person living with young onset dementia must be both capable and willing to interact with the technology. Therefore, becoming an active technology user is critical to getting help from assistive technology. Capacity to become an active technology user is affected by the nature of cognitive impairments and by the person's motivation (Fabricatore et al., 2020). This means that health or care professionals who think a technological solution could be helpful in addressing a particular difficulty need to work with the person with young onset dementia, and perhaps significant others in the household, to consider both the nature and level of cognitive impairment and the person's motivation to use and continue to use any technology that is introduced.

In one Danish study, Busted et al. (2020) interviewed nine people with young onset dementia aged 47–65 years. They found that people with young onset dementia feared losing control, becoming a burden on their family and the thought of a humiliating future. They feared, for example, getting lost one day and felt that wearing a GPS-locator was preferable to the embarrassment of getting lost. They saw no ethical objections to using GPS and were willing to give up privacy in exchange for a sense of safety for both themselves and their family (Busted et al., 2020).

In a study from the UK, Gerritzen et al. (2023) explored the experiences of people with young onset dementia of using online peer support groups during the COVID-19 pandemic. Twenty people living with young onset dementia, from four different support groups, took part. They found online peer support to be of huge importance, even though they felt it could not replace meeting face-to-face in person. Some people had needed support to connect to the video meetings and mentioned that their family members or fellow group members played an important role in helping to set up the meetings, installing Zoom and so on. They spoke of the importance of the group facilitator having enough knowledge to solve technological difficulties, and they messaged and called each other if they were having trouble accessing a meeting. Even so, some group members were unable to join the meetings, and it was thought that cognitive impairment was the main reason for this (Gerritzen et al., 2023).

A young onset dementia and technology study in detail

Some years ago, I led a Norwegian study which explored the needs of people with young onset dementia living in the community for technology to support everyday living (Holthe, 2015). I describe the study in detail here because with research on technology being scarce, it remains significant today. It is influential because we went beyond finding out what technologies people living with young onset dementia wanted. We provided technologies to each individual to help them to achieve their goals and we followed them up over 19 months to find out about their use of the technologies and the impact on people's lives (Holthe et al., 2018).

Twelve people with young onset dementia were recruited from memory clinics in four regions of Norway, together with a family member (spouse, child or parent). The participants were four men and eight women, aged 52–65 years. Ten were diagnosed with Alzheimer's dementia, one with frontotemporal dementia and one with non-specific dementia. All had been diagnosed during the previous 6 months and, according to a cognitive assessment scale, half had moderate dementia and half had mild dementia. None of the participants had been offered technology or any other aids to assist them to live with young onset dementia before entering the project. Four had day care centre services, one had home nursing services, and four had an activity friend. Five had no services at all.

The participants' needs and preferences were to be able to:

- connect with nature;
- undertake training and exercise (outdoor walking, yoga, fishing, visit their cabin, training groups with friends, and so on);

- have social contact with their children and grandchildren, friends and former colleagues; and
- to manage at home for as long as possible and be independent.

Typical daily challenges of living life with young onset dementia were:

- difficulties in finding objects;
- turning the TV on and off and choosing channels;
- using their mobile phone;
- telling the time on a watch;
- remembering appointments;
- remembering to do things (such as taking medicines, doing the gardening, locking the door when leaving home);
- finding their way around outside, or inside a shopping centre; and
- feeling anxious when alone.

Having identified the challenges, the researchers and each individual person with young onset dementia jointly selected technologies and aids that might address those challenges, and which were also matched with the person's abilities and preferences. Nineteen different technologies were evaluated in the project and are grouped into aids with high, medium and low technological complexity in Table 5.1; the table also shows the purposes for which they were chosen. For example, a digital calendar is a high-tech device, a white board is a medium-tech device and a paper calendar is a low-tech device, and all can be used to assist memory. Low-tech devices may not be thought of as technologies because they do not involve automation or the internet but, nonetheless, these simpler, non-digital devices can be of help as they provide ways to overcome the problems cognitive impairment is causing in a person's life. It is hoped the list in Table 5.1 will inspire you to find solutions to common everyday difficulties, whether you are someone living with young onset dementia, a family member or a care professional.

As some people used more than one technology, we evaluated 39 different experiences of using technologies and aids in total. The technologies were of benefit for a certain period of time, which varied from person to person. Technologies with high complexity required more skills. For some, over time, a device was no longer needed due to the progression of dementia. For others, family carer support was needed and this sometimes became too demanding for the two of them, so the technology was no longer used. Average length of use was 6 months for the digital calendars and 12 months for the night-and-day calendar (a calendar that showed whether it was morning, day, evening or night).

The length of use depended not only on the initial level of cognitive impairment and its progression over time but also on the family circumstances and whether the technology was good enough. For example, one couple used the memo planner (a digital calendar). The wife with young onset dementia was

Table 5.1 Nineteen technologies used in the project, grouped by technical complexity and the purposes they may serve

Products	Purposes					
	Activity	Security	Memory	Communication	Orientation	Alerting others
Aids with high technical complexity						
GPS	✓	✓		✓		✓
Cognitass (digital calendar)			✓		✓	✓
Memo planner (digital calendar)			✓		✓	✓
Mobile phone		✓		✓		✓
Electronic door-lock		✓	✓			
Memory clock for verbal reminders			✓		✓	✓
Speaking watch (tells the time)			✓		✓	
Simplified remote TV control	✓					
Cooker timer		✓	✓			
Aids with medium technical complexity						
Verbal reminder			✓			
Whiteboard			✓			
Night and day calendar (with day/month)			✓		✓	
Item locator			✓			
Audio books	✓					
Aids with low technical complexity						
Paper calendar diary	✓		✓		✓	
Labels			✓		✓	
Colour-coded cooker knobs		✓	✓			
Medicine box		✓	✓			
Verbal reminders of key times of the day			✓		✓	
'My time' (speaking device that tells time and day)			✓		✓	

at home on her own while her husband worked long days. He added all his wife's appointments and events to the planner so she could easily look at the screen and be informed about what to do on each day. However, the couple stopped using the device because the husband was very tired when he came home from work and began to forget to add the events and appointments to the calendar, meaning there was no information available to help his wife. In another instance, the husband had retired from work due to health issues which affected his mobility. He still did the shopping and was out of the house for several hours each day. His wife, who was living with young onset dementia, got a memory clock. This reminded her of tasks and when to take her medication when she was at home alone. She had recorded the messages herself, so she would hear her own voice and found the device was supportive and helpful. However, after a while the couple discovered that the device interfered with their radio signal, causing scraping noises and beeping sounds. If they disconnected the power to the memory clock, the noise stopped. Although perhaps this could have been solved by contacting the company who provided the memory clock, the couple no longer had faith in it and stopped using it.

The study showed that technologies can be useful to people with moderate as well as mild cognitive impairment. However, timely access to technologies is particularly important. People need to have access to the right device at the right time. Early diagnosis can allow people to become familiar with any new technologies they might benefit from. The study also identified that assessment of potential technological support is an important and valuable element of post-diagnostic care planning.

The conclusions from this young onset dementia project were:

- Developers of technologies seldom fully understand users' needs, resulting in some products being marketed that are not yet fit for use and others being adapted in ways that are more suitable for children than adults.
- Technologies were introduced too late.
- When it came to user-friendliness, there was a narrow gap between being user-friendly and causing frustration. If people became frustrated using a certain technology, they would give up using it despite its potential.
- Family carers were seen as important to support motivation, daily use and continuity (all the participants in this study had supportive family members).
- Infrastructure and supporting systems in community health services, such as being able to access an occupational therapist, were not always in place (Holthe et al., 2018).

Current situation and new technology

Many more technologies have been developed since this young onset dementia and technology project was carried out 10 years ago. In the Norwegian context, for example, electronic medicine dispensers that are connected to the internet are now quite common as part of community health care (www.evondos.no).

Komp, a screen that allows two-way communication where people can see each other on the screen, has also become widely adopted (www.noisolation.no).

In a systematic literature review of 14 primary studies on technology for people with mild cognitive impairment and dementia, Holthe et al. (2022) found that technologies have shifted from stand-alone-devices in the home to 'wearables'. Wearable technologies, often within mobile phone apps, are worn on the body to monitor body functions, report states or imbalances, and provide reminders and timely support. Three strategies for support seem evident:

1. Prompting and reminding people living with dementia about appointments, daily tasks and so on. Frequent questions to a carer from a person living with dementia is one of the most stressful things experienced by couples. So using a technology that provides reminders may relieve stress for both the person with young onset dementia and their family members. Technology can provide as many reminders as are needed and means the person living with young onset dementia does not have to ask their spouse or child.

2. Monitoring health and safety at home using environmental sensors and bio-sensors. One example of bio-sensors is a study which tested Fitbit applications to monitor physical exercise and sleep quality in ten people living with dementia for 9 weeks (O'Sullivan et al., 2023). Fitbit looks like a normal wristwatch but has bio-sensors that monitor physical activity (such as movements, steps, pulse) and sleep patterns (time awake or asleep at night) over time. Fitbit can therefore provide objective and unbiased data on exercise habits, sleep patterns and aspects of fitness. The findings revealed that people found it challenging to get the application up and running. Since none of the people with dementia in the study had smartphones, the applications were downloaded onto family carers' phones. Only one of the people with dementia kept the Fitbit bracelet on at night. The family carers' responsibility for setting up and following up the data needed to be balanced against its potential utility.

3. Providing safety out of doors by use of GPS to help someone to navigate or to find a person if they should become lost (Holthe et al., 2022).

At the end of the 9 weeks, half the participants wanted to keep the Fitbit device, implying it had been valued (O'Sullivan et al., 2023). But because none had managed to use the Fitbit on their own, it was considered of limited utility. However, this study was not conducted with younger people with dementia, so it might be that people with young onset dementia are more familiar with smartphones and Fitbit applications than older people with dementia. Equally, successive age cohorts will each be more used to high-tech developments and find them easier to incorporate into their everyday living. For sleep monitoring, it would be important for the person with young onset dementia to understand why the watch must be worn overnight. Data on exercise and sleep patterns may be of interest to the user and could also enable health service providers to monitor the person's physical and mental state, prompting timely intervention as needed.

Different needs

Young onset dementia has different aetiologies from later onset dementia, meaning that the disease commonly affects either the frontal or the posterior part of the brain (Mendez et al., 2009). When the disease affects the *frontal* part of the brain, the person may experience difficulties with judgement, sequencing of complex tasks, and experience effects on mood. Sometimes, operating remotes, keys or buttons becomes difficult. One man with young onset dementia explained it like this: *'My hands are no longer doing what I ask of them!'* When the *posterior* part of the brain is affected, this may lead to difficulties in seeing, interpreting visual input and performing; for example, to visually search for the TV remote control, grasp it, direct it towards the TV, and press down on the ON-button. This requires a sequence of steps that must be in the correct order.

Before introducing a new technological device, it is important to investigate how the person with young onset dementia handles and operates devices they are used to, such as the phone, TV, radio and cooker. If the person has any issues operating these devices, it will influence the choice of technology. It is essential to find a device that is suited to a particular cognitive profile, such as one that can be used despite particular visual or sequencing issues and which the person living with dementia can readily control. In other words, it is vital to consider possible difficulties, obstacles, needs and preferences, as well as what support is required when choosing technology to use on a daily basis. (See Chapter 3 for more information on rarer dementias.)

An individual way forward

Coping with daily living and daily tasks is important for people living with young onset dementia, given the expectation of independence in mid-life and the many aspects of life people are likely to be involved in when they develop the condition. When technology is directed at easing those things that cause the most stress and the greatest feeling of being incapable, it can help people to surmount obstacles, maintain independence and self-esteem, and live gracefully, despite cognitive limitations. However, as it takes time, energy and persistence to incorporate technology into everyday routines, identifying the key things to focus on is vital.

Identifying specific daily struggles that demand a lot of energy and affect self-confidence is the main issue here. To understand what makes a task difficult, it is necessary to think through what causes the sense of struggle and leads to feelings of being incapable or stressed. This helps to pinpoint what a technology must be able to address to cope with the task in question and reduce that stressful feeling. Figure 5.1 reproduces a problem-solving sheet of questions that can be used to assist people living with young onset dementia to unpick the nature of daily struggles to inform whether a technological solution might be of help.

Figure 5.1 Problem-solving questions to help identify where to focus use of technology

Considerations	My answers
What do you struggle with in a normal day?	
Describe what happens	
Where does it happen?	
When does it happen?	
Under what circumstances does it happen?	
How does it happen?	
How often does it happen?	
Why do you think it's happening?	
How do you experience this?	
How does your spouse/family member experience this?	
Do you see this differently from your spouse or family member? How?	
Is the problem always present? If not, what is the difference between when it is present and absent?	
Has the situation where the problem occurs already been adapted in some way?	

Source: Problem-solving sheet from Høeg and Jensen (2004). Published with the permission of the authors.

Technology to assist daily living

This final section presents some technologies that are readily available to buy. They are key technologies that may help with maintaining autonomy, identity and relationships. I describe here the technologies and their functions, while weblinks to current products are available in the appendix.

Technology to maintain autonomy

Some technologies aim to support independence in people with young onset dementia. Independent living is very important for most people. The term is associated with self-determination, equal opportunities and self-respect, with regard to being in control of your own life, in the same way as before diagnosis. It could be mistaken as meaning you have to do everything by yourself but as pointed out by the Independent Living Institute (https://www.independentliving. org), it is actually about having choices and control.

Much of our identity is embodied in the way we do everyday things, in our habits and routines. So, for example, most people are used to choosing when to get up, what to have for breakfast and so on. We have a preference for tea or coffee, strong or weak, black or white. At the point of diagnosis, these things do not change, and continuing with a familiar routine is one way of retaining a sense of identity. This is sometimes referred to as 'normalcy'. Daily routines and habits are ingrained. Often, we can do things without thinking too much because our habits are over-learned motor patterns – that is, they are engrained and we can do them automatically. Maintaining established routines and familiar ways of doings things is an advantage in the face of progressive cognitive impairment.

Therefore, technology that enables daily habits and routines to be maintained is an important way of helping to maintain autonomy. The following are examples of technologies which can be purchased or accessed, and which can support independence in daily tasks. These address the type of issues that have been found to be important to people living with young onset dementia that were listed earlier in this chapter. In this section, I address those living with young onset dementia directly with the use of 'you'.

Watching TV

Using a TV remote control can be challenging, especially if you have to get used to a new one. You can obtain an infra-red (IR) remote TV control with a simple interface that overcomes the difficulty of following multiple steps. You can add preferred TV channels and easily click on the one you want. The remote has bigger buttons, which are easy to click on and off, and volume is easy to control. The device allows you to add control buttons for other functions too, such as turning the lights or music on and off, and opening the door and windows. However, it is wise not to add too many functions since the idea is to make things simpler, not more confusing.

Keeping appointments

One way to keep a better track of appointments is to take steps to personalise any online calendar, such as Outlook, that you are familiar with using. This can make it easier to read and easier for the user to locate what they are looking for. For those without an account already, one can be created for free, allowing you access to both a calendar and to email from your phone as well as from a tablet or computer.

Also, to help with keeping track of activities and appointments, there are technologies that pair a digital calendar that provides reminders with a bracelet that gives the wearer alerts with icons, sound, vibration and light when out of the house. This is a little like a 'smart' watch.

Many people are accustomed to having a calendar on their computer and/or phone. However, sometimes these feel less user-friendly and a separate digital calendar can be a good solution. A digital calendar can help keep track of the day and any appointments, check the weather forecast and read the papers. Some have a 'Please contact me' function, which allows the user to press a button that directs the request to an appointed contact person's phone, so they can call back.

Orientation to time

There are a number of technologies designed to assist with keeping track of the time, date and phase of the day. There are different ones to suit people living with young onset dementia depending on lifestyle and the degree of cognitive impairment. For keeping track of time as well as coordinating appointments within a family, it is possible to buy a digital clock with an integral calendar, some of which show not only the date but also the day, date and year. Digital displays can be helpful if a person finds it hard to read a conventional clock face. Some integrated calendar clocks also allow the addition of icons to show the weather forecast. They can also link remotely with others (e.g. family members who live elsewhere) and, if you enable remote control, family members can add appointments to a calendar which show up on the screen on the day of the appointment.

A range of clocks is also available to help people with more severe disorientation to keep track of day and night.

Light to support circadian rhythms and sleep

People with dementia can have disturbed sleep, finding it hard to get sleep, waking early or awakening several times during the night. Sleep is important for the brain.

A blue light-lamp, which provides natural light during the morning, for example at breakfast time, can help to overcome issues with circadian rhythms as well as winter-depression. You can set the light to suit your individual routine. Although blue-light lamps have been evaluated in a number of studies with promising results, including boosting alertness, helping memory and cognitive function, and elevating mood, more research is needed (Mitolo et al., 2019).

Circadian light that offers light in different colours depending on the hour of day/night has been used in nursing homes in Denmark and Norway, and may improve sleep, general health (in staff as well as care home residents) and reduce depression. This sort of light system can also be installed in private homes and can help with falling asleep and waking up at preferred times.

Computer use

You can source an adapted personal computer with a simple graphical user interface.

It is also possible to simplify your computer desktop screen. An interface that is clear, uses contrast colours and proper placement of the apps will be easier to use. Someone who is computer-skilled can help with this. For example, a single-coloured background will show the apps better and the one you wish to use will be more visible and easier to navigate to.

There are various online programs that allow you to customise your screen.

Locating objects

Searching for lost objects can be a time-consuming and often annoying activity. It is usually a good strategy to keep things in the same place. For example, keeping your keys on a hook in the entrance hall, keeping your wallet in your handbag or in a kitchen drawer, and the mobile by the charger. Sometimes, it may help to lighten up these places with a contrast colour cloth, because it makes it easier to see them. For example, if you have a black mobile phone, it will be more visible on a yellow background than a brown one.

Item locators are small devices used to find objects and come in many different forms. They usually consist of one sender and four or five electronic tags that you can fasten to different items. When you need to locate a device, you press the button on the sender. The tag will answer with a beep, which makes the object easier to locate. For those with an iPhone, there are special tags you can put on devices you often misplace. You can then use your phone to locate the missing objects.

Taking medications

An electronic medicine dispenser is a device that tells you when to take your medications, and some also tell you how to do so. Rather than being a passive device like a box with compartments, these are active dispensers. The dispenser can be programmed by a community nurse on a fortnightly basis. It is stocked with pre-filled pouches of multi-dose medicines. The dispenser is connected to the internet and, at a pre-destined time, it spits out the correct pills in a small plastic bag. In some versions, an instruction then appears in the display telling the individual to take the pills with a glass of water. Others provide alerts using sound, light and text. Some can be paired with the person's phone number or that of a family member and issue them with an alert if medication is not taken.

Virtual assistants

Virtual assistants (e.g. Alexa) have become more widely used since the COVID-19 pandemic. They involve having a speaker in the house which is linked to the internet and are installed via an app on a mobile phone. They can easily be instructed with simple voice comments to remind you of things and appointments or to answer a wide range of questions. One attractive aspect is that they are designed for universal use and so carry no stigma.

Technology to support identity

Technology can support identity by keeping or triggering significant memories, keeping up personally meaningful activities, and providing comfort and well-being at times of upset or stress.

Triggering memories

When cognitive changes make it harder to access memories, then photos, albums and films can be a way to trigger past memories and provide topics for conversations, bringing joy and laughter to the person with young onset dementia, family and friends. Watching digitised pictures and films on a bigger screen can enable a group of people to watch and remember events together.

Some specialist apps have been designed especially to promote reminiscence by gathering collections of trigger materials that are familiar to particular generations or particular social contexts. They might be organised by theme such as school, work, leisure time and maritime life. Some will allow uploading of a person's own photographs to make them even more personal.

Keeping a diary

Daily diaries can help people to take care of or conserve their memories of events and can be revisited to strengthen memories. Sometimes, it may seem easier to write than to speak. Speaking often requires a quick response, whereas when writing you take the time you need, and you can rephrase sentences. You can choose to write with pen and paper or on a personal device.

Taking photos

Almost all mobile phones have a camera these days. Taking photos or videos can be an enjoyable and easy way to save memories from events with family and friends, or what you observe in nature. Later the same day, or the next, you can look at the photos, possibly together with someone else and talk about what they show, naming the people and places to help consolidate memories.

Outdoor activities

For people living with young onset dementia who like to exercise or go for outdoor walks, these activities are important for a sense of bodily well-being and fresh air. Outdoor activity can be assisted by technology, such as Fitbits, biometric sensors, training apps and so on, helping you to continue to take exercise. A GPS-locator, on a smartphone or Apple watch, can support people who are afraid of getting lost. If there is an emergency or you need help to find your way, using the device's panic button will connect you to a family member or a response centre, who can offer help.

Music

Music is comforting for many, especially music and songs that are associated with past memoires and can provoke positive emotions. You can compose your personal playlist with your favourite music on your phone or for use with Alexa.

One innovative product is a soft 'music pillow', which starts to play when it is touched. It is interactive and combines music, touch, movement and sensory stimulation. The pillow can be placed under your head, on your stomach or be held in your hand so you can dance with it. The pillow is linked with a computer, so you can upload preferred music and it can invite you to sing or move.

Technology to feel connected with others

Development of technology that contributes to feeling connected with family and friends is a growing field. Sustaining relationships is important to all, regardless of any dementia diagnosis. Telephones, tablets and personal computers have clear potential to support social communication but need to be better adapted for users who have moderate or severe cognitive challenges.

Phones

Cognitive challenges make it more likely that a person living with young onset dementia will forget to charge their smartphone or forget where they put it. It can be hard to scroll through your list of friends or open the calendar to identify if you have any appointments. The icons are often too small and fail to react as we assume they will. Also, sometimes a person's fingertips can be too dry or cold to work on a touch screen. Sometimes, applications request PIN-codes that are hard to recall or demand you follow complex instructions to perform updates.

Phones are not easy to upgrade. Having a new phone means you have to learn how to use it, because it no doubt has been upgraded. Trying a phone before buying it can help identify the one that works best for you. This can include testing the sound and asking if the screen can be simplified, so it has only the important apps that you need.

There are also adapted phones developed for people who require cognitive support which have a simple interface and allow a supporter to administer and synchronise the content from a PC, tablet or phone. It is also possible to download an app that provides a more usable interface for a phone by having enlarged buttons and texts, which make it easier to read and operate.

Two-way screens

Some devices have been developed specifically for ease of use to promote two-way communication. One consists of a two-way communication tool, involving a big screen in or near your sitting room. Family members and friends can call you, using an app on their mobile phone. If you do not want to receive their call, you press the one and only button at the bottom of the screen. Your friends and family can also send text messages or photos. The disadvantage is that you cannot call your friends, only receive calls.

Mary, Fred, Joe and Iris's technology solutions

Before concluding, we would like to give some brief real-life examples of using technology to try and address key struggles being experienced by four different individuals living with young onset dementia who took part in our study (Holthe et al., 2018). The names used are all pseudonyms.

Mary forgot the coffee

Mary's daily routine was to make coffee for her husband in the morning. For safety reasons they had an automatic switch-off timer device installed, which made the coffee machine switch off after 10 minutes. After Mary had turned the machine on, she forgot about it. After a while, her husband asked: 'Is my coffee ready yet?' Mary gave him a cup but her husband was annoyed because the coffee had become cold. He was irritated and she became frustrated, and this was causing a strain on the couple's relationship.

The study authors suggested installing a verbal reminder device that would give a message when the timer shut off. So, Mary made coffee as usual and after 10 minutes, when the timer switched off, a voice message said: 'The coffee is ready now!' And Mary was able to serve her husband hot coffee. The loudspeaker giving the message was placed in the sitting room, so Mary would hear it clearly. On a follow-up visit, Mary was asked how she felt about the voice message. The researchers thought maybe she would be afraid of suddenly hearing an unfamiliar male voice. '*Well*', she said, '*it helps me a lot, and now we have started to call him Mr. Nelson!*'

Fred forgot to lock the door

Fred, his wife and two children lived in a suburban house near a big city. Fred had impaired vision and young onset dementia. On weekdays, his wife was at work and the kids at school. Fred liked to take a walk every day but he did not always remember to lock the door or manage to keep the key safe in his pocket. His wife was anxious that someone might break in when the door was unlocked.

The authors suggested installing an electronic lock that would always be locked until a tag was within 2–3 metres. Although quite costly to install, Fred could now wear a tag in his pocket, and the door would be open for him, but locked as soon as he was 2 metres away. The kids also had their own tags, so this was an excellent solution for this family, and Fred's wife had peace of mind.

Joe got a new mobile phone

Joe's mobile phone was broken and Peter, his son, wanted him to have a new one. The study's occupational therapist suggested a simpler phone with a flip, but Peter thought it was too 'feminine' and that his father should have a black phone. So Joe got a fairly simple, black phone. Peter practised how to use it with Joe. The key lock turned out to be tricky for Joe to manage, so Peter de-activated it. However, the result was that the phone unintentionally called his wife or Peter ('pocket-calling'), meaning they were worried something was wrong. The study authors concluded that instead of a mobile phone, it would be better for Joe to have a GPS-locator, because he seldom used the phone and the priority was for his wife and son to ensure that he was okay when he was out walking in the woods.

Iris gets to try a GPS-locator

Iris, who was 58 years old, lived alone in a flat in the city. She had retired due to young onset dementia and was supported by her daughter but didn't want to be a nuisance to her. Iris wanted to try and use a GPS to get help if she got lost. The daughter said they could use 'Find my iPhone', but Iris wanted a GPS device connected to a response centre, to avoid being a burden to her daughter.

To ensure Iris took the GPS device out with her, a verbal reminder was set up at her front door. The 'door-speaker' reminded Iris to take the GPS with her. This worked well as she always puts it in her handbag. The response centre was responsible for training both Iris and her daughter in how to use the GPS, and what to do to call for help.

Conclusions

Technology can play an important role in everyday life for people living with young onset dementia and their family members. Technology needs to be personalised to each user's needs and preferences. This is seldom done just once, since most dementias progress. It may be possible to find help to tailor the technology a person prefers to use to solve new challenges that may arise.

When a person starts to use a technology that is unfamiliar, it can be very helpful to have input from someone technologically skilled to install the technology and settings according to the user's preferences. Learning to use and benefit from any technology takes time and patience. If the technology has some benefit, even for a short period of time, it can provide a good way of coping, a way of stimulating the brain and maintaining performance skills, and can assist in maintaining connections, identity and autonomy.

So what does this mean in practice?

If you are diagnosed with young onset dementia

You may find it strange to have a new device or gadget at home and be hesitant to use it. You might think that you do not really need the device and be tempted to put off using it until later. However, it is worth getting used to new devices sooner rather than later. Experience has shown that everybody needs time to learn how to operate a new device or gadget and to include it in their daily routine. Repeated training is often needed, so don't be surprised if you forget how to use the gadget and need help to re-learn to do so.

If you are a family or friend of someone diagnosed with young onset dementia

You can help to support the person with young onset dementia you know to use technology. You can remind them to use a device; explain to them how to use it; show them how to use it; encourage its use; and provide practical help, including with charging or changing batteries, or checking the display to help ensure the information is always correct.

If you are a professional involved in assessing and advising people with young onset dementia

The person living with young onset dementia has a right to have their needs assessed and to access knowledge about technology that may support their everyday living. To enable this, you need to keep up to date with technologies that can support people with young onset dementia; be able to advise people how to get hold of them; know whether there are aids people can access from public services, such as the local authority, or if they must buy the devices themselves. If you cannot guide people with young onset dementia in these matters, you should refer to an occupational therapist or a dementia assessment team.

References

Bannon, S.M., Reichman, M.R., Wang, K., et al. (2022) A qualitative meta-synthesis of common and unique preferences for supportive services among persons with young onset dementia and their caregivers, *Dementia*, 21 (2): 519–39.

Busted, L.M., Nielsen, D.S. and Birkelund, R. (2020) 'Sometimes it feels like thinking in syrup': the experience of losing sense of self in those with young onset dementia, *International Journal of Qualitative Studies on Health and Well-being*, 15 (1): 1734277. Available at: https://doi.org/10.1080/17482631.2020.1734277.

Fabricatore, C., Radovic, D., Lopez, X., et al. (2020) When technology cares for people with dementia: a critical review using neuropsychological rehabilitation as a conceptual framework, *Neuropsychological Rehabilitation*, 30 (8): 1558–97.

Gerritzen, E.V., Kohl, G., Orrell, M., et al. (2023) Peer support through video meetings: experiences of people with young onset dementia, *Dementia*, 22 (1): 218–34.

Holthe, T. (2015) *Mot - håp - tålmodighet. Yngre personer med demens og betydningen av å få kognitive hjelpemidler til støtte i hverdagen* [*Courage, hope and patience: Younger people with dementia and the significance of having cognitive aids for supporting everyday living*]. Tønsberg: Forlaget Aldring og helse.

Holthe, T., Jentoft, R., Arntzen, C., et al. (2018) Benefits and burdens: family caregivers' experiences of assistive technology (AT) in everyday life with persons with young-onset dementia (YOD), *Disability and Rehabilitation: Assistive Technology*, 13 (8): 754–62.

Holthe, T., Halvorsrud, L. and Lund, A. (2022) Digital assistive technology to support everyday living in community-dwelling older adults with mild cognitive impairment and dementia, *Clinical Interventions in Aging*, 17: 519–44.

Høeg, M. and Jensen, L. (2004) Problem solving sheet, in *Hjælpemidler til mennesker med demens* [*Aids to people with dementia*]. Århus: Hjælpemiddelinstituttet Forlaget.

Kottorp, A., Nygård, L., Hedman, A., et al. (2016) Access to and use of everyday technology among older people: an occupational justice issue – but for whom?, *Journal of Occupational Science*, 23 (3): 382–88.

Lancioni, G., Singh, N., O'Reilly, M., et al. (2009) Persons with moderate Alzheimer's disease improve activities and mood via instruction technology, *American Journal of Alzheimer's Disease and Other Dementias*, 24 (3): 246–57.

Lancioni, G., Singh, N., O'Reilly, M., et al. (2010) Persons with Alzheimer's disease perform daily activities using verbal-instruction technology: a maintenance assessment, *Developmental Neurorehabilitation*, 13 (2): 103–13.

Lindqvist, E., Nygard, L. and Borell, L. (2013) Significant junctures on the way towards becoming a user of assistive technology in Alzheimer's disease, *Scandinavian Journal of Occupational Therapy*, 20 (5): 386–96.

Mendez, M.F., Mcmurtray, A.M., Licht, E.A., et al. (2009) Frontal-executive versus posterior-perceptual mental status deficits in early-onset dementias, *American Journal of Alzheimer's Disease and Other Dementias*, 24 (3): 220–27.

Mitolo, M., Tonon, C., La Morgia, C., et al. (2019) Effects of light treatment on sleep, cognition, mood, and behavior in Alzheimer's disease: a systematic review, *Dementia and Geriatric Cognitive Disorders*, 46 (5/6): 371–84.

O'Sullivan, G., Whelan, B., Gallagher, N., et al. (2023) Challenges of using a Fitbit smart wearable among people with dementia, *International Journal of Geriatric Psychiatry*, 38: e5898. Available at: https://doi.org/10.1002/gps.5898.

Appendix: Technology as an aid to independent living – products and websites

This appendix should be read in combination with the text, where the different products are outlined. This appendix gives named examples and web links. We recognise that over time, these will change but have chosen those that are the most well established.

Technology to maintain autonomy

Keeping track of day, date, time and appointments

- Technology that pairs a digital calendar with a bracelet that gives the wearer reminders. See, for example: https://vestfoldaudio.no/en/home/
- A digital calendar for date, appointments, weather and call back. See the Memas calendar here: https://www.youtube.com/watch?v=0ywyUlUe96U
- A digital clock with an integral calendar. See, for example: https://clockaid.com/.
- A day-and-night clock to help with more severe disorientation. See, for example, those at: https://www.alzproducts.co.uk/
- Other devices for cognitive support are shown at: https://www.abilia.com/intl/our-products/cognition-time-and-planning

Computer use

- DUKA adapted personal computer, with a simple graphical user interface: https://www.duka.no/datamaskin-til-seniorer/
- Screen adaptation programmes. See, for example, Canva at: https://www.belightcare.com/

Locating objects

- Item locators. See, for example: https://www.amazon.com/Key-Finder-Wireless-Bluetooth-Tracker/dp/B09MFJYXRJ/ref=sr_1_10?keywords=Finder+Tags&qid=1682940643&sr=8-10
- Apple Air Tags: https://www.apple.com/uk/shop/buy-airtag/airtag

Medicine dispensers

- Internet-connected electronic medicine dispensers. See, for example: Evondos (www.evondos.no.); Medido Clock (https://www.medido.com/nl/); Karie, which can also alert others if medicine is not taken (https://kariehealth.com/)

Virtual assistants

- Amazon Alexa is a widely used example: https://play.google.com/store/apps/details?id=com.amazon.dee.app&hl=en_US
- A two-way communication screen. See, for example, Komp at: https://www.noisolation.com/no. You can ask for English by clicking on the menu

Technology to support identity

Triggering memories

- Apps with online collections of themed photos from particular contexts and times, which also allows you to upload your own photos. See, for example, My House of Memories at: https://www.liverpoolmuseums.org.uk/house-of-memories/my-house-of-memories-app

Outdoor activities

- Outdoor activities may be undertaken with more confidence with use of a smart watch or GPS (global positioning system) device to show where you are and give information about well-being. The Angel watch is an example that has GPS tracking, a falls alert and shows body temperature: https://angelwatchco.com/en-uk/products/angel-watch-series-r-assist

Music

- Personalised playlists. One well-established company is Playlist for Life: https://www.playlistforlife.org.uk/
- Interactive devices, e.g. the INMU music pillow: https://inmutouch.com/de/

Technology to maintain connections

Mobile phones

- Smartphones with a simple interface. See, for example, Handi One + G2: https://www.abilia.com/en
- Easy-to-use phone interfaces. See, for example, Big launcher's BIG Phone and BIG SMS at: http://biglauncher.com/help/en/
- Two-way communication tools. See, for example, Komp: https://www.noisolation.com/about-us

6 Using cognitive rehabilitation to enable independence in daily life

Jackie Pool and Sue Evans

Overview

This chapter describes cognitive rehabilitation, an approach that assists people with young onset dementia to regain or retain independence in everyday activities and stay socially connected. To do so, cognitive rehabilitation uses a range of techniques to restore lost function or compensate for cognitive problems.

This chapter gives a brief summary of the different approaches to addressing cognitive problems in dementia before focusing on cognitive rehabilitation. The aim of cognitive rehabilitation is to restore lost function or to compensate for cognitive deficits. The chapter looks at the place of rehabilitation in current policy and guidance, and summarises evidence for the effectiveness of Goal-Oriented Cognitive Rehabilitation Therapy (known as GREAT CR). The chapter then describes the approach in some depth, including the steps involved, how to set personally meaningful goals, strategies and principles that can be used to help achievement of goals, and how to measure progress. It ends with some examples of application in practice.

Cognitive rehabilitation can be delivered effectively at modest cost in routine services, and is viewed positively by people with dementia, family carers and practitioners. GREAT Cognitive Rehabilitation is recommended in the NICE Dementia Guidelines (2018), the World Health Organisation Global Action Plan (2021) and by the Alzheimer's Society. To fully realise its benefits and achieve widespread and sustainable implementation requires a reorientation of service priorities towards preventive and rehabilitative approaches.

Keywords

Cognition, rehabilitation, function, dementia, reablement.

> **Learning points**
>
> - There is an evidence base for therapeutic approaches that restore lost function relating to cognitive impairment.
> - GREAT Cognitive Rehabilitation is a personalised programme of therapy delivered over six sessions on an individual basis.
> - GREAT Cognitive Rehabilitation uses a range of techniques to overcome cognitive barriers to achieve meaningful personalised goals.
> - Goal-setting is important to provide structure to the GREAT CR programme and acts as a motivator as well as to provide evidence of goal attainment.

Introduction

It is highly important to younger people with dementia (young onset dementia) to maintain independence in day-to-day life but this is difficult in the face of progressive cognitive impairment. This chapter takes an approach informed by cognitive rehabilitation to look at compensatory, restorative and practical approaches that can assist people with young onset dementia to continue to manage activities of daily life and stay socially connected.

If a person has had to give up their work or interests because of cognitive difficulties, this can impact on how others relate to them, as their status in society and in the family changes. For example, if the person has difficulty remembering the sequence of steps needed to operate machinery, they might be at risk or put their work colleagues at risk; or if the person has difficulty finding the right words, is slower in their speech or less able to hold a rapid conversation with friends, this might result in them reducing their social contacts. Such changes are very likely to undermine the person's sense of self-esteem and self-confidence and this, in turn, can further affect their cognitive and everyday activities as they begin to doubt their own capabilities. Not surprisingly, this is likely to have an impact on mental health too and so even the early symptoms of young onset dementia can have a devastating effect.

However, with timely advice and interventions, it might be possible to continue with interests and activities, by learning how to adapt the way they are carried out. The previous chapter reviewed ways that technology can support autonomy. In this chapter, we consider how people with young onset dementia can be supported to use their cognitive capacity most effectively by using strategies based on how learning and other cognitive processes work.

Approaches to managing cognitive impairment

Cognitive training, cognitive stimulation and cognitive rehabilitation techniques are the three major non-pharmacological (i.e. not medication-based) approaches to managing cognitive impairment (Irazoki et al., 2020) and it is important to understand the differences between them.

Cognitive training is commonly referred to as 'brain training'. Cognitive training games are often marketed as enabling people to improve or to slow down the rate of progression of cognitive impairment when they have been diagnosed with a dementia. Such activities can be absorbing and enjoyable. The evidence from six randomized controlled trials (RCTs) is that cognitive training can improve cognition scores in older people without cognitive impairment in the aspect of cognition trained but this does not transfer to other areas (Butler et al., 2018). A word search game, for example, can help the person to increase the speed or quantity of words they can find in a word search table but this doesn't lead to improvements in other skills. Two reviews of RCTs with people with mild cognitive impairment came to contrasting conclusions. Butler et al. (2018) did not find any evidence of benefit on cognition but Zhang et al. (2019) concluded there was evidence for small but significant improvements in aspects of memory and global cognition.

A Cochrane review (a high-quality systematic review of RCTs) of the effectiveness of cognitive training for mild-to-moderate dementia examined the results of 33 trials (Bahar-Fuchs et al., 2019). The review found that cognitive training had a small-to-moderate benefit on global cognition and verbal semantic fluency compared with control groups who did not receive cognitive training. These benefits were maintained 3–12 months later. However, when cognitive training was compared with another intervention, such as reminiscence or mindfulness, there was no evidence it had greater benefits than the other intervention. They found no effects on ability to carry out everyday tasks, mood, or behavioural and psychological symptoms of dementia. Participants in two studies had an average age between 65 and 70 years but in all others the average was in the seventies or eighties. There was no study with people with young onset dementia. In a further review, Hill et al. (2017) found some promising evidence that virtual reality interventions may have potential to improve visuospatial skills, an area that deserves further work.

Cognitive stimulation supports the person to engage through all of their senses in a range of activities that target the main cognitive functions, including thinking, reasoning, perception and judgement. It is usually, but not always, delivered as a group-based activity and so provides opportunities for social interaction and peer support. It takes place according to a set 'topic guide', rather than being directly related to the individual goals of participants. Cognitive stimulation therapy (CST) has a good evidence base when used with people with late onset dementia (Cafferata et al., 2021) and is recommended by NICE (2018). The review by Cafferata et al. (2021) identified 44 relevant randomized controlled trials (considered a gold standard for obtaining evidence). The authors concluded that cognitive stimulation improves global cognition, memory, activities of daily living and depressive symptoms, although the benefits are modest and not sustained when people are followed up after the therapy sessions have finished. However, the average ages of those taking part were 70 years and above, except for one small study, so there is a lack of evidence for the benefits of cognitive stimulation for people living with young onset dementia.

Cognitive rehabilitation (CR) focuses on the specific cognitive difficulties that are impacting on a person's ability to maintain everyday functions by addressing meaningful individual goals. It is usually delivered as a one-to-one programme via a series of individually tailored sessions from a trained CR practitioner. The sessions are used to identify personally meaningful goals which can be achieved using targeted cognitive techniques. We focus on cognitive rehabilitation in this chapter as there is a strong and growing evidence base for its effectiveness (Clare et al., 2018, 2023) alongside limited awareness of the approach.

Policy and guidance on rehabilitation for people living with dementia

There has been increasing emphasis on the potential of rehabilitation approaches in dementia in recent policies. The Global Action Plan on the Public Health Response to Dementia 2017–25 (WHO, 2021) represents the formal commitment by WHO member states to develop comprehensive multisectoral responses to address dementia worldwide. It contributes to WHO's Triple Billion Targets and achieving the United Nations' Sustainable Development Goals (SDGs) by improving timely diagnosis, treatment, (long-term) care and rehabilitation for people with dementia. In chapter 7 of the Global Action Plan, 'Dementia diagnosis, treatment and care', Helen Rochford-Brennan, a Global Dementia Ambassador with the National University of Ireland, is quoted as saying:

> When you are diagnosed, you only think, I'll never do anything again – like drive, cook dinner, or go on holidays. It would be nice to be informed of how we can continue to live and do the things that we did before being diagnosed, and what you really want is for your clinician to give you that information. (WHO, 2021: 141)

The Global Action Plan addresses this by recommending a dementia care pathway rooted in a human rights-based approach. The pathway is designed to be delivered by services from within and outside the health sector, including primary health care, specialist medical care, community-based services, rehabilitation, long-term care and palliative care. The pathway recommends that the person with dementia and their care partner should have access to rehabilitation as part of post-diagnostic support. The Plan concludes with a summary of opportunities to accelerate action in the area of dementia treatment and care, which includes a focus on rehabilitation.

Likewise, in their report, 'A Future for Personalised Care' (2021a), the Alzheimer's Society UK recommends that the UK Government should ensure that interventions, including the GREAT Cognitive Rehabilitation approach, which are effective in improving outcomes for people with dementia are rolled out widely. The current UK NICE guidelines for dementia (NICE, 2018) recommend that cognitive rehabilitation (also known as 'reablement') approaches should be considered for people living with mild-to-moderate dementia.

Evidence for the effectiveness of cognitive rehabilitation

Much of the evidence for effectiveness of cognitive rehabilitation has been gathered in studies with older people but some younger people took part in two major studies which looked at the effectiveness (Clare et al., 2018) and the implementation (Clare et al., 2023) of GREAT CR. The studies built on earlier work, including that of Clare et al. (2010).

The 2018 publication reported a randomised controlled trial which compared cognitive rehabilitation with treatment as usual for 475 people living with mild-to-moderate Alzheimer's, vascular or mixed dementia. The trial found that those who took part in cognitive rehabilitation and their informants (usually a partner or other family member) were significantly more likely to achieve their goals and that this progress was maintained 9 months later.

The 2023 article reported on implementing GREAT CR in 10 NHS Trusts and a care home provider. The study was disrupted by COVID-19 but nonetheless 41 practitioners delivered cognitive rehabilitation to 54 people living with dementia. Goals related to managing using appliances, the internet and devices in the home, as well as everyday activities and tasks. Although there were various organisational barriers to implementation, over 50% of participants fully achieved their first goal and almost all made at least some progress. The people who took part, family members and the therapists were all positive about the intervention.

Experience in the GREAT studies (Clare et al., 2018, 2023) indicated that the approach suited people with mild-to-moderate dementia who had some insight into their level of functioning as well as motivation to improve their everyday functioning. A person who is still very independent or someone who has already developed coping strategies that rely heavily on others might be less motivated, with the consequence that cognitive rehabilitation might not be suitable for them. Whilst the motivators behind the participants' individual goals might differ between younger and older people living with dementia, the same techniques and strategies were appropriate.

We (the chapter authors) were co-investigators in these studies and draw on our knowledge of cognitive rehabilitation and our experience of working with some people with young onset dementia in the detailed descriptions below.

What is cognitive rehabilitation?

Cognitive rehabilitation (CR) is a long- established approach used to support people with cognitive impairments due to brain injury (Wilson, 2002).

The approach uses a range of evidence-based strategies based on knowledge of cognitive functioning, including cued recall techniques (Bird et al., 2001) and errorless learning techniques (Clare et al., 1999). You can read more about these strategies and the underlying 'cognitive science' in *Neuropsychological Rehabilitation and People with Dementia* (Clare, 2008). The intervention strategies can either focus on restoring lost function or on compensating for cognitive deficits by working around them or on both these elements.

GREAT CR utilizes these evidence-based strategies and techniques in a highly personalised programme of therapy and practice delivered by a trained CR practitioner, who has completed dedicated training (see section on resources below). They are usually health or social care professionals, including occupational therapists, clinical psychologists, nurses, senior care assistants and activity professionals. Occupational therapists are well-placed to offer GREAT CR because they are highly skilled in breaking down tasks into their component parts to identify and understand the barriers that prevent independent performance of an activity.

The aim of the practitioner is to collaborate with the individual to address the impact of cognitive impairment on their functional ability. The programme starts with the person with dementia identifying the goal or goals that they want to achieve. The choice of a goal supports the person with dementia to maintain control over their rehabilitation programme. It serves to reinforce sense of identity by maintaining or developing meaningful roles, habits and routines, and people also find it is highly motivating to engage in the intensive programme.

The GREAT CR process is divided into five stages:

Stage 1: Assessment. The first stage is to establish the person's current level of functioning. This involves getting to know the person and establishing a therapeutic relationship between the person with dementia, their care partner and the GREAT CR practitioner. The assessment includes both self-reported and observed completion of everyday activities in order to understand which cognitive impairments are undermining the person's functional ability. This stage also includes discussing the areas of everyday life that the person would like to improve or things they would like to learn to do for the first time

Stage 2: Defining clear goals. The person with dementia works with the GREAT CR practitioner to identify and agree goals that are SMART: Specific, Measurable, Attainable, Relevant and Time-limited. (More information on setting goals is given in the next section.)

Stage 3: Assigning attainment scores. The goal informs the nature and time frame for the intervention. By breaking down the goal into observable milestones (i.e. into small interim steps), each step can be allocated an attainment score that enables measurement of progress and also provides a focus for drawing up a personal rehabilitation plan. The final attainment score measures what the person has achieved.

Stage 4: Developing a personal rehabilitation plan. This is where the GREAT CR practitioner identifies the activities needed to achieve the GREAT CR Goal and any problems that need attention before the goal can be focused on. The practitioner uses their expertise around rehabilitation and their knowledge of the person to select the rehabilitation strategies that are most likely to support the person to achieve their goal.

Stage 5: Carrying out the GREAT CR plan. The personal rehabilitation plan is put into practice over several sessions, usually six weekly one-to-one sessions for approximately one hour each. The sessions guide the person to understand how to use the selected strategies. They are conducted in the home or the task setting to ensure that changes are directly implemented in everyday situations. The GREAT CR practitioner role is to help the individual understand how to use the selected strategies but the individual is responsible for practice and implementation between sessions. Progress towards attaining the goals is evaluated through participant and care partner (where appropriate) reported levels of goal attainment.

Evaluation and re-assessment. Progress towards the goal is monitored at every session. If a selected strategy is not working, the practitioner might suggest an alternative strategy and adapt the plan with the person's input and agreement. When the end of the time for working on the goal is reached, the attainment level is assessed to see how much progress has been made. The person is encouraged to maintain their achievement and also to address further goals, either with ongoing support from the practitioner, or independently, using the strategies that they have learned.

Maintaining control and identity through personal goals

Identifying needs and formulating goals with the person living with dementia is central to GREAT CR and makes this approach truly individual and person-centred. Goal-setting is something that we all do to some degree: having a plan in mind of what we want to achieve, how we are going to go about it and recognising when we have achieved it. This everyday action often goes unrecognised but it provides clarity and motivation for many aspects of our lives. Focusing on goal-setting is a specific way of:

- staying motivated;
- feeling in control of one's own life;
- using the steps towards achievement of the goal as a means of measuring success; and
- helping to maintain a sense of hope and purpose.

As the goals set in GREAT CR are tailored to the individual's lifestyle, interests and routines, working towards them also helps the person to maintain their sense of identity and their feeling of control over their own actions and the consequences of those actions.

A helpful tool to set and monitor goals and their attainment is the short version of the Bangor Goal–Setting Interview, or BGSI (Clare et al., 2016). It offers a structured format for obtaining individual goals and rating the person's attainment in relation to the identified goals in a quick and straightforward manner, at the beginning and the end of an intervention, thus evidencing change in performance. The attainment of the goal is rated on a 10-point scale that is presented visually. A score of 1 indicates the person cannot do or is not successfully achieving the behaviour that is their goal. A score of 10 indicates the person can and is achieving their goal very successfully. A sad and happy face at either end provide cues to assist with providing a rating.

The BGSI is completed jointly by the GREAT CR practitioner and the person with dementia, using a conversational format. There are three steps involved, essentially reflecting the stages of a problem-solving process: (1) identifying areas to work on, (2) setting SMART goals and assigning targets for achievement, and (3) completing ratings of readiness to change and level of attainment

Identifying areas to work on

This step is part of the initial assessment and identifies the broad area that the person with dementia would like to improve in, within three pre-specified domains:

1. Managing in the home.
2. Keeping in touch with family and friends.
3. Engaging in meaningful and enjoyable activities.

The GREAT CR practitioner uses prompts to help the person to identify their own goals by discussing if there is something that they would like to start doing, resume doing, or do more of. The discussion also considers if there are areas that the person would like to manage better or that are challenging to do because of their particular cognitive difficulty. For people with young onset dementia, the goal might reflect issues related to middle age, such as their employment or a parenting role.

The person's cognitive difficulty might also be further impacted by mental health needs, as depression and anxiety are common. Without support, mental ill health can affect a person's confidence and motivation. This has a knock-on effect on the person's energy level, concentration and optimism, all of which undermine the ability to function in everyday actions. If the person begins to do less, they can quickly lose the skills needed. It is not hard to see how there is a risk of a downward spiral of mental ill health combined with a faster progression in functional disability.

It might be the case that a person's goal relates specifically to managing their mood in order to positively impact on their functional ability and reverse this downward spiral. The GREAT CR programme includes simple management techniques for reducing anxiety and, as mentioned above, the setting of a goal in itself provides a sense of hopefulness which is further enhanced as the steps towards the goal are achieved. However, if the person has severe mental health needs, the CR practitioner would encourage them to seek professional help and provide signposting for this.

Setting SMART goals and assigning targets for achievement

Goal statements are brief declarations about an action that the person wishes to carry out or achieve – for example, '*I will walk to the shop on my own to buy a newspaper four times a week*'. This often involves developing a broadly expressed objective into a precise and focused goal statement conforming to SMART principles. They should be framed as statements about specific, observable, measurable behaviour. It is important that the goals are realistic and potentially achievable within the time period that the person and their GREAT CR practitioner agree and define as relevant.

Achieving the goal would be 100% attainment. From this, you can break down the goal into manageable steps that provide half-way and quarter-way descriptions of achievement to the entire goal – for example, '*I will walk to the shop on my own to buy a newspaper once a week*' (25% attainment), then '*I will walk to the shop on my own to buy a newspaper twice a week*' (50% attainment). The attainment levels can also be described by the level of independence rather than the frequency, for example a first step might be: '*I will walk to the shop with my friend*'.

These goal attainment ratings are used to assess the extent and direction of progress. They support the development and review of the suitability of the cognitive rehabilitation strategies and the techniques that are selected to work towards the goal. They are completed at the initial visit and at the end of the agreed number of sessions.

Completing ratings of readiness to change and level of attainment

In addition to setting a goal and the target steps towards its achievement, it is helpful to identify the person's motivational level for achieving the goal. A person living with young onset dementia might be highly motivated because of their family and relationship circumstances. It is important to ensure that the goal is not over-influenced by others. It must be the individual's goal if they are to be motivated to work towards it. For example, a partner might want the person living with young onset dementia to focus on learning how to operate the TV remote but the individual might have very little interest in watching television programmes and their goal might be to maintain their interest in a well-loved and long-established hobby.

By asking the person to rate their readiness to make improvements to the problem, on a 10-point visual rating scale, the CR practitioner and the person can identify how important the goal is, whether this is one to address, and if it is relevant and realistic.

Cognitive rehabilitation principles and methods

Key principles

Two key principles to gain maximum benefit from the GREAT CR programme are:

- to use errorless learning combined with
- effortful processing.

Errorless learning breaks down the action or information into very small steps so that each step is achievable without error. The approach also uses positive language to guide the person rather than focusing on any errors made. In addition to being more motivating, errorless learning and positive instructions have the benefit of not leaving the person with the 'undesirable' information or action in their memory. For example, *'remember to turn right at the Post Office'* supports the desired learning, whereas *'don't turn left at the Post Office'* might be unhelpful.

Effortful processing involves conscious, explicit attention to the task at hand as well as the processing of the information or action through more than one cognitive process. So, for example, the person will write down the steps and speak out loud what they are doing as they perform an action, or they will write down and say out loud the information that they are learning.

Key methods

Cognitive rehabilitation methods may include: the use of compensatory strategies, procedural learning of skills and actions, methods for learning or re-learning information.

Compensatory strategies

These are techniques that help the person get around the difficulty without having to re-learn the method for overcoming it. For example, rather than being able to memorise a direction, the person instead refers to a set of notes or, rather than learn how to operate a dishwasher, they use coloured dots to know which button to press next. Even so, a compensatory method will often involve some simple (re-)learning in order to use the aid or equipment effectively.

Compensatory strategies support the person to achieve the goal of completing an everyday activity without having to restore the lost cognitive ability that is getting in the way of achieving it. A strategy is used to get round the impaired cognitive ability (e.g. planning, sequencing, way-finding or maintaining attention). An example of using a compensatory strategy is illustrated in the story 'Gareth sells collectibles' below, where Gareth was supported to attach a keyboard to his tablet rather than learn how to type on the desktop.

Acquiring new skills or re-learning forgotten ones requires a lot of commitment and effort on the part of the person living with dementia. Therefore, it is usually best to use compensatory approaches for goals that are less important to the person. This releases them to focus their energy to work on the more intensive approach to achieve the more meaningful goals. These might be relating to family relationships, such as knowing the names of grandchildren or being able to use a computer to stay in touch, or they could be important goals relating to the person's work or well-loved hobbies.

On the other hand, possibly some of those who are living with young onset dementia might have more energy and resilience than those with late onset dementia to make this commitment. So some people with young onset dementia might prefer to attempt new learning or re-learning first before resorting to compensatory approaches.

Learning of skills and actions

Enhanced learning techniques for engaging in activities are used for acquiring new skills or re-learning forgotten ones. They require an action-based approach that enables the procedural memory, also known as 'motor skill', to be developed through repetition. This ultimately leads to an automatic action that does not require conscious attention. The person is shown how to complete each step and then encouraged to do it. Verbal or physical prompts might be used initially and these are gradually faded out as the person achieves the step. The steps toward the full goal are gradually added through the use of 'expanding rehearsal', which means that the practice of the actions is repeated at increasing intervals up to the point when the action is learned well enough to be performed any time it is required. An example comes from the story of Gareth below. Gareth needed to learn to use eBay. Expanded rehearsal helped him engrain his new learning around how to search for items. He practised searching once, repeated the process 30 seconds later, then one minute later, then 2 minutes later, then 4 minutes later and so on, until there was a 32 minute gap. This process helps encoding of effective learning.

Learning or re-learning information

This involves techniques that optimise the use of memory and other cognitive skills for the manipulation of information. Learning or re-learning information is different from learning or re-learning activities. For example, learning the names of everyone in a book club (information learning) is different from re-learning how to use a remote control for the TV (action learning).

In order to manage information so that it is easier to store and recall, mnemonics or memory devices such as acronyms, rhymes and alliteration are used. The person with young onset dementia will be encouraged to find their own mnemonic that has personal meaning as this will be more easily held and recalled. An example of this is illustrated in Judith's story below, where Judith made use of her existing knowledge of her bedroom number in order to devise a means of knowing the number of the bus she needed to catch to and from the library.

There are also some similarities between techniques for (re-)learning activities and for (re-) learning information. Just as re-learning an activity involves breaking down the goal into smaller steps, information learning utilises 'chunking' of the information to be (re-) learnt into bite-size sections. Similarly, expanding rehearsal is used in information learning as well as in activity learning. In the case of information learning, usually this begins with an immediate repetition of the information after having heard it, followed by recall after 15 seconds, then 30 seconds and continuing with a doubling of the time frame until an interval of 20 minutes results in successful recall. The length can then be further extended, possibly setting a recall once or twice a day as 'homework' in between the cognitive rehabilitation practice sessions.

There is a lot of individual variability in how people respond to different strategies. Different people learn best in different ways, so personal preference as well as ability must be taken into account for the GREAT CR programme to be as effective as possible.

Individual differences

People who are living with young onset dementia are likely to have a younger and, therefore, larger social group than older people. This leads to greater potential for support and encouragement from others to engage in cognitive rehabilitation 'homework' between sessions with the GREAT CR practitioner. It is important that all who are involved in supporting the person with dementia are aware of the methods being used. This enables the learning to be embedded so that the errorless learning and effortful processing approaches are continued beyond the therapy sessions. This education of, and support from, family and others can be a key element of the GREAT CR practitioner role.

People with young onset dementia have different and often complex needs and issues compared with older people. It is often the case that they have taken many years to get a diagnosis. Therefore, when they are in a position to receive cognitive rehabilitation therapy, their disability might already be advanced in its progress and they and their family and other carers might have developed coping strategies that get in the way of a rehabilitation approach. This, of course, makes the case for early diagnosis and treatment of young onset dementia, including the use of rehabilitation therapy. The GREAT CR programme not only includes the focus on skills and information learning but equally the focus on mental health and mood, making it a positive therapeutic model for younger people who will benefit from this holistic approach to meet their complex needs.

Learning from people living with young onset dementia

Because of the lack of age-specific services, people with young onset dementia often receive services that have been developed with older people's needs in mind. They might have more in keeping with those who are delivering the service than they do with other users. For example, staff and those with young onset dementia may be of a similar age, have young dependents and be in paid employment. They might also have more experience of information technology and expect to be able to engage and communicate using mobile devices more than those who are older. The Angela Project, which is the largest study of services for people living with young onset dementia undertaken in the UK to date, reinforces that key outcomes important to people living with young onset dementia are to maintain control over their own lives, retain a sense of identity and feel connected with others (Stamou et al., 2022). The GREAT CR goals that are uniquely meaningful to the individual are likely to be a reflection of their need for continuing their sense of identity, being connected with others and maintaining control over their own lives. The stories below illustrate how the goals of some individuals with young onset dementia were achieved during the GREAT study, and the GREAT-into Practice study, using CR methods.

Gareth sells collectibles

Gareth took part in the GREAT trial (Clare et al., 2018). At the time of the cognitive rehabilitation intervention Gareth was 59 years old, and received his diagnosis of young onset Alzheimer's disease approximately one year prior to taking part in the trial.

Gareth had previously worked as a solicitor, and had first noticed his cognitive difficulties at work. He is now medically retired. He lives with his wife in a small town, and his two adult children live away. Both Gareth and his wife continue to support their own mothers, who live locally, with practical and household tasks.

The CR practitioner visited Gareth at home. She and Gareth collaboratively set a SMART goal to focus the cognitive rehabilitation strategies onto a personally relevant task. Gareth described feeling guilty about his unplanned early retirement, especially as his wife continued to work. He also described struggling with structure and purpose to his week. Throughout his life Gareth had enjoyed collecting various items – stamps, coins, memorabilia – and had a vast, varied collection. Gareth felt he was not deriving pleasure from some collections anymore, and he could raise some income to support the household. Therefore, Gareth's SMART goal was:

To sell a collectable item online within 10 weeks.

The BGSI was used to establish Gareth's perception of his current attainment on this goal prior to the start of the cognitive rehabilitation. Gareth scored his attainment of this goal as 3/10, as he had already sorted through some of his collectables and identified some to sell.

The CR practitioner initially focused the intervention upon using a tablet and familiarity with the online platform eBay, which Gareth intended to use to sell his collectables. He had not used eBay before. He was also finding elements of using a tablet difficult, particularly when wanting to type. He had previously used a desktop computer at work but wished to use the digital camera element on the tablet.

The CR practitioner introduced Gareth and his wife to a range of restorative and compensatory cognitive rehabilitation techniques to support Gareth's new learning of using a tablet and eBay:

- A shortcut icon for eBay was placed on the tablet home screen, allowing Gareth to see this immediately upon opening the tablet, and have one-touch access.
- The CR practitioner graded the activity by splitting the task into steps (accessing eBay, searching for an item, and listing an item).
- The CR practitioner modelled the actions involved in each step. Gareth was then supported in immediately repeating the action himself.
- To ensure errorless action-based learning, verbal instructions were given by the CR practitioner to Gareth as he repeated each step.
- This was reinforced using expanding rehearsal, where Gareth was encouraged to repeat the actions with a small time gap (30 seconds initially), which increased by doubling the time gap between practices.
- New learning was further supported by Gareth writing his own instructions to refer back to in home practice, an effortful processing technique.
- Practice was supported by Gareth's wife between the weekly cognitive rehabilitation sessions.

Each step was introduced, practised and mastery demonstrated by Gareth before proceeding to the next step. In addition to these cognitive rehabilitation techniques, a clip-on keyboard was purchased allowing Gareth to use his established skills of typing, thus reducing the need for re-learning tablet-based typing.

Several sub-tasks were involved in selling each item, including background research for price and listing, photograph, listing and checking the auction. Scheduling these activities and jointly setting a realistic timeline assisted

Gareth with initiating, focusing on one aspect of the task, and completing. Use of a dedicated file (also on shortcut on the home screen) to store facts from background research helped with recall and organisation.

At the end of 10 cognitive rehabilitation sessions, Gareth had listed one item on eBay independently, although it was yet to sell. In addition, Gareth had, through his background research, made contact with a collectible coin dealer, and had negotiated and completed a sale of his entire collection of coins. He recognised that a lack of knowing how to go about selling the collectables had been as significant a barrier as learning how to set up the eBay account and post an item for auction. He felt he had improved in both these aspects. He reported that he was also using the tablet a lot more for general tasks, as his confidence had improved. He re-rated his goal attainment on the BGSI as 7/10. This was an improvement in score of 4 from the 3/10 he had given himself at the outset.

Judith visits the library

Judith took part in the GREAT implementation study (Clare et al., 2023). At the time, Judith was a 63-year-old woman with a diagnosis of young onset mixed dementia, which she had received 4 years previously. She had recently moved into residential care in her home town, making the decision after finding it increasingly challenging to live alone. Judith had a range of friends she used to meet up with regularly before she moved. She was also an avid reader, reporting enjoying trips to her local library to borrow books but had not resumed this since moving.

The CR practitioner visited Judith at the residential home and after discussion with Judith, and then discussion and agreement with the residential home care team regarding risk management, a collaborative SMART goal was established:

> *To catch a bus from the 'home' to the library and back again once a week by the end of the intervention.*

Before commencing the CR intervention, Judith described knowing the location of the library in relation to the town's bus station. She was used to catching a bus. She did not know the bus route or details such as stops close to the residential home or the timetable. She stated she had not caught a bus for about 4 months. Judith rated her initial attainment of her goal on the BGSI as 2/10.

The CR practitioner started by breaking down the task of catching the bus:

- Learn the bus number, route, bus stops and timetable.
- Way-finding in the area local to the residential home to navigate between home and bus stops.

- Establish and initiate a plan to go to town.
- Safety aspects: (1) remember to inform care staff at time of leaving; (2) develop an emergency action plan and ensure Judith can recall this.

The CR practitioner worked alongside Judith to understand and get around the difficulties Judith experienced with these steps. A laminated card, with details of bus times and numbers and emergency information for the care home, was placed in her bus pass wallet. Use of this was practised during bus use sessions through modelling what to do – that is, the therapist showed Judith, so she could then copy what she saw. The technique of action-based learning was also used, meaning Judith did not just listen to instructions on what to do but she performed the actions as well (see the description above). A red bus pass wallet proved useful to allow Judith to check for it easily in her handbag. A prompt card was placed in the staff office to remind them to prompt Judith to take her mobile phone.

Judith was supported in finding her way to the bus stop by being accompanied by the CR practitioner and encouraged to identify her own personal landmarks to ensure she had effortfully attended to the route. The bus stop was 'after the red post box' and 'before the church'. The same landmarks were used to help identify the bus stop on the return journey and the way back to the residential home. These were reinforced in sessions through expanding rehearsal of repeating the visual cues back to the CR practitioner at gradually expanding short time periods, until Judith was able to recall them.

The route number was learnt through a mnemonic developed by Judith: her room number in the home was 1, and the bus route number was 23, hence her mnemonic of 123. This was practised through expanding rehearsal until Judith was able to recall between sessions. Checking the timetable at the bus stop was modelled during bus catching sessions, with immediate encouragement to Judith to repeat the action herself, until the process became habitual.

Practical bus catching sessions were graded, with Judith undertaking more of the bus journey and the walk from and to the home to the bus stop independently, each session. To assist with initiation and planning, Judith identified Thursday as the weekday she would attend the library, and stuck to this. This routine supported both Judith and the residential home staff.

At the end of the 20 sessions, Judith was catching the bus to the library every Thursday independently. She had also arranged with friends to meet her there. She reported gaining a sense of independence and achievement that she was engaging in activities outside of the care home. She gave herself a BGSI score of 9/10, as she occasionally required a prompt from the residential home staff that it was Thursday and to take her phone with her.

Francis keeps track of his plans

At the time he took part in the GREAT study (Clare et al., 2018), Francis was 60 years old and recently diagnosed with an unspecified young onset dementia. He first noticed problems with his recall and cognitive functions when he retired from work as a bricklayer for a local building firm when he was 57. Francis lived with his wife, who reduced her working hours to part time to support him. He had engaged with the local Alzheimer's Society group, alongside attending a monthly peer support group at the memory clinic, both of which he attended by himself. He also attended the local town's home football games with his friends during the season.

When the CR practitioner visited Francis at home, it was quickly established that a range of strategies to assist his memory were in place such as a calendar, notepad and to-do lists, but which were often used by his wife on his behalf. Francis used an electronic clock to identify the day and date. He knew elements of his weekly routine, such as football on Saturday, but identified that he had problems which he found frustrating when something was out of routine, such as dentist appointments or the monthly peer support group. Francis therefore identified his SMART goal as:

> *To know what I've got planned for the week, by the end of May.*
> (CR intervention commenced in early April)

He rated his baseline BGSI attainment as 5/10, due to his ability to recall routine events in the week.

The CR practitioner worked with Francis over a period of 10 sessions. Time was spent reviewing the monthly calendar used by his wife and identifying the pattern of activities throughout a 'usual' week. Expanding rehearsal, gradually increasing a very short recall time, was used to link certain activities to certain days of the week, which worked well. Use of semantic elaboration or a mnemonic was attempted to support this, but Francis found those techniques cumbersome. Instead, the links were supported by fading prompts whenever he was asked by his wife to recall them. In other words, the level of support was highest at the start and was gradually reduced over time. Initially, when Francis asked what events were planned, his wife would tell him to look at the calendar and point it out to him. Gradually, she replaced this instruction with just pointing, and then finally with a question of '*where do you look to find out?*' This approach enabled Francis to learn how to find out the information he needed.

When more routine weekly events were able to be recalled by Francis, the focus shifted to the non-routine events such as GP, dentist, monthly peer group and visits by/to his children or grandchildren. Using the monthly calendar initially, the CR practitioner and Francis concluded that a month was an overwhelming amount of information for Francis to process. Therefore, after discussion, a whiteboard was placed in the kitchen, with the days of the week and the activities for each day to be used as a daily visual cue by Francis.

To reinforce its use, using an effortful processing approach, Francis completed this every Sunday with support from his wife, by referring to the calendar.

At the end of May (after eight of the 10 cognitive rehabilitation sessions), Francis was able to verbally list his routine daily activities. He was referring to the whiteboard daily and it was successful in supporting Francis to attend the non-routine activities. His wife reported that the whiteboard was working well for her too. She reported that Francis was completing it on a Sunday with minimal assistance from her. Francis re-rated his attainment at session 10, with a BGSI score of 10/10.

Resources for GREAT Cognitive Rehabilitation

To fully realise the benefits and achieve widespread and sustainable implementation requires sufficient resources and a reorientation of service priorities towards preventive and rehabilitative approaches. The authors are hopeful that readers of this chapter who are either users or providers of health and social care services, will see this as a 'call to action' to ensure that they provide or receive equity in reablement approaches.

Recognising that the availability of sufficient practitioners with the skills and experience to provide GREAT CR is essential to future implementation, the University of Exeter has developed a foundation-level training course in an e-learning format. This incorporates educational videos prepared jointly with NHS Education for Scotland. These are available to NHS practitioners via the NHS Learning Hub. The course is titled: 'Enabling people with dementia through GREAT goal-oriented cognitive rehabilitation'. It is freely available on the NHS Learning Hub (https://learninghub.nhs.uk/) where it can be accessed by anyone in the UK with an NHS or university email address.

For those outside the UK, and for people without an NHS or UK university email address, the same e-learning course can be accessed, free of charge, via the University of Exeter website (https://sites.google.com/exeter.ac.uk/great-cr/for-practitioners/elearning-course?authuser=0). This version does not save the learner's progress but is otherwise the same.

People living with young onset dementia who cannot currently access the support of a CR practitioner or who wish to work on their goals on their own, can access an easy-to-use, practical guide through the Alzheimer's Society website. It is called 'My Life, My Goals' (Alzheimer's Society, 2021b) and has been created by people with dementia, with input from the GREAT Cognitive Rehabilitation programme researchers at the University of Exeter. There are also short films that accompany the written guide in order to illustrate how to make changes and use achievable strategies. The aim of the guide is to provide people who are living with dementia with a sense of hope that there are ways of managing difficulties, there are solutions to problems and that it is possible to live a good life with dementia. The guide is full of ideas to help the person to think about their goals and create their own plan to achieving those goals.

Conclusions

This chapter reveals the importance of providing re-enabling interventions like GREAT CR to as many people with young onset dementia as possible. Currently, there are few reablement services on offer, mainly because of organisational barriers that reflect the lack of knowledge about the approach and its effectiveness. However, the potential for rehabilitation/reablement is becoming more widely recognised. A research briefing for the Social Care Institute for Excellence (Francis et al., 2011) stated we should maximise the potential for reablement of people living with dementia. Since then, the research evidence for the effectiveness of cognitive rehabilitation has increased significantly.

So what does this mean in practice?

If you are diagnosed with young onset dementia

Consider how cognitive rehabilitation could benefit you and those close to you? Are there tasks/goals you would like to improve, achieve or learn? Ask your dementia worker if cognitive rehabilitation is available. Advocate for cognitive rehabilitation to be provided by your service. The practical, self-help guide 'My Life, My Goals' (Alzheimer's Society, 2021b) could be useful to support you with setting goals, learning and applying cognitive rehabilitation strategies to your everyday life.

If you are a family or friend of someone diagnosed with young onset dementia

Ask them if this is an approach they would like to try? Support them and yourself by finding out more information about cognitive rehabilitation through the 'My Life, My Goals' self-help guide mentioned above. Consider how you could support them with practising and implementing the cognitive rehabilitation strategies to achieve their goals in their everyday life. Support them in advocating for cognitive rehabilitation from their dementia service.

If you are a professional working with people with young onset dementia

There is probably the need for two distinctly focused reflections. First, *service provision* – reflect upon your current service provision. Does it offer a reablement approach and/or cognitive rehabilitation to those you work with? Why should you offer this? How could you offer this approach routinely? What would need to change to enable this? Second, *competencies* – do you and/or your staff have the experience, confidence and skills to offer cognitive rehabilitation? Consider engaging in the e-learning package 'Enabling people with dementia through GREAT goal-oriented cognitive rehabilitation' (https://learninghub.nhs.uk/), visiting the GREAT CR website, offering the time for others to complete, and setting up peer supervision/support within your localityto support the learning, application and evaluation of this approach.

References

Alzheimer's Society (2021a) A *future for personalised care: A discussion paper on reform and the quality of social care*. London: Alzheimer's Society.

Alzheimer's Society (2021b) *Living with dementia: My Life, My Goals*. Available at: https://www.alzheimers.org.uk/sites/default/files/2021-09/my-life-my-goals-workbook.pdf.

Bahar-Fuchs, A., Martyr, A., Goh, A.M., et al. (2019) Cognitive training for people with mild to moderate dementia, *Cochrane Database of Systematic Reviews*, 3: CD013069. Available at: https://doi.org/10.1002/14651858.CD013069.pub2.

Bird, M. (2001) Behavioural difficulties and cued recall of adaptive behaviour in dementia: experimental and clinical evidence, *Neuropsychological Rehabilitation*, 11 (3/4): 357–75.

Butler, M., McCreedy, E., Nelson, V. A., et al. (2018) Does cognitive training prevent cognitive decline?, *Annals of Internal Medicine*, 168 (1): 63–68.

Cafferata, R.M.T., Hicks, B. and von Bastian, C. C. (2021) Effectiveness of cognitive stimulation for dementia: a systematic review and meta-analysis, *Psychological Bulletin*, 147 (5): 455–76.

Clare, L. (2008) *Neuropsychological Rehabilitation and People with Dementia*. Hove: Psychology Press.

Clare, L., Wilson, B.A., Breen, K., et al. (1999) Errorless learning of face–name associations in early Alzheimer's disease, *Neurocase*, 5 (1): 37–46.

Clare, L., Linden, D.E., Woods, R.T., et al. (2010) Goal-oriented cognitive rehabilitation for people with early-stage Alzheimer's disease: a single-blind randomized controlled trial of clinical efficacy, *American Journal of Geriatric Psychiatry*, 18 (10): 928–39.

Clare, L., Nelis, S.M. and Kudlicka, A. (2016) *Bangor Goal-Setting Interview Manual Setting goals with the BGSI Version 2*. Centre for Research in Ageing and Cognitive Health, University of Exeter. BGSI-Short version available at: https://medicine.exeter.ac.uk/v8media/facultysites/hls/healthandcommunitysciences/documents/The_Bangor_Goal-Setting_Interview_Version_2.2_Manual_(BGSI_v.2.2)_March_2022.pdf.

Clare, L., Kudlicka, A., Oyebode, J.R., et al. (2018) Individual goal-oriented cognitive rehabilitation to improve everyday functioning for people with early-stage dementia: a multicentre randomised controlled trial (the GREAT trial), *International Journal of Geriatric Psychiatry*, 34 (5): 709–21.

Clare, L., Kudlicka, A., Collins, R., et al. (2023) Implementing a home-based personalised cognitive rehabilitation intervention for people with mild-to-moderate dementia: GREAT into practice, *BMC Geriatrics*, 23: 93. Available at: https://doi.org/10.1186/s12877-022-03705-0.

Francis, J., Fisher, M. and Rutter, D. (2011) *Reablement: A cost-effective route to better outcomes*, SCIE Research Briefing 36. Available at: https://lx.iriss.org.uk/sites/default/files/resources/briefing36.pdf.

Hill, N.T.M., Mowszowski, L., Naismith, S.L., et al. (2017) Computerized cognitive training in older adults with mild cognitive impairment or dementia: a systematic review and meta-analysis, *American Journal of Psychiatry*, 174 (4): 329–40.

Irazoki, E., Contreras-Somoza, L.M., Toribio-Guzmán, J.M., et al. (2020) Technologies for cognitive training and cognitive rehabilitation for people with mild cognitive impairment and dementia: a systematic review, *Frontiers in Psychology*, 11: 648. Available at: https://doi.org/10.3389/fpsyg.2020.00648.

National Institute for Health and Care Excellence (NICE) (2018) *Dementia: Assessment, management and support for people living with dementia and their carers*, NICE Guidance NG97. Available at: https://www.nice.org.uk/guidance/ng97.

Stamou, V., La Fontaine, J., O'Malley, M., et al. (2022) Helpful post-diagnostic services for young onset dementia: findings and recommendations from the Angela Project, *Health and Social Care in the Community*, 30 (1): 142–53.

Wilson, B.A. (2002) Towards a comprehensive model of cognitive rehabilitation, *Neuropsychological Rehabilitation*, 12 (2): 97–110.

World Health Organisation (WHO) (2021) Dementia diagnosis, treatment and care, in *Global status report on the public health response to dementia*. Geneva: WHO. Available at: https://www.who.int/publications/i/item/9789240033245.

Zhang, H., Huntley, J., Bhome, R., et al. (2019) Effect of computerised cognitive training on cognitive outcomes in mild cognitive impairment: a systematic review and meta-analysis, *BMJ Open*, 9: e027062. Available at: https://doi.org/10.1136/bmjopen-2018-027062.

7 Legal and financial aspects of young onset dementia[1]

Calum Macdonald

Overview

Young onset dementia impacts all aspects of an individual's life. Two of the areas where this impact is often first and most keenly felt (usually long before diagnosis) is in their financial and legal affairs. However, both of these areas have historically received relatively limited attention in post-diagnosis care and planning despite the number of challenges they can pose and the clear benefits if they are well managed.

This chapter sets out the legal framework relevant to those with young onset dementia and their caregivers. It then considers the legal and financial considerations for those living with a young onset dementia diagnosis and their carers and explores issues raised by a young onset dementia diagnosis thematically under the headings of: (1) planning and preparation, (2) problem-solving and (3) protection vs. autonomy.

Keywords

Young onset dementia, Alzheimer's, finances, money, legal, advance planning, Living Wills, social care, paying for care, Lasting Powers of Attorney, mental capacity.

Learning points

- Know about the key pieces of legislation that give rights and protections to those living with young onset dementia and their family carers.
- Be aware of several tools that can be used to help people with young onset dementia to manage their affairs and ensure care is in line with their wishes after they have lost mental capacity.
- Understand more about entitlements to provision and funding of health and social care.

- Appreciate the importance and challenges of advance consideration and planning for those living with young onset dementia around financial and legal matters.
- Know about some of the resources that can help with problem-solving in relation to legal and financial issues.

Introduction

Numerous studies have identified that dementia can cause problems in individuals' financial management years before first diagnosis (Giebel et al., 2019; National Institute on Aging, 2021). One study found that the ability to manage finances, from making bank transactions to using a cash machine and paying in shops or virtually online, was one of the first complex daily activities to deteriorate in dementia – occurring up to 10 years prior to a diagnosis (Peres et al., 2007). However, whilst the symptoms and effects of young onset dementia often first present in an individual's finances, employment and legal affairs, available evidence indicates that these aspects of an individual's life receive relatively limited focus and resourcing in the aftermath of a young onset dementia diagnosis (Giebel et al., 2023).

This chapter begins by setting out the legal framework relevant to those with young onset dementia (and indeed those with dementia/illnesses experiencing cognitive degeneration more generally). Through this framework, the legal rights, protections and tools that are relevant to the financial and legal affairs of those with young onset dementia are explored. The remainder of the chapter then considers financial and legal issues for those with young onset dementia under three headings: (1) planning and preparation, (2) problem-solving and (3) protection vs. autonomy.

The legal framework

Three main pieces of legislation (not dementia-specific) provide the core legal framework which enables and protects those living with young onset dementia and their carers. A majority of the key legislation applies across the UK. However, where this differs for constituent parts of the UK, this is noted with the position under English law explained in this chapter. In addition, many other general areas of law are of potential relevance and can assist with legal and financial issues – these are summarised as applicable.

Equalities legislation

The Equality Act 2010 applies across the UK (excluding Northern Ireland[2]) and is designed to empower those living with 'protected characteristics'.

Disability is one of the protected characteristics and is defined as any impairment (physical and/or mental) that has a substantial and long-term adverse effect on an individual's ability to carry out day-to-day activities.[3] Young onset dementia is such an impairment and so those with young onset dementia are entitled to the protections granted by the Equality Act.

Importantly, for progressive conditions (such as young onset dementia) the Equality Act also states that if progressive illness has an effect on an individual's day-to-day activities but the effect is not yet substantial, then it can still be treated as a disability if it is likely to result in a substantial impairment in the future.[4] The effect of this is that an individual diagnosed with young onset dementia gains the rights and protections provided by the Equality Act from the point of their diagnosis even if they themselves (or others) regard their illness as still being relatively mild/not yet a disability.

The Equality Act prohibits direct and indirect discrimination in a wide range of circumstances. These circumstances include where an individual with young onset dementia is in employment, a consumer or customer; a user of public services (these could range from social services to transport); buying or renting property and/or a member of a club or association.[5]

Direct discrimination is defined by the Equality Act as any situation where one person (A) treats someone with a protected characteristic (B) less favourably than they would others.[6] Indirect discrimination is defined as any situation where A puts in place a rule or practice which puts people with B's characteristic at a particular disadvantage and where A cannot objectively justify the rule or practice.[7]

The Equality Act also prohibits discriminating against an individual because of their association with someone with a protected characteristic.[8] This is of particular relevance for caregivers of those with young onset dementia who must not be discriminated against simply by virtue of them performing that role.

In addition, disability discrimination also includes situations where A treats B unfavourably because of something arising as a result of B's disability and where A is unable to objectively justify the treatment as being proportionate.[9] This could, for example, include discriminating against an individual because they had to take time off work for doctors' appointments or where they were experiencing side effects from medication. Notably, this additional prohibition does not apply if A can show they did not know (and could not reasonably have known) that B had the disability.[10] This is one of several reasons why securing and disclosing a young onset dementia diagnosis is particularly important to ensure that an individual gains the full benefit of legal protections.

The Equality Act also includes a duty to make reasonable adjustments to assist those with disabilities.[11] In particular, it imposes general requirements that where arrangements put B at a substantial disadvantage to others, A must take reasonable steps to avoid the disadvantage. Similarly, where an auxiliary aid could remove B's substantial disadvantage, A must take reasonable steps to provide that aid. Where these requirements relate to the provision of information, reasonable steps include ensuring that information is provided in an accessible format.

Protections afforded by the Equality Act are of particular significance for those with young onset dementia in the employment context. Potential workplace discrimination is a considerably more significant issue for those with young onset dementia (and/or their carers). One study found that 18% of people diagnosed with young onset dementia continue to work after their diagnosis (Alzheimer's Society, 2017), many are still employed at the time of diagnosis (Kilty et al., 2023), and many carers must juggle caregiving with continuing work commitments. The effect of the Equality Act is that a young onset dementia diagnosis should not result in an automatic dismissal or early retirement. Individuals with young onset dementia wishing to continue working are generally advised to discuss with their employers (Alzheimer's Society, 2023), in particular to address stigma or employers mistaking impaired performance for other issues (Dementia UK, 2023).

One challenging area which often impacts employment is that a young onset dementia diagnosis must be notified to the Driver and Vehicle Licensing Agency (DVLA).[12] They – as for other driving impairments – will decide (potentially with medical consultation) whether an individual's license is to be revoked. Anecdotally, many individuals with young onset dementia choose to surrender their license upon or soon after diagnosis.

Mental capacity legislation

The Mental Capacity Act 2005[13] establishes general rules for dealing with and protecting individuals who are unable to make some or all decisions themselves. The Mental Capacity Act sets out five statutory principles that guide the approach to dealing with anyone where there is a concern as to their mental capacity[14] (these are set out in the appendix to this chapter). The starting point is that a person must be assumed to have mental capacity unless it is established that they lack capacity.

If there is doubt about a person's capacity, a trained health or social care professional can carry out a Mental Capacity Assessment. A person will be assessed to lack capacity in relation to a matter if at the material time they are unable to make a decision for themselves because of an impairment of, or a disturbance in the functioning of, the mind or brain (this may be permanent or temporary).[15] Importantly, a person's capacity to make a decision relates specifically to their ability to make a particular decision at that particular time. Simply because an individual has lacked capacity to make one specific decision in the past, does not mean they will necessarily lack capacity to make all types of decisions now or in the future. If another significant decision needs to be made, another Mental Capacity Assessment may be required (albeit this must be interpreted in the context of a degenerative illness such as young onset dementia).

The Mental Capacity Act states that a person is unable to make a decision if they cannot:

(a) understand information relevant to the decision;
(b) retain that information;

(c) use or weigh up that information in making a decision; and/or
(d) communicate their decision.[16]

If an individual with young onset dementia lacks capacity, the Mental Capacity Act sets out a number of considerations a decision-maker (including someone exercising a Lasting Power of Attorney) must have regard to when making decisions in the 'best interests' of the person with young onset dementia. These include whether and when the person might have capacity to make the decision in the future and (to the extent they are reasonably ascertainable) the person's past and present wishes, beliefs, values and any other factors the person would be likely to consider.[17]

The decision-maker must also take into account (if it is practicable and appropriate to consult them) the views of any individual named by the person, any caregiver and anyone exercising a Lasting Power of Attorney or deputyship on their behalf (see below). Further, when making any decision on another's behalf, the decision-maker must, as far as reasonably practicable, permit and encourage the person to participate as fully as possible in any act done for them and any decision affecting them.[18]

The Mental Capacity Act Code of Practice[19] also provides further guidance on making decisions when an individual cannot make them for themselves. The Mental Capacity Act requires certain people to follow the Code of Practice;[20] including anyone acting under a Lasting Power of Attorney.

Finally, within the framework of the Mental Capacity Act, the Deprivation of Liberty Safeguards (DOLS) 2009 exist to protect those who lack capacity and who need to be deprived of their liberty to protect them from harm (and set out the formal procedures for doing so).

Decision-making tools and powers relevant to those with young onset dementia

The operation of the Mental Capacity Act highlights the importance of making appropriate plans, including who will take decisions with and/or on behalf of an individual with young onset dementia in order to reduce uncertainty and to avoid potential disputes. Importantly, there is no presumption in English law that a spouse or civil partner can manage the affairs of their partner. Similarly, one person's status in another person's will (for example, as executor or main beneficiary) does not give them legal power to manage another person's affairs while they are still alive.

There are several tools which those with young onset dementia can use to help manage their care and affairs and to ensure that decisions are made by those they trust in accordance with their wishes after they have lost mental capacity. These include Advance Care Plans, Advance Decisions and Lasting Powers of Attorney. In addition, there are various legal safeguards which can be relied upon where a person with young onset dementia has not made provision for their care and has lost mental capacity to do so: these powers are administered by the Court of Protection and include a legal arrangement known as deputyship. Also relevant are independent advocates (in circumstances where there is no-one to consult as to the person's wishes).

Advance Care Plans

An Advance Care Plan (also referred to as an Advance Statement) is any document which sets out an individual's preferences regarding future care and support (NHS, 2023a). Although Advance Statements are not legally binding, they must be taken into account by anyone acting in the individual's best interests in circumstances where the individual has lost mental capacity. There is no prescribed content for an Advanced Statement. However, several young onset dementia charities offer templates that can be helpful to ensure that an Advanced Statement covers all matters important to the person.[21] Whilst there are no formalities for an Advance Statement (for example, that it be signed or witnessed), certain practical steps such as dating the document and informing others of its existence are recommended.

Advance Decisions ('Living Wills')

An Advance Decision to Refuse Treatment (an 'ADRT', often called a 'Living Will' or simply an Advance Decision) is a decision to refuse certain medical or clinical treatment in the future. Importantly, a valid Advance Decision will take precedence over decisions made in an individual's best interests by others (this is the normal position once an individual with young onset dementia has lost mental capacity). Although under UK law both assisted suicide and euthanasia are illegal,[22] an individual may make an ADRT which refuses life-sustaining treatment such as ventilation, cardiopulmonary resuscitation (CPR) or antibiotics (NHS, 2023b).

In contrast to an Advance Care Plan, an Advance Decision is legally binding provided it complies with certain formalities. In summary, it must be:

- made by the individual with young onset dementia when they had mental capacity;
- in writing;
- signed by the individual in question;
- witnessed and, if an individual is choosing to refuse life-sustaining treatment, it must also include a statement that the ADRT applies even if their life is at risk.[23]

In addition to an ADRT, all adults also have the right to make a specific decision in respect of whether they wish to receive CPR – this is referred to as a 'DNACPR'. This is a recommendation not to attempt CPR, made and recorded in advance, to guide those present if a person subsequently suffers a cardiac arrest.[24]

Lasting Powers of Attorney

A regular power of attorney is simply a legal document granting one person (called an attorney) power to do specific acts on behalf of another person (the donor). Lasting Powers of Attorney are a broader, longer-lasting legal tool created by the Mental Capacity Act.[25] They apply to England and Wales and replaced Enduring Powers of Attorney.[26]

There are two types of Lasting Power of Attorney (LPA) relating to: (1) property and affairs and (2) health and welfare.[27] An individual can choose to make one or both types of LPA and nominate different attorneys for each. The important distinction between the two (other than the areas they cover) is that a health and welfare LPA can only come into operation once an individual with young onset dementia has lost mental capacity (see above), whilst a property and affairs LPA can be used by the attorney whilst the individual still has mental capacity (with their permission) to assist in managing their affairs.

Certain legal formalities must be complied with when making an LPA. If these formalities are not complied with, the LPA is invalid. It is therefore generally recommended to seek advice/assistance when preparing the document.[28] Once an LPA has been made, it must be registered with the Office of the Public Guardian if it is to have effect.[29] This process currently can take several months.[30] Importantly, if a health and welfare LPA is intended to grant an attorney power to refuse life-sustaining treatment. then this must be explicitly indicated on the relevant form.

The Court of Protection

The Court of Protection is a specialist judicial body that deals with issues relating to mental capacity and decision-making. Its role is often highly relevant to those with young onset dementia and their carers in the event difficulties or disputes arise in respect of care or a person's financial or legal affairs arise. The Court of Protection has general powers in considering matters relating to the Mental Capacity Act.[31] For instance, it can decide what is in an individual's best interests and intervene if there is a dispute regarding the use of an LPA or between attorneys and others.

Deputyship

In some instances, if there is a discrete matter relating to someone with young onset dementia who has lost mental capacity, it may be appropriate to apply to the Court of Protection for a one-off decision. However, if the individual has not made an LPA and no longer has capacity to do so, then it is often desirable to apply to the Court of Protection to appoint one or more deputies who have similar powers and responsibilities to attorneys.[32] Deputies may be appointed for property and affairs or, very occasionally, for personal welfare.[33]

Independent Advocates

Independent Mental Capacity Advocates (IMCAs) are a legal safeguard created by the Mental Capacity Act for people who lack the capacity to make specific important decisions, including making decisions about where they live and about serious medical treatment options.[34] IMCAs are mainly instructed to represent people where there is no-one independent of service providers, such as a family member or friend, able to represent the person. Similar provisions exist under the Care Act (see below) requiring individuals to be provided with an independent advocate where they may have substantial difficulty understanding, making or communicating a decision.[35]

Care legislation and funding of care

The position relating to the funding of care needs (both health and social care) arising as a result of young onset dementia (and dementia more generally) is often considered to be unsatisfactory and unnecessarily complex. The Health and Social Care Select Committee (House of Commons Library, 2021: 3) described it as a 'a bureaucratic maze that patients and their families are expected to navigate at their most vulnerable and when in need of swift and effective support'.

The reasons for this are several. First, the law (particularly in England and Wales[36]) draws a distinction between health and social care needs that often appears artificial and to treat dementia as distinct from most other illnesses. Generally speaking, where young onset dementia (or consequences of the illness) can be said to be primarily a healthcare need, it is covered under the UK's universal right to free health care. However, symptoms of young onset dementia are often viewed or assessed as a social care need (particularly at earlier stages of the illness). Rights to publicly funded social care and the processes for applying for such care vary across the UK, and will normally depend on whether an individual meets eligibility criteria and the severity of their needs and impairment caused by young onset dementia. Separate social care assessments apply to both an individual with young onset dementia and their carer(s).

Secondly, even where individuals are in principle eligible for social care support, financial means testing applies. There is a common misconception that social care is government-funded as part of the NHS. The applicable thresholds are relatively low and recent proposed and then postponed reforms to funding have only added to confusion.

Thirdly, individuals with young onset dementia (dependent on healthcare needs) may receive free, non-means-tested care under NHS Continuing Healthcare provisions if their illness is judged to be a primary healthcare need. Carers may receive specific assistance under a carer's assessment. Individuals with young onset dementia and their carers are also likely to be eligible for various social benefits and welfare (see below). Whilst additional support is positive, in many cases these schemes have separate applications and assessment criteria, thus adding to the complexity.

Social care: eligibility

The Care Act 2014 (England only)[37] simplified previous legislation on the provision of care and support by local authorities. It sets out local authorities' general responsibilities, how they should assess and meet individuals' care needs. The Care Act (and regulations made under it) also sets out when and how individuals with young onset dementia and their carers will be eligible for local authority-funded social care and support.

When exercising social care functions, a local authority's general duty is to promote the individual's well-being.[38] Well-being is defined broadly and includes personal dignity, emotional and mental health, domestic, family and personal relationships and their contribution to society. Similar to the Mental Capacity Act principles, when acting under the Care Act, a local authority must have regard to certain matters (these are set out in the appendix to this chapter).

The type of support a local authority is obliged to provide depends on the individual's circumstances and may include care home accommodation, or care at home or in the community. Where it appears that an adult may have care and support needs, a local authority must conduct a 'needs assessment'.[39] In conducting a needs assessment, the local authority must involve the individual, any carer they have and any person the individual asks the local authority to involve.[40,41]

Under the Care Act, an individual is eligible for local authority social care if they have care and support needs as a result of a physical or a mental condition and because of those needs, they cannot achieve two or more of certain specified outcomes causing a significant impact on their well-being. These specified outcomes are set out in the Care and Support (Eligibility Criteria) Regulations 2015 (DHSC, 2015). In summary, the outcomes relate to the ability to perform basic day-to-day activities such as nutrition, personal hygiene, toileting, personal safety, clothing and maintaining relationships.

Importantly, the Care Act also creates a specific obligation on local authorities to support caregivers by requiring them to assess whether a carer has needs requiring support (or is likely to in the future) and what those needs are.[42] The duty to carry out a carer's assessment applies irrespective of the local authority's view of the financial resources of the carer or the adult needing care. Records of both the needs and carer's assessments must be provided in writing to the relevant individual and any other person they request.[43]

Social care: funding

Once an individual's eligible needs are established, a financial assessment (often referred to as means testing) will be conducted by the local authority to establish what, if anything, an individual must contribute towards their cost of care. Generally, the financial thresholds applied are relatively low. In England,[44] at the time of writing, the position is that an individual must pay for their social care from their savings if they have more than £23,250 in assets (called the upper capital limit). If an individual has less than £14,250 in assets (the lower capital limit), then their savings will be disregarded. Between these two limits, funding contributions from assets are made based on a sliding scale. It is notable that these limits have remained frozen for more than a decade despite inflation and cost of living increases (House of Commons Library, 2021).

Even if below the upper capital limit, individuals are still required to contribute to the cost of their social care from their income (including wages, pensions and non-means-tested benefits). Although local authorities have a level of discretion as to this contribution, at a minimum individuals must be left with a Personal Expenses Allowance (currently £25.65 a week) if they are in residential care. If they are receiving care and support at home, then under the Care Act, individuals receive a Minimum Income Guarantee intended to leave them a sum for basic living expenses (this figure varies considerably dependent on age and circumstances).

In addition, certain exemptions and presumptions apply to means testing, particularly when calculating assets and income. These are contained in the Care and Support (Charging and Assessment of Resources) Regulations 2014. Of note, where there are joint assets, the rule is to generally assume a 50% share for calculating assets[45] and where an individual is receiving care in their home, the home is excluded from the financial assessment. Where an individual enters residential care, their home will be counted towards assets from 12 weeks after admission. However, where an individual with young onset dementia's partner or other qualifying relative (e.g. a child) continues to live in the family home, it will continue to be disregarded for the purposes of calculating assets – this applies regardless of whether the couple are married or whose name the property is in.[46]

In September 2021, the UK Government introduced a White Paper which set out a number of significant reforms to the funding of social care. However, in the 2022 Autumn Statement, the government delayed introduction of reforms to social care funding until October 2025 (HM Treasury, 2022). Further changes to this area appear likely.

Health and social care: other forms of assistance

In addition to social care, NHS continuing health care (CHC) may also be available to individuals in England and Wales with young onset dementia. Crucially, this is not means-tested and may cover part or all of an individual's residential or non-residential care needs if they are judged to have a primary healthcare need.

The continuing healthcare assessment process is relatively complex.[47] The assessment process will generally involve an initial assessment and, if that is passed, a full assessment by a multidisciplinary team of healthcare professionals. The assessment criteria used are different (although involve considerable overlap) from those used to determine social care eligibility under the Care Act. Needs are considered under headings including breathing, nutrition, continence, mobility and communication. The criteria and decision-making framework (known as the Decision Support Tool) used for NHS continuing healthcare assessments can be difficult to navigate for individuals and ordinarily is strictly applied – the majority of all applications for continuing health care (irrespective of illness) are rejected (Taylor, 2022).

As part of the continuing healthcare assessment process, if an individual is assessed as ineligible for continuing health care but is assessed as requiring nursing care in a care home, then they will be eligible to have NHS-funded nursing care. In addition, in certain circumstances, care packages may involve both health and social care needs referred to as 'joint packages' of care with elements provided by both the local authority and the NHS. Further details of this approach are set out in the National Framework 2022 (DHSC, 2022).

In addition to the above forms of social support, individuals with young onset dementia and their carers are normally eligible for certain benefits, particularly if they are no longer able to work. These vary based on circumstances. The most common benefits available include Personal Independence Payments (PIPs), Access to Work grants, council tax reductions[48] (or exemptions) and the Carer's Allowance. Many individuals (with or without young onset dementia) do not claim their full social entitlement and certain benefits are mutually exclusive: as a result, using a benefits calculator and/or seeking advice is recommended.

Whilst a level of health and social care financial support exists for those with young onset dementia and their carers and is to be welcomed, it is by no means comprehensive. In addition, as the above demonstrates, the system is unhelpfully complex. Individuals with young onset dementia and their carers can face up to half a dozen assessments to determine eligibility for support, often with different criteria, sometimes conducted by different public bodies. A person newly diagnosed with young onset dementia is often unfamiliar with most or all of these support options (Jones et al., 2018). Added to the fact that many assessments must be reviewed annually, it is unsurprising that individuals with young onset dementia report confusion as to which assessment is being conducted. The result is that a system intended to assist is often confusing and can be overwhelming.

Other legislation/regulation

Whilst the Equality Act, Mental Capacity Act and Care Act are the primary sources of statutory rights and protections, many other pieces of legislation (whilst not young onset dementia-specific) are also of help to those with young onset dementia. These include general employment law protections, particularly the rights against unfair and constructive dismissal.

In addition, the Human Rights Act 1998 requires public bodies to act in a manner compatible with individuals' human rights.[49] Of particular relevance are Article 8 (rights to a private and family life) and Article 14 (protection from discrimination). These can, in appropriate circumstances, be used as an alternative legal argument if specific protections/safeguards under specific legislation do not apply.

In relation to individuals' financial affairs, there are specific rules relating to the treatment of customers by financial services firms. The Financial Conduct Authority (FCA) regulates such firms and has created various rules and guidance in relation to 'vulnerable' customers.[50] Broadly speaking, the effect of these rules is that financial services firms should be able to understand the needs of vulnerable customers, embed fair treatment of vulnerable customers across their workforce, and take practical action to ensure product design, customer service and communications are appropriate for vulnerable customers. Similar vulnerability requirements apply to most utility providers – this can be particularly helpful if an individual with young onset dementia is threatened with cutting off of a utility for accidental non-payment of a bill (Alzheimer's Society, 2018c).

Guidance and non-legal tools

Whilst the UK's legal framework relevant to those with young onset dementia is relatively well-developed, there is inevitably a limit to what legislation can achieve on its own. Guidance, awareness and non-legal tools play an essential role in helping ensure there is appropriate support to manage the legal and financial impacts of a young onset dementia diagnosis. Additional solutions also include business training and education, support groups, industry codes of conduct, best practice guides and new technologies (see Chapter 9 for more on employment issues).

Financial institutions are becoming increasingly aware of the role they can play in supporting individuals with dementia. Significant sources of industry guidance issued in recent years include the Dementia Friendly Financial Services Charter (Alzheimer's Society, 2013), the Dementia Friendly Finance and Insurance Guide (Alzheimer's Society, 2018) and the Dementia-Friendly Guide for Insurers (Chartered Insurance Institute, 2019).

However, despite these positive steps, the themes emerging from the following sections indicate that there is still significant work to be done in creating a legal and financial environment in which those with young onset dementia and their carers are appropriately supported, assisted and protected in managing their financial and legal matters and in resolving related challenges which arise as a result of their diagnosis.

Planning and preparation

The financial impact of a young onset dementia diagnosis on an individual and their family is invariably significant. Careful advance planning of one's legal and financial affairs is therefore essential to live as well as possible with young onset dementia.

It is clearly desirable for those with young onset dementia to make arrangements for their financial and legal affairs earlier rather than later. However, in reality, these often receive limited attention and a significant minority of individuals do not make important legal provisions at all. For example, the Alzheimer's Society (2011) found that of those surveyed (persons with dementia generally), only 72% had an LPA in place, whilst 82% had made a will. A failure to make a will is particularly concerning given that, if an individual has lost the specific mental capacity required to make a will, then default inheritance provisions apply, which may not reflect their wishes.

Of similar concern, Mayrhofer et al. (2021) found that only around half of individuals receiving a young onset dementia diagnosis had conducted any kind of financial review. The closest to a financial review individuals conduct will often be the financial assessment conducted as part of a needs assessment. However, the purpose of this is simply to determine whether an individual meets the financial criteria for social support. It is not intended to consider issues of long-term financial planning, money management or, more generally, if the legal and financial affairs of an individual with young onset dementia are arranged in their best interests.

There are various relatively simple steps that can be taken to facilitate easier money management for those with young onset dementia. These include:

- current and savings accounts (for instance, considering whether a joint account would be or remains appropriate);
- assessing whether account spending and credit limits remain appropriate;
- increased use of standing orders/direct debits;
- use of a chip and signature card (which avoids the need to remember a PIN); and
- taking a full inventory of financial products and services used.

Problem-solving

Individuals with young onset dementia and their carers frequently encounter challenges and difficulties when managing legal and financial affairs – even where plans have been put in place.

There has been some progress in this area over the past decade. One of the commitments of the UK Government's 2020 Dementia Challenge (DHSC, 2019) was that all businesses were to be encouraged and supported to become dementia friendly, with all industry sectors developing dementia friendly charters[51] and working with business leaders to make individual commitments. In addition, Dementia Friendly Businesses was created by the Alzheimer's Society to encourage businesses to focus on how people, processes and places can become dementia friendly. Technological innovations (e.g. mobile apps) also increasingly assist people living with young onset dementia and their family members and carers to support and monitor their finances. Recently, the first debit card and app aimed specifically at those with dementia was launched.[52]

However, there is still much to be done. For example, the Alzheimer's Society (2018a) reported low awareness of LPAs across the financial services sector. In one recent study (Giebel et al., 2023), nearly all carers reported no support in managing their relative's finances: whilst carers knew how to manage their own finances, there were additional layers of complexity when managing their relative's finances, including LPAs and liaising with banks regarding access to a person's bank account and a separate debit card, as well as receiving copies of any financial communications.

Young onset dementia also poses challenges beyond the financial services sector. For example, a person with dementia may forget to pay a utility bill or have difficulty interacting with utility providers. This can result in missed payments and, in cases where a customer has not been identified as vulnerable (for example, because they haven't disclosed their condition), their energy supply could be cut off. Confusion and forgetfulness can also mean that people with dementia struggle to manage their energy usage (Alzheimer's Society, 2018c).

Some paid services exist to assist carers and care providers. For example, the Money Carer Foundation offer a money management service and assistance with appointeeships and deputyships.[53] Similarly, independent financial advisers can offer advice and assistance on long-term planning (a list of specialist advisers is maintained by the Society of Later Life Advisors[54]). Free services include the Equality Advisory Service, MoneyHelper and Citizens Advice, although these are not young onset dementia-specific.

Often individuals with young onset dementia encountering problems can negotiate for better treatment and/or challenge unfavourable treatment from business or organisations without needing to go to court. However, where this is not possible, the UK operates a relatively comprehensive ombudsman scheme. This provides flexible, low- or no-cost dispute resolution mechanisms by an independent adjudicator.[55] The specialist expertise offered by these ombudsman services can be particularly beneficial for those with young onset dementia and their caregivers, offering guidance and clarity through the resolution process.

There is a significant need for greater knowledge and signposting of these tools and resources for those with young onset dementia and their carers (as well as availability of resources themselves).

Autonomy vs. protection

A final recurring theme with young onset dementia and individuals' financial and legal affairs is the need to balance an individual with young onset dementia's autonomy to manage their own affairs (particularly in the earlier stages of the illness) against the need to protect them from financial abuse or exploitation.

Financial abuse includes theft, fraud, exploitation, and pressure in connection with wills, property or inheritance or financial transactions, or the misuse or misappropriation of property, possessions or benefits (Department of Health, 2000). It can also include rogue traders and, increasingly, internet-based and similar frauds (such as mobile phone push payment frauds). In one study, 15% of carers reported that the person they cared for had been subject to some form of financial abuse and nearly two-thirds had been approached by unsolicited salespeople or cold callers (Alzheimer's Society, 2011).

Whilst those with young onset dementia are often not uniquely/individually targeted, the Financial Abuse Evidence Review (Davidson et al., 2015: 7) noted that 'those who have dementia or reduced cognitive function are the subgroup of people who are most at risk of being victims of financial abuse'. Research also indicates that people with Alzheimer's disease are already at increased risk of financial exploitation prior to their diagnosis (Fenton et al., 2022).

Having a dementia diagnosis is likely to put an individual at greater risk of financial risk or exploitation for multiple reasons. These may include a reduced ability to judge risk and profound changes to their personal circumstances which make them more vulnerable. This risk can also be heightened for individuals with young onset dementia as a dementia diagnosis may often not be considered by many due to age, thus making it less likely for third parties to suspect that financial abuse is occurring.

Other practical steps typically recommended to older/more vulnerable individuals can also assist those with young onset dementia. These include registration with the telephone preference service and opting out of unaddressed (junk) mail, which both reduces the volume of post and the risk that an individual with young onset dementia may mistakenly sign up to goods or services they do not in fact require.[56] Familiarity with basic consumer protection measures can also assist in reducing risks of financial abuse. For instance, checking financial services providers are authorised on the FCA Register, using approved local traders and understanding limits and restrictions on cold calling[57] and, in the case of a mistaken or unwanted purchase, the right to return/cancel goods and services sold at a distance (generally for 14 days after a purchase).[58]

In addition to fraud by third parties, there exists the complex and challenging area of familial and/or carer financial abuse and exploitation. The Alzheimer's Society report 'Short Changed: Protecting People with Dementia from Financial Abuse' noted that:

> people with dementia may avoid speaking out against relatives for fear of losing their support network. The person with dementia may also have low expectations for themselves, and feel too grateful for services to question potentially abusive situations. (2011: 45)

These findings speak to the importance of also considering the risk of financial abuse/exploitation from a safeguarding perspective. One study found that 25% of adult safeguarding referrals for adults living in their own home concerned financial abuse (Cambridge et al., 2006). Limited dementia-specific data appear to be available, although for safeguarding alerts reported across the

Alzheimer's Society from April to September 2011, 20% were reported to have an element of financial abuse (Alzheimer's Society, 2011). Notwithstanding these risks, people with young onset dementia understandably wish to maintain financial independence (or a degree thereof) for as long as possible. The same report summarised the dilemma (and a potential solution) as follows:

> Cognitive impairment can have a huge impact on someone's ability to look after their finances. However, we know that people with dementia, even in the later stages, want to stay involved with their money wherever possible. For people to do so while protecting themselves from abuse, they must feel comfortable and empowered to talk about financial issues openly, before and after diagnosis. (Alzheimer's Society, 2011: v)

Conclusions

Dementia is the costliest illness both from a macroeconomic perspective – it cost the UK an estimated £25 billion in 2021 (Luengo-Fernandez and Landeiro, cited in Alzheimer's Research UK, 2023) and from an individual perspective – people with dementia typically spend at least £100,000 on their care (Alzheimer's Society, 2018b).

Beyond reinforcing the benefits of timely diagnosis, the conclusions which emerge from considering the legal and financial aspects of dementia illustrate the need for:

- greater resourcing of and a more proactive approach to supporting people with young onset dementia to plan these areas of their lives to enable them to live better with their illness and in accordance with their wishes;
- specialist resources and assistance to address barriers to early planning of the legal and financial affairs of persons with young onset dementia;
- more education and guidance for organisations and carers to either avoid financial and legal difficulties in the first place or to resolve them efficiently when they do arise;
- a more integrated, consistent and rational approach to health and social care provision and funding and greater certainty on the long-term funding of social care.

Those living with young onset dementia may have certain advantages over older individuals with dementia (such as familiarity with technology) which can assist independent living. However, in most cases, this is outweighed by the fact that their financial situations are likely to be considerably much more complex.

Whilst the UK legal and regulatory framework for protecting and enabling those with young onset dementia is relatively well developed, it is essential that an understanding of the rights and protections for those with young onset dementia (and dementia more generally) is embedded within relevant organisations through non-legal tools such as education, training and codes of conduct.

Finally, as a young onset dementia diagnosis progresses, careful thought needs to be given to balancing financial independence against protecting individuals with the condition from financial abuse and exploitation – again, more specialist support and education is needed in this area.

In this context it is clear that, although legal tools and financial assistance for those with dementia are available, they are currently inadequate; and all the more so for the complex challenges facing those with young onset dementia. Whilst there are significant hurdles to addressing the issues identified in this chapter, if they can be successfully addressed in the context of a young onset dementia diagnosis, the impact will be far greater. As the Dementia-Friendly Financial Services Charter put it:

> The barriers and impact of dementia are so broad that the learning and progress made under the dementia umbrella will simultaneously tackle a number of barriers associated with a wide range of mental capacity issues and provide a framework to address other types of disability or vulnerability in the future. (Alzheimer's Society, 2013: 6)

So what does this mean in practice?

If you are diagnosed with a type of young onset dementia

- Make arrangements to review your financial and legal affairs as soon as you are able to.
- Make sure that your finances are fit for the future and you are receiving all the support you are entitled to.
- Ensure you have put in place a Lasting Power of Attorney (property and financial affairs) and decided whether a health and welfare LPA is also needed.
- Consider putting in place an Advance Care Plan and/or an Advanced Decision.
- Discuss with someone you trust how to protect yourself from financial abuse and how you would like to maintain your financial independence.

If you are a family or friend of someone living with young onset dementia

- Reflect on the role that you want to have in setting up and administering a Lasting Power of Attorney and/or an Advance Care Plan.
- Help the person you support set out their wishes as clearly as possible.
- Discuss how to balance protecting the person you support with maintaining their autonomy and participation in their financial and legal affairs.

> **If you are a professional or supporter involved in assessment or advising people living with young onset dementia**
>
> - Do you know about key pieces of legislation and legal tools such as the Equality Act, Mental Capacity Act, Advance Care Plans, Advance Decisions and Lasting Powers of Attorney?
> - Do you take appropriate steps to help people with young onset dementia to manage their affairs and ensure care is in line with their wishes after they have lost mental capacity?
> - Do you know about resources that can help with problem-solving in relation to legal and financial issues?

References

Alzheimer's Research UK (2023) *The economic impact of dementia*, Dementia Statistics Hub. Available at: https://dementiastatistics.org/statistics/the-economic-impact-of-dementia/#:~:text=In%202021%20the%20estimated%20cost,(World%20Alzheimer%20Report%202018) (accessed 10 November 2023).

Alzheimer's Scotland (2022) *Information sheet: Powers of Attorney*. Available at: https://www.alzscot.org/sites/default/files/2022-10/Powers%20of%20attorney_October%202022.pdf (accessed 10 November 2023).

Alzheimer's Society (2011) *Short changed: Protecting people with dementia from financial abuse*. Available at: https://www.alzheimers.org.uk/sites/default/files/migrate/downloads/short_changed_-_protecting_people_with_dementia_from_financial_abuse.pdf (accessed 12 November 2023).

Alzheimer's Society (2013) *Dementia-Friendly Financial Services Charter*. Available at: https://www.alzheimers.org.uk/sites/default/files/migrate/downloads/dementia_friendly_financial_services_charter.pdf (accessed 8 November 2023).

Alzheimer's Society (2017) *Dementia-friendly business guide*. Available at: https://www.alzheimers.org.uk/sites/default/files/2018-04/Alzheimer_s_Society_NEW_Business_guide_Web.pdf (accessed 2 November 2023).

Alzheimer's Society (2018a) *Dementia-friendly finance and insurance guide*. Available at: https://www.alzheimers.org.uk/sites/default/files/2019-07/AS_DF_NEW_Finance_Insurance_Guide_Online_09_07_19.pdf (accessed 4 November 2023).

Alzheimer's Society (2018b) *Dementia – the true cost: Fixing the care crisis*. Available at: https://www.alzheimers.org.uk/sites/default/files/2018-05/Dementia%20the%20true%20cost%20-%20Alzheimers%20Society%20report.pdf (accessed 10 November 2023).

Alzheimer's Society (2018c) *Dementia-friendly utility guide*. Available at: https://www.alzheimers.org.uk/sites/default/files/2019-07/AS_NEW_DF_Utilities_Guide_Online_09_07_19.pdf (accessed 6 November 2023).

Alzheimer's Society (2023) *Working with dementia: How the law helps and how to talk to your employer about your diagnosis*. Available at: https://www.alzheimers.org.uk/blog/work-dementia-how-tell-employer-diagnosis (accessed 4 November 2023).

Cambridge, P., Beadle-Brown, J., Milne, A., et al. (2006) *Exploring the incidence, risk factors, nature and monitoring of adult protection alerts*. Canterbury: Tizard Centre. Available at: https://research.kent.ac.uk/tizard/wp-content/uploads/sites/2302/2019/01/cambridge_2006_tizardadultprotection.pdf.

Chartered Insurance Institute (2019) *Good practice guide: Dementia-friendly guide for insurers*. Available at: https://www.cii.co.uk/media/10121999/dementia-frienfly-gpg-insurers.pdf (accessed 6 November 2023).

Davidson, S., Rossall, P. and Hart, S. (2015) *Financial abuse evidence review, November 2015*, Age UK. Available at: https://www.ageuk.org.uk/globalassets/age-uk/documents/reports-and-publications/reports-and-briefings/money-matters/financial_abuse_evidence_review-nov_2015.pdf (accessed 10 November 2023).

Dementia UK (2023) *Dealing with stigma and discrimination*. Available at: https://www.dementiauk.org/wp-content/uploads/dementia-uk-understanding-and-challenging-stigma-discrimination.pdf (accessed 10 November 2023).

Department of Constitutional Affairs (2007) *Mental Capacity Act 2005: Code of Practice*. Available at: https://assets.publishing.service.gov.uk/media/5f6cc6138fa8f541f6763295/Mental-capacity-act-code-of-practice.pdf (accessed 11 November 2023).

Department of Health (2000) *No secrets: Guidance on developing and implementing multi-agency policies and procedures to protect vulnerable adults from abuse*. Available at: https://assets.publishing.service.gov.uk/media/5a7af2a640f0b66a2fc03f4d/No_secrets__guidance_on_developing_and_implementing_multi-agency_policies_and_procedures_to_protect_vulnerable_adults_from_abuse.pdf (accessed 11 November 2023).

Department of Health and Social Care (2014a) *Care and Support (Charging and Assessment of Resources) Regulations*. Available at: https://www.gov.uk/government/publications/care-act-statutory-guidance/care-and-support-statutory-guidance#charging-and-financial-assessment (accessed 31 December 2023).

Department of Health and Social Care (2014b) *Care and Support Statutory Guidance*, updated 5 October 2023. Available at: https://www.gov.uk/government/publications/care-act-statutory-guidance/care-and-support-statutory-guidance (accessed 4 November 2023).

Department of Health and Social Care (2015) *Care and Support (Eligibility Criteria) Regulations 2015*. Available at: https://www.legislation.gov.uk/uksi/2015/313/introduction/made (accessed 31 December 2023).

Department of Health and Social Care (2019) *Dementia 2020 Challenge: 2018 Review phase 1*. Available at: https://assets.publishing.service.gov.uk/media/5c6ed7bee5274a0ec174cd6b/dementia-2020-challenge-2018-review.pdf (accessed 4 November 2023).

Department of Health and Social Care (2022) *National Framework for NHS Continuing Healthcare and NHS Funded Nursing Care*. Available at: https://assets.publishing.service.gov.uk/government/uploads/system/uploads/attachment_data/file/1170290/National-Framework-for-NHS-Continuing-Healthcare-and-NHS-funded-Nursing-Care_July-2022-revised_corrected-July-2023.pdf (accessed 12 November 2023).

Director of Public Prosecutions (DPP) (2014) *Suicide: Policy for Prosecutors in Respect of Cases of Encouraging or Assisting Suicide*. The Code for Crown Prosecutors. Available at: https://www.cps.gov.uk/legal-guidance/suicide-policy-prosecutors-respect-cases-encouraging-or-assisting-suicide (accessed 4 November 2023).

Fenton, L., Weissberger, G.H., Boyle, P.A., et al. (2022) Cognitive and neuroimaging correlates of financial exploitation vulnerability in older adults without dementia: implications for early detection of Alzheimer's disease, *Neuroscience and Biobehavioral Reviews*, 140: 104773. Available at: https://doi.org/10.1016/j.neubiorev.2022.104773.

Financial Conduct Authority (FCA) (2015) *Consumer vulnerability*, Occasional Paper No. 8, February. https://www.fca.org.uk/publications/occasional-papers/occasional-paper-no-8-consumer-vulnerability.

Financial Conduct Authority (FCA) (2017) *Ageing populations and financial services*, Occasional Paper 31. Available at: https://www.fca.org.uk/publication/occasional-papers/occasional-paper-31.pdf#6 (accessed 12 November 2023).

Financial Conduct Authority (FCA) (2021) *Guidance for firms on the fair treatment of vulnerable customers*, FG21/1. Available at: https://www.fca.org.uk/publications/finalised-guidance/guidance-firms-fair-treatment-vulnerable-customers (accessed 12 November 2023).

Giebel, C., Flanagan, E. and Sutcliffe, C. (2019) Predictors of finance management in dementia: managing bill and taxes matters, *International Psychogeriatrics*, 31 (2): 277–86.

Giebel, C., Halpin, K., O'Connell, L., et al. (2023) The legalities of managing finances and paying for future care in dementia: a UK-based qualitative study, *Aging and Mental Health*, 27 (12): 2403–9.

Government Equalities Office and Equality and Human Rights Commission (2013) *Equality Act 2010: guidance*, updated June 2015. Available at: https://www.gov.uk/guidance/equality-act-2010-guidance (accessed 4 November 2023).

HM Treasury (2022) *Autumn Statement 2022*, Cm 751. Available at: https://www.gov.uk/government/publications/autumn-statement-2022-documents (accessed 14 November 2023).

House of Commons Library, Foster D. (2021) *Adult social care: Means-test parameters since 1997*, 11 June. Available at: https://researchbriefings.files.parliament.uk/documents/CBP-8005/CBP-8005.pdf (accessed 14 November 2023).

Jones, B., Gage, H., Bakker, C., et al. (2018). Availability of information on young onset dementia for patients and carers in six European countries, *Patient Education and Counseling*, 101 (1): 159–65.

Kilty, C., Cahill, S., Foley, T., et al. (2023) Young onset dementia: implications for employment and finances, *Dementia*, 22 (1): 68–84.

Mayrhofer, A.M., Greenwood, N., Smeeton, N., et al. (2021) Understanding the financial impact of a diagnosis of young onset dementia on individuals and families in the United Kingdom: results of an online survey, *Health and Social Care in the Community*, 29 (3): 664–71.

Millenaar, J., Van Vliet, D., Bakker, C., et al. (2014) The experiences and needs of children living with a parent with young onset dementia: results from the NeedYD study, *International Psychogeriatrics*, 26 (12): 2001–10.

National Institute on Aging (2021) *Dementia may cause problems with money management years before diagnosis*. Available at: https://www.nia.nih.gov/news/dementia-may-cause-problems-money-management-years-before-diagnosis (accessed 5 November 2023).

NHS (2023a) *Health A to Z: Advance statement about your care wishes*. Available at: https://www.nhs.uk/conditions/end-of-life-care/planning-ahead/advance-statement/ (accessed 10 November 2023).

NHS (2023b) *Health to Z: Advance decision to refuse treatment (living will)*. Available at: https://www.nhs.uk/conditions/end-of-life-care/planning-ahead/advance-decision-to-refuse-treatment/ (accessed 10 November 2023).

Peres, K., Helmer, C., Amieva, H., et al. (2007) Natural history of decline in instrumental activities of daily living performance over the 10 years preceding the clinical diagnosis of dementia: a prospective population-based study, *Journal of the American Geriatrics Society*, 56 (1): 37–44.

Taylor, R. (2022) Record numbers of chronically ill patients are being denied vital NHS funding for their care, *Mail on Sunday*, 11 June. Available at: https://www.dailymail.co.uk/health/article-10906803/Continuing-Healthcare-crisis-Record-numbers-chronically-ill-patients-denied-NHS-care-funding.html (accessed 10 November 2023).

Notes

1   This chapter provides a summary of the law as at 10 November 2023. Nothing in this chapter should be considered to be legal and/or financial advice, a financial promotion or a recommendation of a particular product or service.
2   For Northern Ireland, see the Disability Discrimination Act 1995.
3   Section 6, Equality Act 2010.
4   Schedule 1, paragraph 8 to the Equality Act 2010.
5   For a useful summary, see Government Equalities Office and Equalities and Human Rights Commission (2013, updated 2015).
6   Section 13(1), Equality Act 2010.
7   Section 19, Equality Act 2010.
8   This is because in the wording of section 13(1), a protected characteristic is not specific to an individual.
9   Section 15, Equality Act 2010.
10   Section 15(2), Equality Act 2010.
11   Section 20, Equality Act 2010.
12   See https://www.gov.uk/dementia-and-driving – Form CG1
13   Applies in England and Wales. Note that similar provisions exist in Scotland under the Adults with Incapacity (Scotland) Act 2000 and in Northern Ireland under the Mental Capacity Act (Northern Ireland) 2016.
14   Section 1, Mental Capacity Act 2005.
15   Section 2, Mental Capacity Act 2005.
16   Section 3, Mental Capacity Act 2005.
17   Section 4, Mental Capacity Act 2005.
18   Section 4(4), Mental Capacity Act 2005.
19   See Department of Constitutional Affairs (2007).
20   A breach of the Mental Capacity Code of Practice does not carry a specific sanction but can be used as evidence in any criminal or civil proceedings.
21   See, for example: https://www.dementiauk.org/information-and-support/financial-and-legal-support/advance-care-planning/.
22   Assisting suicide is a specific offence under the Suicide Act 1961. In addition, the act of deliberately ending a person's life (irrespective of whether it is at an individual's request to relieve suffering) may either be regarded as manslaughter or murder under English law depending on the circumstances and the individual's mental state. For further information, see Director of Public Prosecutions (2014).
23   Section 25, Mental Capacity Act 2005.
24   See Resuscitation Council UK guidance for further information: https://www.resus.org.uk/home/faqs/faqs-decision-making-cpr and https://www.resus.org.uk/library/publications/publication-decisions-relating-cardiopulmonary (accessed 10 November 2022).
25   Section 9, Mental Capacity Act 2005.
26   In Scotland, the equivalent legal tools are called Continuing (Financial) Powers of Attorney and a Welfare Power of Attorney (see Alzheimer's Scotland, 2022). In Northern Ireland, Enduring Powers of Attorney still exist: see https://www.justice-ni.gov.uk/articles/information-enduring-powers-attorney-epa for further guidance. In England and Wales, any valid Enduring Power of Attorney made before the Mental Capacity Act came into force on 1 October 2007 still has legal effect.
27   Section 9, Mental Capacity Act 2005.

28 See Schedule 1 to the Mental Capacity Act 2005 for full specifics of the formalities required.

29 Schedule 1, Part 2 and section 9(2), Mental Capacity Act 2005.

30 See https://www.gov.uk/power-of-attorney/register (accessed 10 November 2023).

31 Section 16, Mental Capacity Act 2005.

32 Section 19, Mental Capacity Act 2005.

33 The Mental Capacity Act Code of Practice (at 8.38) states that health and welfare deputies will only be appointed in the 'most difficult' cases. Although more recent case law has indicated this is a stricter test than the Mental Capacity Act actually requires: see *Re Lawson, Mottram and Hopton, Re (appointment of personal welfare deputies)* [2019] EWCOP 22.

34 Section 35, Mental Capacity Act 2005.

35 Section 67, Care Act 2014.

36 There are relatively significant differences to the funding of health and social care in Scotland.

37 For equivalent provisions outside England, see the Social Services and Well-being (Wales) Act 2014, Social Work (Scotland) Act 1968, Carers (Scotland) Act 2016 and the Carers and Direct Payments Act (Northern Ireland) 2002.

38 Section 1, Care Act 2014.

39 Section 9, Care Act 2014.

40 Section 9(5), Care Act 2014.

41 Further requirements when conducting a needs assessment are contained in the Care and Support (Assessment) Regulations 2014. For additional guidance, see also Chapter 6 of the Care and Support Statutory Guidance (Department of Health and Social Care, 2014b).

42 Section 10, Care Act 2014.

43 Section 12, Care Act 2014.

44 The position is the same in Northern Ireland. The upper capital limit is £32,750 in Scotland and £50,000 in Wales.

45 See Department for Health (2014a).

46 Schedule 2 to the Care and Support (Charging and Assessment of Resources) Regulations 2014.

47 https://www.nhs.uk/conditions/social-care-and-support-guide/money-work-and-benefits/nhs-continuing-healthcare/ (accessed 12 November 2023).

48 A different system applies in Northern Ireland.

49 Section 6, Human Rights Act 1998.

50 See, for example, FCA (2021) *Guidance for firms on the fair treatment of vulnerable customers*, FG21/1, February. And previously, FCA (2018) *Approach to consumers*, July; FCA (2017) *Ageing population and financial services*, September; FCA (2015) *Consumer vulnerability*, Occasional Paper No. 8, February 2015.

51 See, for example, the Dementia Friendly Financial Services Charter (2013).

52 See https://www.mastercard.com/news/europe/en-uk/newsroom/press-releases/en-gb/2023/new-debit-card-and-app-launches-to-help-those-living-with-dementia-to-safely-manage-spending/.

53 See https://moneycarer.org.uk/.

54 See https://societyoflaterlifeadvisers.co.uk/.

55 See, for example, the Scottish Public Services Ombudsman, the Northern Ireland Public Service Ombudsman, the Public Services Ombudsman for Wales, and relevant Ombudsmen in England depending on the sector, including the Parliamentary and Health Service Ombudsman and the Local Government and Social Care Ombudsman.

56 The Royal Mail operates a specific opt-out service for unaddressed mail whilst other postal services are signed up to the 'Your Choice' preference scheme run by the Data and Marketing Association.

57 Telephone 'cold calling' (i.e. unsolicited marketing phone calls) is generally prohibited for claims management services and pensions services. The UK Government is currently consulting on whether to extend this cold calling ban to all financial services products. Cold calls are also generally prohibited if an individual's number is registered with the TPS. There is no general rule against in-person/doorstep cold calling.

58 See the Consumer Contracts (Information, Cancellation and Additional Charges) Regulations 2013.

Appendix

Mental Capacity Act Principles (section 1, Mental Capacity Act 2005)

(a) A person must be assumed to have capacity unless it is established that they lack capacity.

(b) A person is not to be treated as unable to make a decision unless all practicable steps to help them to do so have been taken without success.

(c) A person is not to be treated as unable to make a decision merely because they make an unwise decision.

(d) An act done, or decision made, under the Mental Capacity Act for or on behalf of a person who lacks capacity must be done, or made, in their best interests.

(e) Before the act is done, or the decision is made, regard must be had to whether the purpose for which it is needed can be as effectively achieved in a way that is less restrictive of the person's rights and freedom of action.

Section 1 of the Care Act 2014

(1) The general duty of a local authority, in exercising a function under this Part in the case of an individual, is to promote that individual's well-being.

(2) 'Well-being', in relation to an individual, means that individual's well-being so far as relating to any of the following –

    (a) personal dignity (including treatment of the individual with respect);

    (b) physical and mental health and emotional well-being;

    (c) protection from abuse and neglect;

    (d) control by the individual over day-to-day life (including over care and support, or support, provided to the individual and the way in which it is provided);

    (e) participation in work, education, training or recreation;

    (f) social and economic well-being;

    (g) domestic, family and personal relationships;

    (h) suitability of living accommodation;

    (i) the individual's contribution to society.

(3) In exercising a function under this Part in the case of an individual, a local authority must have regard to the following matters in particular –

    (a) the importance of beginning with the assumption that the individual is best placed to judge the individual's well-being;

    (b) the individual's views, wishes, feelings and beliefs;

    (c) the importance of preventing or delaying the development of needs for care and support or needs for support and the importance of reducing needs of either kind that already exist;

    (d) the need to ensure that decisions about the individual are made having regard to all the individual's circumstances (and are not based only on the individual's age or appearance or any condition of the individual's or aspect of the individual's behaviour which might lead others to make unjustified assumptions about the individual's well-being);

    (e) the importance of the individual participating as fully as possible in decisions relating to the exercise of the function concerned and being provided with the information and support necessary to enable the individual to participate;

    (f) the importance of achieving a balance between the individual's well-being and that of any friends or relatives who are involved in caring for the individual;

    (g) the need to protect people from abuse and neglect; and the need to ensure that any restriction on the individual's rights or freedom of action is kept to the minimum necessary for achieving the purpose for which the function is being exercised.

Note: The Mental Capacity Act is available under the Open Government Licence v3.0: https://www.nationalarchives.gov.uk/doc/open-government-licence/version/3/.

The Care Act is available under the Crown Copyright/Open Government Licence v3.0: https://www.nationalarchives.gov.uk/doc/open-government-licence/version/3/.

8 Having a voice in planning services

Andrea M. Mayrhofer

Overview

Although this chapter draws extensively from the body of international literature, it is written primarily from a UK perspective. It focuses on voluntary and statutory sector collaboration to establish services for people affected by young onset dementia, on the role of practitioners in introducing consultation and joining up services, and on people affected by young onset dementia bringing their experience to bear on service planning and policy. The chapter highlights that whilst the impetus for dementia research came from policy, the planning and development of services has been largely driven by third sector organisations and was directly informed by younger people with dementia and their family members. This involved collaboration between the voluntary and statutory sector and has led to the improvement of specialist and clinical services during referral, assessment and diagnosis. User involvement in service planning is imperative to help plan, develop, commission and implement services that are sustainable in the longer term, both at the national and community level. This chapter summarises the evidence that intersectoral collaboration, and having a voice in service planning, are effective approaches to supporting younger people diagnosed with dementia to maintain autonomy.

Keywords

Young onset dementia, service planning, service development, service implementation, co-design, collaboration.

Learning points

- Service planning, development and implementation need to focus on:
  - establishing specialist services for people living with young onset dementia;

- o establishing coherent referral pathways for people with young onset dementia to clinical and community-based services that cover pre- and post-diagnostic support;
  - o developing local, place-based, sustainable support services and networks for people with young onset dementia.
- Services must be informed by individuals and families affected by young onset dementia.
- This requires multilevel collaboration between statutory and voluntary sector organisations in relation to policy and commissioning.

Introduction

The fact that the support needs of people diagnosed with dementia at a younger age differ considerably from those of people who develop dementia in later years is well documented (The King's Fund, 2009; Davies-Quarrell et al., 2010; Bakker et al., 2013; Sansoni et al., 2014; Westera et al., 2014; Richardson et al., 2016; Mayrhofer et al., 2018; Mitchell and Wharton, 2018; Baptista et al., 2019; Hutchinson et al., 2020; Stamou et al., 2021a). Initial post-diagnostic support for younger people with dementia included various models and initiatives (Davies-Quarrell et al., 2010; Hewitt et al., 2013; Robertson et al., 2013), primarily provided by the voluntary sector through a mix of direct funding and/or local authority commissioning (Frost et al., 2020). Such funding was often short term, ad-hoc and unsustainable in the longer term. What was lacking were national standards for young onset dementia (Rodda and Carter, 2016) to facilitate a joint approach to developing defined clinical referral pathways, support services, and strategies for their implementation (Van Vliet et al., 2013; Draper et al., 2016; Carter et al., 2018; Revez et al., 2018). The implementation of dementia care for younger people with dementia specifically, and dementia care more widely (Wheatley et al., 2021), requires targeted collaboration between statutory and voluntary organisations. The following section sets out the collaboration required to plan, implement and deliver improved services for people who are diagnosed with dementia at a younger age.

Collaboration as an effective approach to ensuring clinical services

In the UK, planning for clinical services for people with dementia of all ages has recently been based on the National Health Services (NHS) Transformation Framework (NHS England, 2016) and addresses prevention, diagnosis, support and end-of-life care. Services for younger people with dementia have been conceptualized as pre-diagnostic, post-diagnostic and longer-term support.

Pre-diagnostic clinical support

People affected by young onset dementia emphasise that their support needs start before diagnosis, to help mitigate the changes caused by unexplained symptoms that affect everyday activities and therefore relationships, finances and work. The difficulties with diagnosing dementia at a younger age are well known (see Chapters 2 and 3; also Van Vliet et al., 2013; Draper et al., 2016; Millenaar et al., 2016; Cations et al., 2021; O'Malley et al., 2021a). To address this, the Young Dementia Network, clinicians, and consultants in old age psychiatry have worked with general practitioners (GPs) to develop a pilot decision-making tool for GPs (Young Dementia Network, 2017) and to set out a Young Onset Care Pathway (Young Dementia Network, 2018). The Young Dementia Network is a community of younger people diagnosed with dementia, affected family members, and professionals. Non-professionals make up about 40% of this community. This collaboration between the voluntary and statutory sectors resulted in recommendations for the improvement of clinical services. These are echoed in a 2018 publication (Carter et al., 2018), which called for GPs to:

- listen more carefully to a younger person's description of symptoms;
- carry out relevant assessments;
- provide appropriate information to those with young onset dementia and their families; and
- refer to specialist services for further assessment.

These are important steps to ensure that people with young onset dementia and rare dementias receive a timely diagnosis (Crutch et al., 2018; National Collaborating Centre for Mental Health, 2018; Royal College of Psychiatrists, 2018; Rare Dementia Support, 2023). A timely diagnosis helps to lessen anxiety about the symptoms that a person experiences. It allows adjustment to living with the condition, enables potential benefit from timely drug treatments, and allows those affected to plan ahead.

The need to improve specialist and clinical services in relation to referral, assessment and diagnostic processes was also highlighted by a Delphi study (O'Malley et al., 2021b) and subsequent audit of NHS held data, which examined current practice around diagnosis. The audit showed that there was considerable variation in clinical practice across the UK (O'Malley et al., 2022). Variation in care, also referred to as a 'postcode lottery', is frequently reported in the literature (Bhattacharya et al., 2015; Lithgow and Boyd, 2019; Stamou et al., 2021b; Talbot and Coulson, 2023), and in personal communication (Rook and Mayrhofer, 2023). This highlights the need for 'commissioners to review current provision and to configure services to meet specific requirements for people with young onset dementia' (Booth, 2022: 66), and the need to involve people living with young onset dementia to inform service development.

Specialist services and clinical practice

Literature internationally has called for the establishment of specialist services for younger people with dementia (Millenaar et al., 2016; Revez et al., 2018; Stamou et al., 2021b). Services, referred to as a 'single point of access' for young onset dementia, employ staff who:

- receive specialist training;
- can offer information on young onset dementia;
- are equipped to refer onward; and
- can facilitate access to post-diagnostic support immediately after diagnosis, both for the person diagnosed with young onset dementia and affected family members.

In the Angela Project survey, it was found that specialist young onset dementia services outperformed other service configurations on all quality indicators; almost all those with young onset dementia seen in specialist services reported that they had continuity in care, and saw the same professional at each attendance, whereas only just over 50% reported continuity of care if discharged to primary care for ongoing care. Three-quarters of those seen in specialist young onset dementia services reported having a key worker, whereas this was the case for less than 33% of survey respondents overall. Moreover:

> Those diagnosed in specialist young onset dementia services were more likely to receive a follow-up appointment within the first 6 weeks of diagnosis and more likely to have ongoing care management appointments at least quarterly. (Stamou et al., 2021b: 421)

Currently, specialist services for young onset dementia in the UK are scarce. In the above-mentioned survey, 20% of respondents reported receiving care from a specialist service (Stamou et al., 2021b). To be effective, the planning, development and/or improvement of services and support pathways need to be informed by individuals and families affected by young onset dementia (Rook and Mayrhofer, 2023).

Post-diagnostic support immediately after diagnosis

Being diagnosed with dementia at a young age constitutes a life-changing event. Individuals and their families need to come to terms with the ramifications of what a diagnosis means for them and need all the information and support possible (Bakker et al., 2022). Post-diagnostic support ideally starts at the point of diagnosis and requires an integration of formal and informal approaches to enhance the physical, psychological and emotional well-being of both the person diagnosed with young onset dementia and their family (Bamford et al., 2021).

This includes clinical services, adult social care, dementia-focused third sector organisations, and community-based support. Currently, such services are not joined up, which is bewildering for anyone, especially for someone newly diagnosed. To coordinate services, the National Institute for Health and Care Excellence (NICE) recommended that people diagnosed with dementia:

> Should be provided with a single named health or social care professional who is responsible for coordinating their care. This should include providing information about available services and how to access them, developing a care plan, specifying how often this plan should be reviewed, and involving the person's family members or carers in the support and decision making. (NICE, 2018: 157)

These recommendations echo the ambitions of the Clive Project, which had begun two decades previously (The King's Fund, 2009). The Clive Project supported young people with dementia and their families and was started in 1998. It became Young Dementia UK in 2010, and established the Young Dementia Network in 2016. In 2020, Young Dementia UK merged with, and is now hosted by, Dementia UK (Dementia UK, 2023a). It took many years of persistent work, including the voice of people with young onset dementia and their families, to get to this point. The Young Dementia Network (2023) and Dementia UK (2023a) have published recommendations that support the implementation of NICE guidelines. To implement the guidance provided, collaboration between a range of different organisations at national, regional and local levels is imperative.

Longer-term support and services

As younger people with dementia adjust to new ways of living, one of the most important elements of the journey is to establish connections to people who understand, have similar experiences, and can help to maintain autonomy (Oyebode, 2022; Stamou et al., 2023). This has been expressed consistently by people living with young onset dementia (Roach and Drummond, 2014; Harding et al., 2019; O'Malley et al., 2021b; Huizenga et al., 2022). While initial post-diagnostic services might be coordinated based on consultation, the establishment of locally based peer groups does not usually involve clinicians or practitioners but, rather, the voluntary sector. However, practitioners can play a critical role in signposting people to both clinical and community-based support in their local area.

Practitioners' roles in introducing community support: joining up services?

Locally agreed young onset dementia referral care pathways (Carter et al., 2018) are yet to be widely implemented in the UK, which makes the 'array' of services often seem confusing and fragmented. However, practitioners at

GP surgeries and specialist services are in a good position to share insights from practice with commissioners, with a view to promoting the joining up of services, possibly through joint commissioning. There are many different roles that can initiate signposting to non-medical support. These include memory clinic staff, GP practice staff, Admiral Nurses (Dementia UK, 2023b), social prescribers (Chatterjee et al., 2018; Social Prescribing Academy, 2023), Dementia Coordinators (Alzheimer's and Dementia, 2022), community link workers and/or care navigators (Bernstein et al., 2019; Hagan, 2020; Kokorelias et al., 2022). Such roles are variously hosted by primary care networks (i.e. clusters of GP surgeries) and a range of different charities. Practitioners' roles vary accordingly.

The purpose of these various 'navigation' roles is to help people through the maze of services by consulting with memory clinics, health and social care (Davies et al., 2020; Frost et al., 2020; Giebel et al., 2021), community-based voluntary organisations (Age UK, 2023b) and organisations that are members of Local Dementia Action Alliances. The Dementia Action Alliances consist of a range of local organisations across health care, social care, local authorities, the third sector, and organisations such as banks, supermarkets and any local business or charity that wishes to become a member. Their broader aim is to facilitate the development of Dementia Friendly Communities in which pre-diagnosis, post-diagnosis and longer-term dementia care services are informed by local need (Woodward et al., 2019) and can be coordinated effectively. Whilst such alliances do not have a specific remit around young onset dementia, much of their work does include, and is directly informed by, younger people with dementia. However, the current status and indeed existence of Dementia Action Alliances is quite variable and fragile in terms of local champions changing jobs and moving on.

Strategies that assist in the implementation of formal post-diagnostic support include working across services and sectors, and building strategic alliances with key stakeholders in health care, social care, the voluntary sector and community organisations (Wheatley et al., 2021). Nationally known voluntary organisations that focus on dementia and offer support for people with young onset dementia include the Alzheimer's Society (2023a), Age UK (2023a), Dementia UK (2023a), Innovations in Dementia (2023e) via the DEEP Network (DEEP UK Network, 2023), Together in Dementia Everyday (TIDE, 2023a) and the Citizen's Advice Bureau/Legal Aid (Citizen's Advice Bureau, 2023), the latter especially in relation to legal and financial issues. Although local representation of such organisations is variable, many offer channels for younger people with dementia to establish connections and join or form locally based peer support groups.

The space in which support for people with young onset dementia is discussed is quite active. It involves organisations across the statutory, voluntary and private sectors, draws on public and voluntary funding, and involves a range of newly created staff roles. The problem, however, is that 'support' does not equate to a formal service so has remained largely uncoordinated, fragmented and shows little permanency as funding, and therefore staff contracts, are short-term in nature. Expertise and connections are lost when people move on. What is needed is for services to be funded, staffed and coordinated with longer-term benefits in mind.

The following section explores how people with young onset dementia and their families can bring their experience to bear on policy aimed to plan and develop joined-up service provision.

How can younger people with dementia influence service planning and policy?

Raising awareness

While initiatives such as the Alzheimer's Society's Dementia Friends, Dementia Champions and Dementia Ambassadors were launched to raise awareness about dementia more generally, such initiatives were largely informed by younger people with dementia and their carers/supporters. Their input was also evident at national dementia conferences, the annual UK Dementia Congress, and similar events. The Young Dementia Network is a registered charity in England/Wales and Scotland, and members were instrumental in contributing to various fora, both via the Network and via the Alzheimer's Society (Alzheimer's Society Nothern Ireland, Alzheimer's Society Wales, Alzheimer Scotland). Internationally, the Alzheimer European Dementia Working Group (Alzheimer Europe) and Dementia Alliance International engaged in debates, issued policy statements, and gave voice to people with young onset dementia (Roberts et al., 2020). Local, national and international platforms were integral to ensuring that people's voices were heard, so to speak, and for the public to learn what it meant to live with dementia and young onset dementia. 'Young onset dementia' soon became a separate thread in online fora such as Talking Point (Alzheimer's Society, 2023b), and addressed topics that are unique to younger people with dementia and their families. These early steps were followed by innovative initiatives such as online diaries, online dialogue and virtual support groups.

Ongoing dialogue – online

Ongoing dialogue is provided through national fora such as online 'Dementia Diaries' (Innovations in Dementia, 2023a), the DEEP Network (DEEP UK Network, 2023), 'Dementia Enquirers' (Innovations in Dementia, 2023b), Together in Dementia Everyday (TIDE, 2023a) across the UK, and TIDE in Scotland (TIDE, 2023c). Various initiatives, such as the Dementia Arts Festival in Edinburgh (Deepness Dementia Arts, 2024), provide opportunities for younger people with dementia to share what it is like to be diagnosed at a younger age, and to discuss associated, unique support needs. Both nationally and internationally, some contributors became activists for better dementia care

(Swaffer, 2016; Mitchell and Wharton, 2018; Oliver et al., 2020; Davies et al., 2022). An independent evaluation of the Dementia Diaries Project found that participants' contributions had influenced social media reporting, changed the public's perception of young onset dementia, and educated professionals about what was important in dementia care (Woodall et al., 2016), such as the need for care pathways for people with young onset dementia (Rodda and Carter, 2016).

Dementia Enquirers: what is important to us?

Further impact on influencing service planning and policy can be expected as an outcome of the Dementia Enquirers Project, which supported about 20 DEEP Network groups to undertake their own enquiries into themes that are important to them (Innovations in Dementia, 2023b). Topics included post-diagnostic support (Forget-Me-Nots, 2022), the particular needs of those living alone without a constant care partner (York Minds and Voices, 2021), and associated issues pertaining to lasting power of attorney and ongoing consent (Davies et al., 2022). Project reports are available on the Dementia Enquirers website (Dementia Enquirers, 2023) and in a recent publication on co-producing research through the Dementia Enquiries Model (Litherland and Hare, 2024). Dementia Enquirer groups have also produced 'Gold Standards for Co-Research' (Innovations in Dementia 2023c) and 'Gold Standards for Ethical Research' (Innovations in Dementia, 2023d), to guide researchers wanting to include people with young onset dementia in the co-production of research.

Strategic involvement

Due to an emphasis on 'Public Involvement and Community Engagement' (PICE) more widely, younger people with dementia are also involved in project advisory committees, are co-chairs of Lived Experience Advisory Panels, and co-chair a range of steering groups. At the Young Dementia Network, young people with dementia and affected family members have been on the Network's steering group and part of their work streams since the Network started in 2016. Some were founders of the Network. They read, comment on and help co-design funding applications and research projects and are becoming increasingly involved in co-produced research (Oliver et al., 2020; Parkes et al., 2022; Rook and Mayrhofer, 2023). Many such activities and consultations are channels through which younger people with dementia contribute directly and indirectly to service planning, policy and research (Oliver et al., 2020). In their role of research participants who are interviewed for a study, younger people with dementia contribute to discussions around specific topics such as driving (Gouldsborough et al., 2023), finances (Mayrhofer et al., 2021; Kilty et al., 2023), housing developments (Barrett et al., 2016), or adapting meeting centres to local needs (Evans et al., 2020). In addition, national charities offer opportunities for research engagement through research networks (Alzheimer's Association, 2023). TIDE (2023b) promotes its 'Dementia Policy

Influencing Toolkit' to encourage people with dementia and carers' groups to help shape dementia policy.

However, not all programmes are necessarily public facing. Innovations in Dementia and the DEEP Network run a course for younger people with dementia with a recent diagnosis. The course is facilitated by younger people with dementia who have lived with their diagnosis for some time. The impact of this course is positive, encouraging, uplifting and gives hope to participants (Innovations in Dementia and the DEEP Network, 2023). Much of the work that goes on in small, informal peer support groups is not publicised.

What are the next steps?

Voluntary and online organisations appear to be the activist groups that drive service development for younger people with dementia. The stated aim of the Young Dementia Network's national online community is that they are

> ... intent on influencing improvements in services for people with young onset dementia and their families wherever they live in the UK. The steering group, active workstreams and wider membership are a collaborative blend of people with lived experience and professionals working in the field. As such, they prioritise the challenges identified by people affected and harness diverse expertise, experience and multiple networks to ensure a young onset perspective is explicitly addressed in service development and provision. (Tessa Gutteridge, personal communication, 2023)

Members of the Young Dementia Network collaborate with statutory, third sector and community-based stakeholders. They lobby governments and have begun to influence policy around pre-diagnostic and post-diagnostic support for younger people with dementia, and encourage their inclusion in research and policy development. In Scotland, people with lived experience were remunerated for their contribution to the development of Scotland's new dementia strategy, which is a 10-year plan for change (Scottish Government, 2023). Internationally, younger people with dementia and their families interact with professional bodies to affect change through collaboration (Alzheimer Europe, 2017) and various working groups (Dementia Alliance International, 2021; Alzheimer Europe, 2024). Although this is an active space, service provision is not distributed equitably, and much work remains to be done.

Conclusions

As various countries develop different pathways to supporting individuals diagnosed with dementia at a younger age (Carter et al., 2018; Jones et al., 2018; Cations et al., 2021; Loi et al., 2022, 2023; Novek and Menec, 2023), the

UK context highlights an encouraging development over the last decade or so. Of particular note is the collaboration between the voluntary sector and the statutory sector in the design of diagnostic clinical pathways as well as post-diagnostic support services at the community level.

The involvement of younger people with dementia in various committees, steering groups, advisory boards, research-related activities and community-based groups has influenced public discourse and informed service development (Young Dementia Network, 2017, 2018, 2023). However, although some specialist services have been set up in the UK, there is still a long way to go to making these available more equitably throughout the country.

Clinicians, practitioners and people affected by young onset dementia need to continue to work together to develop and enhance pathways to timely diagnosis, to pre- and post-diagnostic clinical support, and to the development of longer-term, sustainable community-based services. In the interim, supported by a larger discourse of community involvement and co-production, the voluntary sector in this country continues to provide a platform for people with young onset dementia, affected families and carers to influence changes in policy and practice.

So what does this mean in practice?

If you are diagnosed with a type of young onset dementia

Could you and/or your family have a role in service development, policy and research?

Although the involvement of younger people with dementia in various committees, steering groups, advisory boards, research-related activities and community-based groups has influenced public discourse and informed service development, there is still a long way to go to making pre- and post-diagnostic services available more equitably throughout the country. Younger people with dementia and their families are therefore encouraged to join online fora to contribute their views. Researchers undertaking secondary data analysis can use communication threads to identify topics and themes that are important to people with lived experience and their families. Charities have designed webpages that invite individuals into research studies in various roles. Overall, the voluntary sector in the UK provides a welcoming platform for people with young onset dementia and their families to help influence changes in policy and practice.

If you are a professional involved in working with people with young onset dementia

Professionals at diagnostic clinics are well placed to contribute to the design of diagnostic clinical pathways through working with other clinicians, and creating evidence through involvement in primary research and evaluation studies. At the community level, practitioners such as social prescribers affiliated with GP practices are ideally placed to signpost individuals and families to post-diagnostic services offered by voluntary sector organisations. This is often the first step on the journey of adjustment when learning how to manage living with dementia at a younger age.

References

Age UK (2023a) *Age UK know what to do*. Available at: https://www.ageuk.org.uk/our-impact/how-we-help/ (accessed 3 April 2023).

Age UK (2023b) *Dementia Coordinators*. Available at: https://www.ageuk.org.uk/hernebayandwhitstable/our-services/dementia-co-ordinators/ (accessed 11 April 2023).

Alzheimer Europe (2017) *Alzheimer Europe collaboration with other organisations*. Available at: https://www.alzheimer-europe.org/policy/positions/alzheimer-europe-collaboration-other-organisations.

Alzheimer Europe (2024) *European Dementia Carers Working Group*. Available at: https://www.alzheimer-europe.org/about-us/european-dementia-carers-working-group.

Alzheimer's Association (2023) *Alzheimer's and dementia in the United Kingdom*. Available at: https://www.alz.org/uk/dementia-alzheimers-uk.asp (accessed 3 April 2023).

Alzheimer's and Dementia (2022) *Dementia Coordinators*. Available at: https://www.alz-dem.org/dementia-coordinators/?utm_source=rss&utm_medium=rss&utm_campaign=dementia-coordinators (accessed 11 April 2023).

Alzheimer's Society UK (2023a) *Dementia and Alzheimer's research*. Available at: https://www.alzheimers.org.uk/research/get-involved/our-research-network-volunteers (accessed 10 April 2023).

Alzheimer's Society UK (2023b) *Dementia Talking Point*. Available at: https://forum.alzheimers.org.uk/ (accessed 3 April 2023).

Bakker, C., de Vugt, M.E., van Vliet, D., et al. (2013) The use of formal and informal care in early onset dementia: results from the NeedYD study, *American Journal of Geriatric Psychiatry*, 21 (1): 37–45.

Bakker, C., Verboom, M. and Koopmans, R. (2022) Reimagining postdiagnostic care and support in young-onset dementia, *Journal of the American Medical Directors Association*, 23 (2): 261–65.

Bamford, C., Wheatley, A., Brunskill, G., et al. (2021) Key components of post-diagnostic support for people with dementia and their carers: a qualitative study, *PLoS One*, 16 (12): e0260506. Available at: https://doi.org/10.1371/journal.pone.0260506.

Baptista, M.A., Santos, R.L., Kimura, N., et al. (2019) Differences in awareness of disease between young-onset and late-onset dementia, *Alzheimer Disease and Associated Disorders*, 33 (2): 129–35.

Barrett, J., Atkinson, T. and Evans, S. (2016) *Exploring views of people living with dementia in housing with care settings and their carers*, Housing and Dementia Research Consortium Summary Report, University of Worcester. Available at: https://housingdementiaresearch.files.wordpress.com/2019/10/service-users-consultations_report-for-alzsoc-1.pdf.

Bernstein, A., Harrison, K.L., Dulaney, S., et al. (2019) The role of care navigators working with people with dementia and their caregivers, *Journal of Alzheimer's Disease*, 71 (1): 45–55.

Bhattacharya, R., Rickards, H. and Agrawal, N. (2015) Commissioning neuropsychiatry services: barriers and lessons, *British Journal of Psychiatry Bulletin*, 39 (6): 291–96.

Booth, J. (2022) Specialist services for people with young-onset dementia (YOD) are associated with better postdiagnostic care quality and satisfaction, *Evidence-Based Nursing*, 25 (2): 66.

Carter, J., Oyebode, J. and Koopmans, R. (2018) Young-onset dementia and the need for specialist care: a national and international perspective, *Aging and Mental Health*, 22 (4): 468–73.

Cations, M., Loi, S.M., Draper, B., et al. (2021) A call to action for the improved identification, diagnosis, treatment and care of people with young onset dementia, *Australian and New Zealand Journal of Psychiatry*, 55 (9): 837–40.

Chatterjee, H.J., Camic, P.M., Lockyer, B., et al. (2018) Non-clinical community interventions: a systematised review of social prescribing schemes, *Arts and Health*, 10 (2): 97–123.

Citizen's Advice Bureau (CAB) (2023) *Advice for citizens*. Available at: https://www.citizensadvice.org.uk/ (accessed 3 April 2023).

Crutch, S.J., Yong, K.X., Peters, A., et al. (2018) Contributions of patient and citizen researchers to 'Am I the right way up?' study of balance in posterior cortical atrophy and typical Alzheimer's disease, *Dementia*, 17 (8): 1011–22.

Davies, S., Hughes, J., Ahmed, S., et al. (2020) Commissioning social care for people with dementia living at home: findings from a national survey, *International Journal of Geriatric Psychiatry*, 35 (1): 53–59.

Davies, T., Houston, A., Gordon, H., et al. (2022) Dementia enquirers: pioneering approaches to dementia research in UK, *Disability and Society*, 37 (1): 129–47.

Davies-Quarrell, V., Higgins, A., Higgins, J., et al. (2010) The ACE approach: promoting well-being and peer support for younger people with dementia, *Journal of Mental Health Training, Education and Practice*, 5 (3): 41–50.

Deepness Dementia Arts (2024) *Dementia-friendly arts festival in Edinburgh*. Available at: https://www.deepnessdementiaarts.co.uk/dementia-arts-festival-edinburgh.

DEEP UK Network (2023) *The UK Network of Dementia Voices*. Available at: https://www.dementiavoices.org.uk/ (accessed 3 April 2023).

Dementia Alliance International (2021) *Young onset dementia: Identifying the signs and diagnosis must-dos*. Available at: https://dementiaallianceinternational.org/blog/young-onset-dementia-identifying-the-signs-and-diagnosis-must-dos.

Dementia Enquirers (2023) *Dementia Enquirers programme 2018–2023*. Available at: https://dementiaenquirers.org.uk/individual-projects-dementiaenquirers/.

Dementia UK (2023a) *Information and support: young onset dementia*. Available at: https://www.dementiauk.org/about-dementia/young-onset-dementia (accessed 3 April 2023).

Dementia UK (2023b) *What is an Admiral Nurse and how can they help?* Available at: https://www.dementiauk.org/get-support/what-is-an-admiral-nurse/ (accessed 10 April 2023).

Draper, B., Cations, M., White, F., et al. (2016) Time to diagnosis in young-onset dementia and its determinants: the INSPIRED study, *International Journal of Geriatric Psychiatry*, 31 (11): 1217–24.

Evans, S., Evans, S., Brooker, D., et al. (2020) The impact of the implementation of the Dutch combined Meeting Centres Support Programme for family caregivers of people with dementia in Italy, Poland and UK, *Aging and Mental Health*, 24 (2): 280–90.

Forget-Me-Nots (2022) *Forget-Me-Nots Dementia Enquirers Report: What impact has COVID-19 had on my connections with others, especially the Forget-Me-Nots?* Available at: https://dementiaenquirers.org.uk/individual-projects/forget-me-not/ (accessed 10 April 2023).

Frost, R., Walters, K., Wilcock, J., et al. (2020) Mapping post-diagnostic dementia care in England: an e-survey, *Journal of Integrated Care*, 29 (1): 22–36.

Giebel, C., Robertson, S., Beaulen, A., et al. (2021) 'Nobody seems to know where to even turn to': barriers in accessing and utilising dementia care services in England and The Netherlands, *International Journal of Environmental Research and Public Health*, 18 (22): 12233. Available at: https://doi.org/10.3390/ijerph182212233.

Gouldsborough, V., Fairmichael, F., Davison, C., et al. (2023) Driving following a diagnosis of dementia: exploring the views and experiences of people with dementia – a UK survey, *International Journal of Geriatric Psychiatry*, 38 (2): e5874. Available at: https://doi.org/10.1002/gps.5874.

Hagan, R.J. (2020) What next? Experiences of social support and signposting after a diagnosis of dementia, *Health and Social Care in the Community*, 28 (4): 1170–79.

Harding, A.J., Morbey, H., Ahmed, F., et al. (2019) What is important to people living with dementia? The 'long-list' of outcome items in the development of a core outcome set for use in the evaluation of non-pharmacological community-based health and social care interventions, *BMC Geriatrics*, 19: 94. Available at: https://doi.org/10.1186/s12877-019-1103-5.

Hewitt, P., Watts, C., Hussey, J., et al. (2013) Does a structured gardening programme improve well-being in young-onset dementia? A preliminary study, *British Journal of Occupational Therapy*, 76 (8): 355–61.

Huizenga, J., Scheffelaar, A., Fruijtier, A., et al. (2022) Everyday experiences of people living with mild cognitive impairment or dementia: a scoping review, *International Journal of Environmental Research and Public Health*, 19 (17): 10828. Available at: https://doi.org/10.3390/ijerph191710828.

Hutchinson, K., Roberts, C., Roach, P., et al. (2020) Co-creation of a family-focused service model living with younger onset dementia, *Dementia*, 19 (4): 1029–50.

Innovations in Dementia (2023a) *Dementia Diaries: Giving a voice to people with dementia through audio and video diaries*. Available at: https://dementiadiaries.org/ (accessed 10 April 2023).

Innovations in Dementia (2023b) *Research by younger people with dementia*. Available at: https://dementiaenquirers.org.uk/ (accessed 10 April 2023).

Innovations in Dementia (2023c) *The Dementia Enquirers Gold Standards for Co-Research*. Available at: https://bit.ly/3YQ7sj6 (accessed 10 April 2023).

Innovations in Dementia (2023d) *The Dementia Enquirers Gold Standards for Ethical Research*. Available at: https://bit.ly/3XF6EwW (accessed 10 April 2023).

Innovations in Dementia (2023e) *Inspiring different conversations*. Available at: http://www.innovationsindementia.org.uk/what-we-do/ (accessed 3 April 2023).

Innovations in Dementia and the DEEP Network (2023) *A good life with dementia*. Available at: https://www.youtube.com/watch?v=XRS4Aha068Y (accessed 10 April 2023).

Jones, B., Gage, H., Bakker, C., et al. (2018) Availability of information on young onset dementia for patients and carers in six European countries, *Patient Education and Counseling*, 101 (1): 159–65.

Kilty, C., Cahill, S., Foley, T., et al. (2023) Young onset dementia: implications for employment and finances, *Dementia*, 22 (1): 68–84.

Kokorelias, K.M., Shiers-Hanley, J.E., Li, Z., et al. (2022) A systematic review on navigation programs for persons living with dementia and their caregivers, *The Gerontologist*, 63 (8): 1341–50.

Litherland, R. and Hare, P. (2024) *People with Dementia at the Heart of Research: Co-Producing Research through The Dementia Enquirers Model*. London: Jessica Kingsley.

Lithgow, S. and Boyd, R. (2019) Early diagnosis, in G.A. Jackson and D. Tolson (eds.) *Textbook of Dementia Care: An Integrated Approach*. London: Routledge.

Loi, S.M., Goh, A.M., Mocellin, R., et al. (2022) Time to diagnosis in younger-onset dementia and the impact of a specialist diagnostic service, *International Psychogeriatrics*, 34 (4): 367–75.

Loi, S.M., Cations, M. and Velakoulis, D. (2023) Young-onset dementia diagnosis, management and care: a narrative review, *Medical Journal of Australia*, 218 (4): 182–89.

Mayrhofer, A., Mathie, E., McKeown, J., et al. (2018) Age-appropriate services for people diagnosed with young onset dementia (YOD): a systematic review, *Aging and Mental Health*, 22 (8): 933–41.

Mayrhofer, A.M., Greenwood, N., Smeeton, N., et al. (2021) Understanding the financial impact of a diagnosis of young onset dementia on individuals and families in the United Kingdom: results of an online survey, *Health and Social Care in the Community*, 29 (3): 664–71.

Millenaar, J.K., Bakker, C., Koopmans, R.T., et al. (2016) The care needs and experiences with the use of services of people with young-onset dementia and their caregivers: a systematic review, *International Journal of Geriatric Psychiatry*, 31 (12): 1261–76.

Mitchell, W. and Wharton, A. (2018) *Someone I Used to Know*. London: Bloomsbury.

National Collaborating Centre for Mental Health (NCCMH) (2018) *The Dementia Care Pathway: Full Implementation Guidance*. London: NCCMH.

National Institute for Health and Care Excellence (NICE) (2018) *Dementia: Assessment, management and support for people living with dementia and their carers*, NICE Guideline NG97. Available at: https://www.nice.org.uk/guidance/ng97.

NHS England (2016) *NHS England Transformation Framework: The Well Pathway for Dementia*. Available at: https://www.england.nhs.uk/mentalhealth/wp-content/uploads/sites/29/2016/03/dementia-well-pathway.pdf.

Novek, S. and Menec, V. (2023) Conceptualizing access to community-based supports from the perspectives of people living with young onset dementia, family members and providers, *Dementia*, 22 (1): 180–96.

Oliver, K., O'Malley, M., Parkes, J., et al. (2020) Living with young onset dementia and actively shaping dementia research: The Angela Project, *Dementia*, 19 (1): 41–48.

O'Malley, M., Carter, J., Stamou, V., et al. (2021a) Receiving a diagnosis of young onset dementia: a scoping review of lived experiences, *Aging and Mental Health*, 25 (1): 1–12.

O'Malley, M., Parkes, J., Campbell, J., et al. (2021b) Receiving a diagnosis of young onset dementia: evidence-based statements to inform best practice, *Dementia*, 20 (5): 1745–71.

O'Malley, M., Parkes, J., Stamou, V., et al. (2022) Current UK clinical practice in diagnosing dementia in younger adults: compliance with quality indicators in electronic health records from mental health trusts, *Aging and Mental Health*, 26 (11): 2233–42.

Oyebode, J.R. (2022) The experience of living with young onset dementia, in M. de Vugt and J. Carter (eds.) *Understanding Young Onset Dementia: Evaluation, Needs and Care*. London: Routledge.

Parkes, J., O'Malley, M., Stamou, V., et al. (2022) Lessons learnt from delivering the public and patient involvement forums within a younger onset dementia project, *Dementia*, 21 (7): 2103–16.

Rare Dementia Support (2023) *Rare Dementia Support*. Available at: https://www.raredementiasupport.org.

Revez, A., Timmons, S., Fox, S., et al. (2018) *Dementia Diagnostic Services for Ireland: A literature review*. Tullamore: National Dementia Office. Available at: https://www.hse.ie/eng/dementia-pathways/files/dementia-diagnostic-services-for-ireland-a-literature-review.pdf.

Richardson, A., Pedley, G., Pelone, F., et al. (2016) Psychosocial interventions for people with young onset dementia and their carers: a systematic review, *International Psychogeriatrics*, 28 (9): 1441–54.

Roach, P. and Drummond, N. (2014) 'It's nice to have something to do': early-onset dementia and maintaining purposeful activity, *Journal of Psychiatric and Mental Health Nursing*, 21 (10): 889–95.

Roberts, C., Rochford-Brennan, H., Goodrick, J., et al. (2020) Our reflections of patient and public involvement in research as members of the European Working Group of People with Dementia, *Dementia*, 19 (1): 10–17.

Robertson, J., Evans, D. and Horsnell, T. (2013) Side by Side: a workplace engagement program for people with younger onset dementia, *Dementia*, 12 (5): 666–74.

Rodda, J. and Carter, J. (2016) A survey of UK services for younger people living with dementia, *International Journal of Geriatric Psychiatry*, 31 (8): 957–59.

Rook, G. and Mayrhofer, A. (2023) Young onset dementia services. Personal communication with a group of ten people diagnosed with young onset dementia, 4 April.

Royal College of Psychiatrists (RCP) (2018) *Young-onset dementia in mental health services: Recommendations for service provision*, College Report CR217. Available at: https://www.rcpsych.ac.uk/improving-care/campaigning-for-better-mental-health-policy/college-reports/2018-college-reports/cr217.

Sansoni, J., Duncan, C., Grootemaat, P., et al. (2014) *Younger onset dementia: a literature review*, Centre for Health Service Development, University of Wollongong. Available at: https://ro.uow.edu.au/cgi/viewcontent.cgi?article=1380&context=ahsri.

Scottish Government (2023) *New dementia strategy for Scotland: Everyone's story*. Available at: https://www.gov.scot/publications/new-dementia-strategy-scotland-everyones-story/.

Social Prescribing Academy (2023) *What is social prescribing?* Available at: https://socialprescribingacademy.org.uk/ (accessed 23 April 2023).

Stamou, V., Fontaine, J.L., O'Malley, M., et al. (2021a) The nature of positive post-diagnostic support as experienced by people with young onset dementia, *Aging and Mental Health*, 25 (6): 1125–33.

Stamou, V., La Fontaine, J., Gage, H., et al. (2021b) Services for people with young onset dementia: The 'Angela' project national UK survey of service use and satisfaction, *International Journal of Geriatric Psychiatry*, 36 (3): 411–22.

Stamou, V., Oyebode, J., La Fontaine, J., et al. (2023) Good practice in needs-based post-diagnostic support for people with young onset dementia: findings from the Angela Project, *Ageing and Society*. Available at: https://doi.org/10.1017/S0144686X22001362.

Swaffer, K. (2016) *What the Hell Happened to My Brain? Living beyond Dementia*. London: Jessica Kingsley.

Talbot, C.V. and Coulson, N.S. (2023) 'I found it the only place that spoke the same language': a thematic analysis of messages posted to an online peer support discussion forum for people living with dementia, *Age and Ageing*, 52 (1): afac330. Available at: https://doi.org/10.1093/ageing/afac330.

The King's Fund (2009) *2009 GSK Impact Award winners: The CLIVE Project*. Available at: https://www.kingsfund.org.uk/insight-and-analysis/videos/2009-gsk-impact-award-winners (accessed 30 March 2023).

Together in Dementia Everyday (TIDE) (2023a) *Carer groups*. Available at: https://www.tide.uk.net/ (accessed 3 April 2023).

Together in Dementia Everyday (TIDE) (2023b) *Policy Influencing Toolkit*. Available at: https://www.tide.uk.net/policy-influencing-toolkit/ (accessed 3 April 2023).

Together in Dementia Everyday (TIDE) (2023c) *TIDE in. Scotland.* Available at: https://www.tide.uk.net/tide-in-scotland/ (accessed 3 April 2023).

Van Vliet, D., De Vugt, M., Bakker, C., et al. (2013) Time to diagnosis in young-onset dementia as compared with late-onset dementia, *Psychological Medicine*, 43 (2): 423–32.

Westera, A., Fildes, D., Duncan, C., et al. (2014) *Final report: Literature review and needs and feasibility assessment of services for people with younger onset dementia*, Australian Health Services Research Institute, Wollongong. Available at: https://ro.uow.edu.au/cgi/viewcontent.cgi?referer=&httpsredir=1&article=1378&context=ahsri.

Wheatley, A., Bamford, C., Brunskill, G., et al. (2021) Implementing post-diagnostic support for people living with dementia in England: a qualitative study of barriers and strategies used to address these in practice, *Age and Ageing*, 50 (6): 2230–37.

Woodall, J., Surr, C., Kinsella, K., et al. (2016) *An independent evaluation of 'Dementia Diaries'*, Project Report, Centre for Health Promotion Research, Institute for Health and Wellbeing, Leeds Beckett University. Available at: https://eprints.leedsbeckett.ac.uk/id/eprint/3446/.

Woodward, M., Arthur, A., Darlington, N., et al. (2019) The place for dementia-friendly communities in England and its relationship with epidemiological need, *International Journal of Geriatric Psychiatry*, 34 (1): 67–71.

York Minds and Voices (2021) *York Minds and Voices Dementia Enquirers Report: The pros cons and particular needs of those living alone with dementia and those living with a care partner.* Available at: https://dementiaenquirers.org.uk/wp-content/uploads/2021/05/minds-and-voices-in-york_report.pdf (accessed 10 April 2023).

Young Dementia Network (2017) *Diagnosing dementia in younger people: A decision-making guide for GPs.* Available at: https://www.youngdementianetwork.org/wp-content/uploads/2023/01/V1_YDN_GP_Guide_Leaflet_DL_2022_Web.pdf.

Young Dementia Network (2018) *Young onset dementia pathway: An outline of our recommendations.* Available at: https://www.youngdementianetwork.org/resources/young-onset-pathway/.

Young Dementia Network (2023) *Supporting implementation of the NICE guideline for people with young onset dementia.* Available at: https://www.youngdementianetwork.org/wp-content/uploads/2021/09/NICE-young-onset-dementia-guideline-FINAL.pdf.

Reflections on Part 1

The first part of this book has covered topics connected with maintaining autonomy despite receiving a diagnosis of dementia. Reflecting on the chapters raises some interesting issues.

The initial chapter stressed that a specific diagnosis can make a huge difference to understanding symptoms and therefore to knowing how to accept and manage them. It suggests that professionals working in all-age dementia assessment services should consult or refer on to specialist academic centres for advice or a second opinion when necessary to help them arrive at the specific diagnosis. This raises the wider issue of how best to organise services to meet the needs of those with young onset dementia. There is no easy answer because there are several pathways into services, dependent on the diagnosis the general practitioner thinks most likely and on what services are available locally. If you have possible young onset dementia you may be referred to neurology, memory assessment services or adult psychiatric services. In the Angela Project (Stamou et al., 2021), we found that the most common service in which people had received their diagnosis was an all-age dementia assessment service (i.e. a memory clinic) and the second most common was a neurology service. A smaller proportion were diagnosed by specialist young onset dementia teams. It could be argued that all-age dementia assessment services have the least expertise in diagnosing young onset dementia, and neurology services have the least expertise in providing post-diagnostic dementia services. The best configuration of diagnostic services may be dedicated young onset dementia teams that have the experience and knowledge required to recognise and diagnose the range of dementias, backed up by neurologists and specialist academic centres that can be consulted about complex presentations. These comments relate to the UK context but international comparison could also be helpful. Loi et al. (2022) found that, in Australia, where there was a specialist young onset dementia service, time to diagnosis for those under 65 years was reduced by a year. They called for a young onset dementia multidisciplinary team or 'hub' to be established in each region of Australia.

The second chapter drew directly on consensus from people living with young onset dementias on what is important in the way assessment and diagnosis are conducted. The importance of a relationship-centred approach shines through and supports the holistic stance of our book. Interestingly, another recent study also using Delphi methodology, which looked at best practice in communicating a diagnosis of dementia at any age, also highlighted compassion and empathy as the most important aspects of this process (Armstrong et al., 2024). When we submitted the first draft of this text, one of the series editors commented that the research drawn on, much of which is now 10–12 years old, felt out of date. She asked for it to be updated. Searches of the literature to discover more recent studies revealed only two that were directly relevant, highlighting the lack of young onset dementia research compared to the high volume focused on late onset dementia.

The chapters on using technologies and cognitive rehabilitation exemplify the solution-focused approach. Use of gadgets and cognitive rehabilitation techniques can counteract the images of helplessness that are commonly associated with dementia (Gerritsen et al., 2018). These negative images can lead those diagnosed and those supporting them to feel there is nothing that can be done. However, these approaches help to avoid or overcome disability and social exclusion; they deserve greater investment and a higher profile. It is very positive that advances in disease-modifying treatments are being made but it will be many years before such treatments are routinely available. We owe people who are living with dementia now, access to effective technology and rehabilitation. The chapter on cognitive rehabilitation is based on key UK studies of goal-oriented rehabilitation for dementia. These were restricted to people with Alzheimer's disease, vascular or mixed dementia, or dementia related to Parkinson's disease, as these were the populations for which there was evidence of effectiveness (Clare et al., 2019, 2023; Hindle et al., 2018). Wider work is looking at how to support the cognitive functioning of people with rarer diagnoses, such as finding and testing ways to help those with a diagnosis of posterior cortical atrophy to continue to be able to read (Yong et al., 2015) but more of this sort of work is needed.

In contrast to other chapters, the one on legal and financial issues is not research-based but, rather, gives a summary of important information relevant to everyone who has young onset dementia. Calum MacDonald, the chapter author, urges those affected to gain some control over their future lives by informing themselves about the legal framework governing finances and welfare. Human beings remain reluctant to plan ahead for a time when we lack capacity. Studies of advance care planning in dementia generally show how few people have had advance conversations about what is important to them in their future care (Piers et al., 2018). A recent study of palliative care in young onset dementia found under 33% had made their views known (Maters et al., 2024). A relatively easy way into thinking more about this would be to read Wendy Mitchell's final book, *One Last Thing: Living with the End in Mind* (Mitchell, 2023).

The final chapter in Part 1 is on the importance of those directly affected having a voice in design of services. This chapter is in harmony with our theme of empowering people living with young onset dementia to retain autonomy over their lives. It shows the value of 'dementia activism' that has emerged as a major force to change public attitudes toward dementia and to try to ensure people with dementia get the services they deserve (Cahill, 2018; Shakespeare et al., 2019). I have recently come across the term *epistemic injustice* (Fricker, 2007). This refers to the exclusion and silencing of certain sections of society due to prejudicial views of the majority. People living with dementia have historically been subject to epistemic injustice but this is changing as more of those living with dementia speak out, with those living with young onset dementia having especially strong voices.

Overall, we hope this part of the book gives those living with young onset dementia, and those supporting them, the evidence and ideas they need to meet the need for people with a diagnosis to continue to have control over their lives.

References

Armstrong, M.J., Bedenfield, N., Rosselli, M., et al. (2024) Best practices for communicating a diagnosis of dementia: results of a multi-stakeholder modified Delphi consensus process, *Neurology: Clinical Practice*, 14 (1): e200223. Available at: https://doi.org/10.1212/CPJ.0000000000200223.

Cahill, S. (2018) *Dementia and Human Rights*. Bristol: Policy Press.

Clare, L., Kudlicka, A., Oyebode, J.R., et al. (2019) Goal-oriented cognitive rehabilitation for early-stage Alzheimer's and related dementias: the GREAT RCT, *Health Technol Assess*, 23 (10): 1–242. Available at: https://doi.org/10.3310/hta23100.

Clare, L., Kudlicka, A., Collins, R., et al. (2023) Implementing a home-based personalised cognitive rehabilitation intervention for people with mild-to-moderate dementia: GREAT into Practice, *BMC Geriatrics*, 23 (1): 93. Available at: https://doi.org/10.1186/s12877-022-03705-0.

Fricker, M. (2007) *Epistemic Injustice: Power and the Ethics of Knowing*. Oxford: Oxford University Press.

Gerritsen, D.L., Oyebode, J. and Gove, D. (2018) Ethical implications of the perception and portrayal of dementia, *Dementia*, 17 (5): 596–608.

Hindle, J.V., Watermeyer, T.J., Roberts, J., et al. (2018) Goal-orientated cognitive rehabilitation for dementias associated with Parkinson's disease: a pilot randomised controlled trial, *International Journal of Geriatric Psychiatry*, 33 (5): 718–28.

Loi, S.M., Goh, A.M., Mocellin, R., et al. (2022) Time to diagnosis in younger-onset dementia and the impact of a specialist diagnostic service, *International Psychogeriatrics*, 34 (4): 367–75.

Maters, J., van der Steen, J.T., de Vugt, M.E., et al. (2024) Palliative care in nursing home residents with young-onset dementia: professional and family caregiver perspectives, *Journal of Alzheimer's Disease*, 97 (2): 573–86.

Mitchell W. (2023) *One Last Thing: How to Live With the End in Mind*. London: Bloomsbury.

Piers, R., Albers, G., Gilissen, J., et al. (2018) Advance care planning in dementia: recommendations for healthcare professionals, *BMC Palliative Care*, 17 (1): 88. Available at: https://doi.org/10.1186/s12904-018-0332-2.

Shakespeare, T., Zeilig, H. and Mittler, P. (2019) Rights in mind: thinking differently about dementia and disability, *Dementia*, 18 (3): 1075–88.

Stamou, V., La Fontaine, J., Gage, H., et al. (2021) Services for people with young onset dementia: the 'Angela' Project national UK survey of service use and satisfaction, *International Journal of Geriatric Psychiatry*, 36 (3): 411–22.

Yong, K.X., Rajdev, K., Shakespeare, T.J., et al. (2015) Facilitating text reading in posterior cortical atrophy, *Neurology*, 85 (4): 339–48.

Part **2**

Retaining Identity

The second overarching theme from the Angela Project analysis of survey responses and interviews with people living with young onset dementia and their supporters, reflected that helpful support promotes people to retain their individual identity, even if cognitive impairment affects of some aspects of life. This can be achieved by:

- having access to support that is respectful of each person's cultural identity;
- having guidance and assistance to manage employment;
- availing of opportunities to pursue meaningful hobbies and activities;
- getting involved in research on young onset dementia;
- being listened to as dementia advances to inform person-centred care; and
- having the chance to live in an accepting, validating environment, if you cannot manage at home.

Retaining identity is also relevant for:

- family supporters or carers, who find it helpful to have support that enables them to have time and space to be themselves, as well as to be 'a carer'.

The chapters in Part 2 reflect these themes.

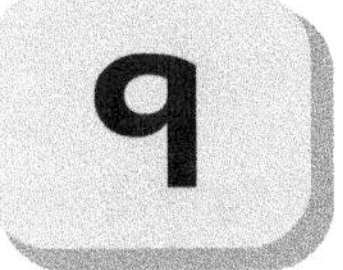

Indigenous dimensions of dementia: considerations for culturally safe dementia care

Pamela Roach and Jennifer Walker

Overview

It is acknowledged that families and societies influence the quality of care that a person living with dementia receives. For Indigenous populations (i.e., the original inhabitants of a specific land/location), this may be more complex and is layered with a lack of services that are culturally safe or accessible. Enhanced health care for Indigenous people requires cultural safety and humility. Recent work with ethnic minority populations living with dementia has similarly demonstrated that commonly used interactive therapies for dementia treatment (e.g. reminiscence therapy) can be inappropriate and culturally unsafe for ethnic minority groups. To mitigate and eliminate potential harm, Indigenous dementia care services must be self-determined and Indigenous-led. The direction is clear for improved culturally safe dementia care services, and that is to shift our paradigm to strengths-based, trauma-informed dementia care. This can provide direction and improved dementia care for all minority groups deserving of health equity globally.

Keywords

Culturally safe care, Indigenous-centred dementia care, traditional knowledge, equity, deserving groups, health equity, self-determination, Indigenous health.

Learning points

- Indigenous populations globally experience disproportionate rates of young onset dementia.

- There is a lack of culturally safe dementia care services for younger Indigenous people living with dementia.
- To improve outcomes for younger Indigenous people living with dementia, services must integrate trauma-informed and strengths-based Indigenous-centred approaches to care.

Introduction

Young onset dementia is used to describe a group of symptoms that affects the memory and cognitive ability of individuals diagnosed under the age of 65 years (Rossor et al., 2010). Indigenous communities (the original inhabitants of a specific land/location) have identified young onset dementia as a priority. First Nations populations in Canada have physician-treated prevalence rates of young onset dementia that are two to three times higher than other populations (Jacklin et al., 2013). Individuals living with young onset dementia face different challenges and issues because of their social constructs and social responsibilities than individuals living with dementia over the age of 65 (Parker, 2014). Because a diagnosis of young onset dementia comes at a time of complexity within family systems (Rolland, 1988, 1994; Roach et al., 2008, 2012, 2014a, 2014b), this creates additional stressors on individuals, families and communities while contributing to a loss of identity on the part of the younger person living with dementia. Despite the realities of family and community impact and Indigenous worldviews that prioritise collectivism, young onset dementia research still typically focuses on individuals and dyads (usually person with dementia and 'carer') rather than larger groups like families and communities. It is crucial to consider evidence that utilises family-centred design in dementia care as it can become a foundation for the conceptualisation of non-individual units of experience in dementia care and research. In other words, it can help us to move from thinking about an individual or couple with dementia to thinking about a wider family or community.

It has long been acknowledged that families have the potential to greatly influence the quality of care that a person living with dementia receives at home and, by implication, their quality of life. Extrapolating this to Indigenous contexts, we know that individuals in communities also do not exist in isolation from one another; they have a shared history, a shared future, shared ways of knowing, and some will have shared biology. We also know that Indigenous people share an experience of ongoing colonisation, accompanied by systemic and interpersonal racism, particularly when accessing health care (Allan and Smylie, 2015; Leyland et al., 2016; McLane et al., 2019; Roach et al., 2023). Views and experiences are shaped by being part of this group (Copeland and White, 1991). The memories, stories and narratives that are constructed by this group may vary from the way that they are constructed by individuals (Roberts, 2002). This is similar to perpetuation of culture, language and traditional knowledge experienced through relationships and stories in Indigenous communities that has persisted despite many systemic attempts at cultural disruption, intergenerational disconnection and genocide (Sium and Ritskes, 2013; TRCC, 2015). Despite this, little research has examined the experience of young onset dementia from Indigenous perspectives.

In 2015, the Truth and Reconciliation Commission of Canada (TRCC) released 94 Calls to Action compelling Canadian society across all public institutions and services (including, but not limited to, education, child welfare, criminal justice and health care) to acknowledge colonisation as the primary driver of population-level health disparities experienced by Indigenous people (TRCC, 2015). Colonisation in Canada included race-based legislation: the Indian Act, which limited participation in society, cultural and spiritual practices, and forced Indigenous children to attend Indian residential schools (segregated boarding schools) and day schools (segregated schools for the purposes of assimilation) that were designed to separate Indigenous children from their families, disrupt the intergenerational transmission of language and culture, and eradicate Indigenous people from the larger Canadian society. It also facilitated the creation of land bases called 'reserves' that were policed by Indian agents who limited movement on and off of them. Segregated hospitals were also used for medical experimentation and mistreatment of Indigenous people.

Though there have been updates to the Indian Act, it remains an active piece of Canadian race-based legislation and impacts the way that different Indigenous groups can access health care. This has led to many ongoing health disparities today for Indigenous people. These disparities encompass dementia and brain health. The Calls to Action (TRCC, 2015) provide actionable strategies to reduce disparities between Indigenous and non-Indigenous health outcomes.

Indigenous dementia care becomes a more urgent Canadian healthcare priority when current population-level data is considered (Canadian Academy of Health Sciences, 2019; Public Health Agency of Canada, 2019). Data show the age-standardised prevalence of dementia in First Nations people to be 34% higher than in non-First Nations people in Alberta (Jacklin et al., 2013). This trend is also evidenced in comparator countries, with data from Australia showing higher incidence rate ratios of dementia for younger Indigenous males and females (27.3 cases per 1000 person-years) between the ages of 45 and 64 years than the non-Indigenous population (10.7 cases per 1000 person-years) (Li et al., 2014). Research on the epidemiology and pathophysiology of young onset dementia experienced by Indigenous people in Canada, Australia and the United States has helped provide more insight into the prevalence, incidence and risk factors (including childhood trauma and colonisation) of dementia (Li et al., 2014).

Culturally safe dementia care

For younger people living with dementia, specialist young onset services have now been repeatedly recommended as best practice (Beattie et al., 2002;

Roach et al., 2008; Carter et al., 2018) and yet guidance as to how these services should look remains sparse. Due to the complexity of the intergenerational relationships often present in these situations, it is crucial that family-centred care is integrated into any new specialist care structure (see also Chapter 15 on family relationships in young onset dementia). Services should consider the needs and experiences of each person's networks, including family, friends and work colleagues, when working with younger people living with dementia (Keady and Matthew, 1997; Hutchinson et al., 2020). Indigenous-specific young onset dementia services also need to consider community roles and relationships. Lack of knowledge of local prevalence has become an unacceptable argument for lack of adequate care for younger people living with dementia (Barker et al., 1997) and Indigenous people living with dementia.

Progress has been evidenced in developing person-centred philosophies towards dementia care practice. However, despite these advances, both literature and families living with young onset dementia still report infrequent referrals of younger people living with dementia to specialist young onset services (Williams et al., 2001; Hutchinson et al., 2018). This is exacerbated for Indigenous people living with dementia due to the compounded impact of the general lack of culturally safe dementia care (Public Health Agency of Canada, 2019) and under-service of health care more broadly (Leyland et al., 2016).

There are likely a variety of reasons for these low referrals to specialist services, including a lack of knowledge on the part of primary care providers and other referring health professionals, a lack of primary care provision generally that does not meet demand, and a frequent lack of service availability. This often leaves the younger person living with dementia and their family with little or no specialist support for the diagnosis once it has been made (Beattie et al., 2004). Once again, these limitations may impact Indigenous people more due to the lack of culturally safe assessments for Indigenous people living with dementia that would prompt a referral from a health professional (Walker et al., 2021a).

Specialist service provision for younger people living with dementia has been recommended as 'best practice' in policy, published and grey literature (Barker et al., 1997; Beattie et al., 2002; Department of Health, 2009; Public Health Agency of Canada, 2019; Alzheimer Society of Canada, 2020). However, due to small population sizes in some geographical contexts, specialist services for dementia care can be challenging to advocate for and to maintain (Tindall and Manthorpe, 1997; Dal Bello-Haas, 2014). This is a particular challenge for Indigenous people living in rural and remote areas of Canada where specialist care is limited (Morgan et al., 2014). For First Nations individuals living with dementia in their home community on reserves, there are further limits to accessing health and social supports due to funding policies that limit access to some services by those under the age of 65 (Standing Committee on Indigenous and Northern Affairs, 2018).

As outlined in other chapters, there are strong arguments that younger people will have more specific needs than an older population, including work or benefits issues; family and parenting roles; the person is likely to be fitter and be more affected by social isolation of peers and colleagues; and are likely to have intimacy issues and sexual needs that may need addressing by services (Beattie et al., 2002; Holdsworth and McCabe, 2018). Such networks would help to counteract the feelings of loneliness and social isolation that are often reported by younger people living with dementia; this is a particular concern with the strong links between isolation and loneliness and cognitive outcomes (Sutin et al., 2020). Appropriate peer support relationships are even more crucial for equity-deserving groups, including Indigenous peoples, to avoid the stigma, racism and discrimination that they may experience in western healthcare systems (Roach et al., 2023). One way forward may be to look at virtual supports for Indigenous people living in rural areas that have proven successful in other contexts (Roach et al., 2022b; Fitzpatrick et al., 2023).

Alzheimer's disease and vascular dementia in younger people are more likely to have a genetic link than in late onset dementia, which can lead to increased anxiety in families experiencing young onset dementia (see Chapter 3 and also Keady, 1996; Department of Health, 2005). As such, genetic counselling may need to become part of service provision, given the emphasis on earlier diagnosis within current government policy (Department of Health, 2009; NHS England, 2019). This need may be compounded by specific documented genetic predisposition in some Indigenous families (Jacklin et al., 2013) but any efforts to provide genetic counselling services related to dementia must carefully also consider the impacts of colonisation for Indigenous peoples, both in Canada and internationally (Walker et al., 2020). Indeed, regarding the availability of culturally safe dementia care for Indigenous people, we must consider the wider context of Indigenous experiences in the health system. There is irrefutable evidence that Indigenous people living in Canada experience racism in the healthcare system (Allan and Smylie, 2015; Leyland et al., 2016; McLane et al., 2019; Roach et al., 2023). This anti-Indigenous racism is associated with direct impacts on physical and mental health outcomes. For example, racism results in reduced access to routine services, increased emergency visits and increased mortality (Paradies et al., 2015; McLane et al., 2019). In addition to interpersonal experiences of racism, the pervasive systemic racism present throughout the Canadian healthcare system (Roach et al., 2022a, 2023) includes services and structures that are inappropriate and culturally unsafe. This further exacerbates existing health conditions.

This experience of racism is layered with the fact that, broadly, families living with young onset dementia report a feeling of stigma that accompanies a diagnosis (Lee, 2003; Bryden, 2005; Ashworth, 2020). Friends, family and community members may disengage from younger people living with dementia and withdraw from their social network, essentially stripping the younger person of their dignity and personhood (Sterin, 2002). Often, because of the age of onset in young onset dementia, a diagnosis can be met with disbelief from friends and loved ones, reinforcing the stigma of diagnosis (McGowin, 1993; Lee, 2003; Rose, 2003; Bryden, 2005; Taylor, 2007). This stigma then intersects with anti-Indigenous bias and racism for younger Indigenous people living with dementia. A recent study reported that for Indigenous people living with young onset dementia, it can be especially difficult navigating health and social supports with a decline in cognitive ability and memory and also encountering systemic and interpersonal racism (Ody et al., 2022). This expectation of encountering racism when seeking care leads to stereotype threat (Aronson et al., 2013). Stereotype threat is a phenomenon which operates when people feel at risk from the stereotype. For example, if a young black man knows he is likely to be seen as aggressive, he may always be alert to situations that are dangerous for him because others may interpret his behaviour as aggressive. This may cause him anxiety and stress his physical health, as well as meaning he constricts his life to avoid situations where there may be a police presence. This is an additional factor causing negative health impacts for Indigenous people.

The need for healthcare services and systems designed and led by and for Indigenous people is necessary to counter the impacts of anti-Indigenous racism and stereotype threat. This is outlined further in health-related Call to Action #22 from the TRCC (2015), and aligns with refined definitions of person-centred care (Vernooij-Dassen and Moniz-Cook, 2016) and principles of relationship-centred care (Nolan et al., 2004) that form the central tenets of ethical dementia service co-design. The Public Health Agency of Canada (2015, 2019) has repeatedly called for ongoing work to improve dementia care services, and this includes services specific to both Indigenous people and younger people living with dementia as a priority.

Recent work with ethnic minority populations living with dementia in the UK has demonstrated that commonly used interactive therapies for dementia treatment (e.g. reminiscence therapy) can be inappropriate and culturally unsafe for Black, Asian and Minority Ethnic (BAME) groups (Truswell, 2020). In an Indigenous context, these interventions are not cognisant of intergenerational trauma, the legacy of residential schools and the effects of colonisation on lived experience and cognition, or of Indigenous ways of knowing. This means that many of these interventions that are commonly utilised in western models of dementia care are inherently unsafe for Indigenous people living with dementia. Reminiscence can risk re-traumatisation, particularly by connecting to potentially traumatic long-term memories such as the Indian Residential Schools or Day Schools experienced by many Indigenous people living in Canada. Strengths-based and trauma-informed dementia care must play a role in enhancing safety and health equity when accessing the healthcare system.

To achieve enhanced healthcare safety for Indigenous people, cultural safety and humility are essential to dementia care planning. This requires developing deep engagement with Indigenous understandings of dementia.

The literature indicates that for some Indigenous communities, cognitive decline or memory loss may be seen as normal for Elders, though this may be different for younger individuals who have a role in the workforce and their communities (Hulko et al., 2010). Traditional understandings of dementia have been described to be holistic, circular and interconnected through generations. In the traditional sense, young onset dementia was seen as a natural way of life or extra ability for visions and deeper understandings of the natural and spiritual world. Having a diagnosis of dementia or any other chronic illness is not necessarily pathological but, for some Indigenous knowledge systems, is considered part of a plan that the Creator has put in place and it is part of a person's journey (Jacklin and Walker, 2020).

A recent study describing the experiences of urban Indigenous people living with young onset dementia reported that there are variable reactions to cognitive changes, as similarly experienced by non-Indigenous people. However, the overarching anxiety about accessing the healthcare system in a culturally safe way was foundational to the experience of younger Indigenous people living with dementia (Ody et al., 2022). The same authors reported that physicians also felt challenged in finding appropriate dementia care services for younger Indigenous people living with dementia to be referred to, and that the complexity of social factors such as lack of secure or affordable housing, income, social isolation and cultural disconnection made it more challenging for younger Indigenous people living with dementia to access health and social care supports (Ody et al., 2022).

Strengths-based approaches to Indigenous-centred dementia care

Given the evidence presented thus far, the direction is clear for improved Indigenous specific dementia care services, and that is to shift to strengths-based, trauma-informed and Indigenous-centred dementia care (Walker et al., 2021b). This shift is still closely aligned with the principles of person-centred dementia care prevalent in dementia care generally, while also incorporating an Indigenous worldview that moves the focus of the care model from individual to community. Previous work has recommended a shift from person-centred to family-centred care (Roach et al., 2008, 2012, 2014a). Indigenous dementia care models must extend that further to the community level and deeply integrate cultural safety, cultural humility and anti-racist approaches.

Previous health research completed with Indigenous people demonstrates that self-determination is an important factor in maintaining well-being and contributes to positive health outcomes (Chandler and Lalonde, 2008). Other work has indicated that a connection to culture can have quantifiable impacts on physical health in diabetes care (Oster et al., 2014), and that connectedness to culture and roles in the community are important to the experience of living with dementia as an Indigenous person (Ody et al., 2022). Knowledge of traditional approaches to wellness and healing, connection to the land, community history and knowledge, all form an important part of promoting good well-being, especially when living with a diagnosis of young onset dementia (Browne et al., 2017; Ody et al., 2022). This means that self-determination in health care is a collective right and is indeed enshrined in international law adopted by the United Nations in 2008 (UN, 2008). Healthcare systems and leaders must consider sovereignty of Nations and Indigenous-led approaches to health care for all individuals when undertaking service design, delivery and evaluation.

Related to this right of self-determination, there remains an ongoing challenge connected to healthcare resourcing and structuring. There need to be sufficient resources to support Indigenous people living with young onset dementia in their home communities, and to counteract the lack of cultural safety outside of those communities (Browne et al., 2017). Limited primary care capacity, inconsistency in healthcare professionals practising in the community, and culturally unsafe supportive living and/or long-term care facilities are all reported barriers to providing appropriate care to people living with young onset dementia (Ody et al., 2022).

Traditional healing methods have been discussed in the literature. These include building care models on community-based practices, attending ceremony, connecting to the land and having access to Elders who are familiar with these traditional ways of healing (Browne et al., 2017). This is in contrast to the way Indigenous people living with dementia may describe western practices. They may perceive conventional services as aimed at mitigating symptoms and treating individuals as a diagnosis, rather than treating them holistically as a person who is part of a larger community with roles and obligations to that community (Browne et al., 2017; Jacklin and Walker, 2020).

There is a need, and indeed a requirement, to respond to Call to Action #22 (TRCC, 2015), which asks for healthcare services to find a way to promote both western and Indigenous ways of knowing and healing. To fulfil this, healthcare professionals need to be able to access effective cultural safety training. An example of a community-based and Indigenous-led clinic is Maamwesying, a North Shore Community Health Services clinic that is working in partnership with communities and researchers to implement culturally safe memory clinic service models (Maamwesying, 2021). This is one example of healthcare design and delivery being led by the individuals accessing the care so that services are culturally safe and meaningful. Involvement in service design echoes the call to action in Chapter 8 but is of even greater importance to Indigenous peoples.

We conclude our chapter with the example of an indigenous woman's experiences when she developed young onset dementia. She is described in 'Alice's story' and you will find our reflections on this below.

Alicia's story

Alicia, a pseudonym, comes from a small rural First Nations reserve in western Canada where she grew up practising her culture. She has been living in the city for the last 20 years; Alicia moved to the city for university when she was 18 and has moved back home to her reserve a couple of times but came back to the city to stay when she was about 26. Alicia has been working for a local non-profit organisation for the last 8 years where she has worked her way up to a management position. She now leads a staff of 12 and has a large annual budget. She's been very busy both at work and with her two high-school-aged children and their sports activities. This means that she doesn't get back to her home community as much as she'd like and has become somewhat disconnected from practising her traditional cultural teachings. About a year ago Alicia started noticing that she was becoming disoriented in familiar settings, sometimes even while driving on the way home from work. She also noticed she started getting confused when working on the financial data at work. Her staff have also started to notice changes but are very supportive of Alicia and her leadership. Her team have been helping support her in these challenges and double-checking her work to prevent errors, so her director isn't aware of any changes so far. Alicia is generally well-liked and admired by her team, other leaders and customers.

Alicia's sister, Rose, visited her in the city about 6 months ago and also started noticing some changes. One evening Alicia and Rose went out for dinner and when Alicia went to get the car after, she became disoriented and lost on the way to the car park. Rose eventually found Alicia four blocks away from the restaurant being questioned by a police officer who assumed Alicia's disorientation and confusion were the result of intoxication and was attempting to arrest her. The situation escalated and both Alicia and Rose were taken into custody. Ultimately, no charges were laid but the officer did send child protective services to Alicia's home. Alicia then had to navigate the family services system, which impacted her ability to maintain her hours at work, her relationship with her children, and her stress and anxiety levels. Eventually, child protective services indicated there were no concerns but this further delayed Alicia connecting with health services to address her cognitive symptoms as she felt overwhelmed by the multiple appointments and professionals coming into her home.

Rose has stayed in more consistent contact with Alicia and her children since this incident and convinced Alicia to seek help and mention it to her doctor. When Alicia mentioned it to her family doctor, the doctor asked her about drug use and when Alicia said she doesn't use drugs or alcohol, the doctor told her that the symptoms she was noticing were likely due to anxiety and stress and suggested taking anti-anxiety medications. Alicia agreed but went back to her doctor when there were no signs of improvement after taking the medication for a number of weeks. At this point Alicia's family doctor referred her to a cognitive clinic for assessment.

At Alicia's appointment at the cognitive clinic, the Mini Mental State Examination (MMSE) was administered and Alicia felt the questions were a bit strange and difficult to answer; the results of the MMSE, along with the rest of the assessment, resulted in a diagnosis of young onset dementia, and more specifically, probable Alzheimer's disease. Alicia's mother and her grandmother had both experienced memory difficulties later in life, though they never received a diagnosis, and were supported to live in their community until the end of life. Alicia's employer has been very understanding and has offered to reduce her hours to alleviate stress and make it easier to attend appointments, but this has increased financial stress for her family as she is the primary income earner to pay the rent and other expenses while also trying to save for two children to attend university in the coming years. Alicia has expressed a desire to the neurologist at the cognitive clinic and to her family doctor to access traditional healing but needs to stay in the city to continue working at her current job and for her children to continue in their school.

Reflections on Alicia's story

Alicia's experience was similar in some ways to the experience of non-Indigenous people living with young onset dementia, such as difficulty getting a diagnosis and complexities of having a career and a young family. Alicia's story also illustrates some of the specific challenges she experiences due to stereotyping and anti-Indigenous bias in the health, social and justice systems. These stereotypes and racist generalisations resulted in the inappropriate involvement of family services and therefore her mental health and work performance were additionally impacted. Some important considerations for health professionals when referring Alicia to any specialist support services include the cultural safety of those services, their history of working with Indigenous people, and their understanding of historical impacts to current Indigenous health outcomes.

Alicia and her family experience some challenges that are similar to other ethnic minority groups when seeking care for young onset dementia. For all populations, the use of cognitive assessment tools that are culturally appropriate and/or translated into multiple languages is important when trying to determine a diagnosis. Making an effort to understand social supports and cultural priorities and traditions in conceptualising dementia for different groups is important to improve cultural safety for all people living with dementia. Cultural humility also means asking about these parts of someone's life to better understand when clarity is needed and not making assumptions about what may or may not be helpful. These approaches can lead to improved diagnosis, treatment and ongoing support for ethnic minority groups.

Conclusion

Dementia strategies around the world are recognising the diverse needs and experiences of Indigenous communities in relation to dementia and acknowledge the importance of supporting Indigenous communities in culturally appropriate and culturally safe ways (Alzheimer Society of Canada, 2020). This includes treatment and care provision for families and communities but also diagnosis, as standardised cognitive testing has been shown to be less accurate for Indigenous people, possibly resulting in misdiagnosis (LoGiudice et al., 2006; O'Connell et al., 2020; Walker et al., 2021a). However, national dementia strategies are not young-onset dementia-specific (Canadian Academy of Health Sciences, 2019; Public Health Agency of Canada, 2019) and certainly in a Canadian context, when they do include Indigenous peoples, they focus more on the populations of the Indigenous people that live in non-urban settings (Canadian Academy of Health Sciences, 2019; Public Health Agency of Canada, 2019).

So what does this mean in practice?

If you or someone you know is living with young onset dementia

There are critical components to culturally safe dementia care and this has been highlighted through work with many ethnic minority groups. These components may include dedicated funding for culturally safe dementia services, research initiatives specifically for culturally relevant dementia care, the development and implementation of culturally safe interventions, and innovative approaches to supporting families and communities (Alzheimer Society of Canada, 2020; Truswell, 2020). Ask what is available for you and how you can access these types of supports.

If you are a policy-maker

There is a need to include more of the experiences of Indigenous people with young onset dementia who live in all geographic areas, which also aligns with Call to Action #20 (TRCC, 2015). Acknowledging the cultural, socioeconomic and past experiences of Indigenous individuals with young onset dementia seeking support is critical to Indigenous-centred dementia care. A collaborative approach to creating healthcare services for Indigenous people can account for the heterogeneity of Indigenous peoples and specific community needs.

If you are a professional working with younger people living with dementia

Culturally safe health and social supports for younger Indigenous people living with dementia can also include cultural supports, access to Elders and traditional healing, circles with peers and trauma-informed mental health supports for Indigenous people living with dementia, their families and their communities. Increased understanding of how ethnicity, intersectionality and identity are directly related to health enables us to better understand the care needs of under-represented groups.

Though this chapter is dedicated to Indigenous experiences of young onset dementia, there are parallels to some of the same social drivers and determinants of health that impact cognition and ageing in minority ethnic or under-represented populations in other countries around the world. Indeed, cultural humility and person-centred dementia care can provide ways for us to proceed in safe ways to provide better care and improve the lives for people living with dementia in all groups. Through solidarity and humility, we can embrace other ways of knowing, to approach young onset dementia care with new paradigms that holistically incorporate equity to improve outcomes for all communities.

References

Allan, B. and Smylie, J. (2015) *First Peoples, second class treatment: The role of racism in the health and well-being of Indigenous peoples in Canada.* Toronto, ON: The

Wellesley Institute. Available at: https://www.wellesleyinstitute.com/wp-content/uploads/2015/02/Summary-First-Peoples-Second-Class-Treatment-Final.pdf.

Alzheimer Society of Canada (2020) *Race and dementia*. Available at: https://alzheimer.ca/en/about-us/national-statements.

Aronson, J., Burgess, D., Phelan, S.M., et al. (2013) Unhealthy interactions: the role of stereotype threat in health disparities, *American Journal of Public Health*, 103 (1): 50–56.

Ashworth, R. 2020. Perceptions of stigma among people affected by early- and late-onset Alzheimer's disease, *Journal of Health Psychology*, 25 (4): 490–510.

Barker, W., Barrett, K., Bingley, W., et al. (1997) *Mental Health Services: Heading for Better Care. Commissioning and providing mental health services for people with Huntington's disease, acquired brain injury and early onset dementia*. London: HMSO.

Beattie, A.M., Daker-White, G., Gilliard, J., et al. (2002) Younger people in dementia care: a review of service needs, service provision and models of good practice, *Aging and Mental Health*, 6 (3): 205–12.

Beattie, A., Daker-White, G., Gilliard, J., et al. (2004) 'How can they tell?' A qualitative study of the views of younger people about their dementia and dementia care services, *Health and Social Care in the Community*, 12 (4): 359–68.

Browne, C.V., Ka'opua, L.S., Jervis, L.L., et al. (2017) United States Indigenous populations and dementia: is there a case for culture-based psychosocial interventions?, *The Gerontologist*, 57 (6): 1011–19.

Bryden, C. (2005) *Dancing with Dementia: My Story of Living Positively with Dementia*. London: Jessica Kingsley.

Canadian Academy of Health Sciences (CAHS) (2019) *Improving the quality of life and care of persons living with dementia and their caregivers*. Ottawa: CAHS. Available at: https://cahs-acss.ca/improving-the-quality-of-life-and-care-of-persons-living-with-dementia-and-their-caregivers/.

Carter, J.E., Oyebode J.R. and Koopmans R.T.C.M. (2018) Young onset dementia and the need for specialist care: a national and international perspective, *Aging and Mental Health*, 22 (4): 468–73.

Chandler, M.J. and Lalonde, C.E. (2008) Cultural continuity as a moderator of suicide risk among Canada's First Nations, in L. Kirmayer and G. Valaskakis (eds.) *Healing Traditions: The Mental Health of Aboriginal Peoples in Canada*. Vancouver: University of British Columbia Press.

Copeland, A. and White, K. (1991) *Studying Families*. Newbury Park, CA: Sage.

Dal Bello-Haas, V., Cammer, A., Morgan, D., et al. (2014) Rural and remote dementia care challenges and needs: perspectives of formal and informal care providers residing in Saskatchewan, Canada, *Rural and Remote Health*, 14 (3): 192–204.

Department of Health (2005) *Everybody's business. Integrated mental health services for older adults: A service development guide*. London: Department of Health.

Department of Health (2009) *Living Well with Dementia: A national dementia strategy*. London: Department of Health.

Fitzpatrick, K.M., Ody, M., Goveas, D., et al. (2023) Understanding virtual primary health-care with Indigenous populations: a rapid evidence review, *BMC Health Services Research*, 23 (1): 303. Available at: https://doi.org/10.1186/s12913-023-09299-6.

Holdsworth, K. and McCabe, M. (2018) The impact of younger-onset dementia on relationships, intimacy, and sexuality in midlife couples: a systematic review, *International Psychogeriatrics*, 30 (1): 15–29.

Hulko, W., Camille, E., Antifeau, E., et al. (2010) Views of First Nation elders on memory loss and memory care in later life, *Journal of Cross-Cultural Gerontology*, 25 (4): 317–42.

Hutchinson, K.A., Roberts, C. and Roach, P. (2018) Feeling invisible and ignored: families' experiences of marginalisation living with younger onset dementia, in G. Macdonald and J. Mears (eds.) *Dementia as Social Experience: Valuing Life and Care*. London: Routledge.

Hutchinson, K.A., Roberts, C., Roach, P., et al. (2020) Co-creation of a family-focused service model living with younger onset dementia, *Dementia*, 19 (4): 1029–50.

Jacklin, K.M. and Walker, J.D. (2020) Cultural understandings of dementia in Indigenous peoples: a qualitative evidence synthesis, *Canadian Journal on Aging*, 39 (2): 220–34.

Jacklin, K.M., Walker, J.D. and Shawande, M. (2013) The emergence of dementia as a health concern among First Nations populations in Alberta, Canada, *Canadian Journal of Public Health*, 104 (1): 39–44.

Keady, J. (1996) The experience of dementia: a review of the literature and implications for nursing practice, *Journal of Clinical Nursing*, 5 (5): 275–88.

Keady, J. and Matthew, L. (1997) Younger people with dementia, *Elderly Care*, 9 (4): 19–23.

Lee, J.L. (2003) *Just Love Me: My Life Turned Upside Down by Alzheimer's*. West Lafayette, IN: Purdue University Press.

Leyland, A., Smylie, J., Cole, M., et al. (2016) *Health and health care implications of systemic racism on Indigenous peoples in Canada*. Mississauga, ON: College of Family Physicians of Canada. Available at: https://www.cfpc.ca/CFPC/media/Resources/Indigenous-Health/SystemicRacism_ENG.pdf.

Li, S.Q., Guthridge, S.L., Aratchige, P.E., et al. (2014) Dementia prevalence and incidence among the Indigenous and non-Indigenous populations of the Northern Territory, *Medical Journal of Australia*, 200 (8): 465–69.

LoGiudice, D., Smith, K., Thomas, J., et al. (2006) Kimberley Indigenous Cognitive Assessment tool (KICA): development of a cognitive assessment tool for older indigenous Australians, *International Psychogeriatrics*, 18 (2): 269–80.

Maamwesying (2021) *Annual Report 2020–2021*. Cutler, ON: North Shore Community Health Services Inc. Available at: https://maamwesying.ca/wp-content/uploads/2022/07/Annual-Report-2021-complete-compressed.pdf.

McGowin, D.F. (1993) *Living in the Labyrinth: A Personal Journey through the Maze of Alzheimer's*. New York: Dell Publishing.

McLane, P., Bill, L. and Barnabe, C. (2019) *Emergency Department Experiences and Concerns Participants' Report*, Alberta First Nations Information Governance Centre, Alberta, Canada.

Morgan, D., Crossley, M., Stewart, N., et al. (2014) Evolution of a community-based participatory approach in a rural and remote dementia care research program, *Progress in Community Health Partnerships: Research, Education, and Action*, 8 (2): 337–45.

NHS England (2019) *The NHS long term plan*. Available at: https://www.longtermplan.nhs.uk/.

Nolan, M.R., Davies, S., Brown, J., et al. (2004) Beyond 'person-centred' care: a new vision for gerontological nursing, *Journal of Clinical Nursing*, 13 (s1): 45–53.

O'Connell, M.E., Walker, J.D., Jacklin, K., et al. (2020) Classification accuracy of the English version of the Canadian Indigenous Cognitive Assessment (CICA) in a majority culture memory clinic sample, *Alzheimer's and Dementia*, 16: e040029. Available at: https://doi.org/10.1002/alz.040029.

Ody, M., Rodrigues, C., Banwait, P., et al. (2022) Urban Indigenous experiences of living with early onset dementia: a qualitative pilot study in Calgary, Alberta, Canada, *Journal of Neurology Research*, 12 (2): 69–75.

Oster, R.T., Grier, A., Lightning, R., et al. (2014) Cultural continuity, traditional Indigenous language, and diabetes in Alberta First Nations: a mixed methods study, *International Journal for Equity in Health*, 13: 92. Available at: https://doi.org/10.1186/s12939-014-0092-4.

Paradies, Y., Ben, J., Denson, N., et al. (2015) Racism as a determinant of health: a systematic Review and meta-analysis, *PLoS One*, 10(9): e0138511. Available at: https://doi.org/10.1371/journal.pone.0138511.

Parker, R.M. (2014) Dementia in Aboriginal and Torres Strait Islander people, *Medical Journal of Australia*, 200 (8): 435–36.

Public Health Agency of Canada (2015) *Ways Tried and True: Aboriginal Methodological Framework for the Canadian Best Practices Initiative.* Ottawa: Public Health Agency of Canada.

Public Health Agency of Canada (2019) *A Dementia Strategy for Canada: Together We Aspire.* Ottawa: Public Health Agency of Canada.

Roach, P., Keady, J., Bee, P., et al. (2008) Subjective experiences of younger people with dementia and their families: implications for UK research, policy and practice, *Reviews in Clinical Gerontology*, 18 (2): 165–74.

Roach, P., Keady, J. and Bee, P. (2012) 'It's easier just to separate them': practice constructions in the mental health care and support of younger people with dementia and their families, *Journal of Psychiatric and Mental Health Nursing*, 19 (6): 555–62.

Roach, P., Keady, J. and Bee, P. (2014a) Family-AiD: a family-centred assessment tool in young onset dementia, *Quality in Ageing and Older Adults*, 15 (3): 136–50.

Roach, P., Keady, J., Bee, P., et al. (2014b) 'We can't keep going on like this': identifying family storylines in young onset dementia, *Ageing and Society*, 34 (8): 1397–1426.

Roach, P., Hernandez, S., Carbert, A., et al. (2022a) Anti-Indigenous bias of medical school applicants by application status: a cross-sectional study, *BMC Medical Education*, 22: 683. Available at: https://doi.org/10.1186/s12909-022-03739-3.

Roach, P., Ody, M., Campbell, P. (2022b) Access, relationships, quality and safety (ARQS): a qualitative study to develop an Indigenous-centred understanding of virtual care quality, *BMJ Open Quality*, 11: e002028. Available at: https://doi.org/10.1136/bmjoq-2022-002028.

Roach, P., Ruzycki, S.M., Hernandez, S., et al. (2023) Prevalence and characteristics of anti-Indigenous bias among Albertan physicians: a cross-sectional survey and framework analysis, *BMJ Open*, 13: e063178. Available at: https://doi.org/10.1136/bmjopen-2022-063178.

Roberts, B. (2002) *Biographical Research.* Buckingham: Open University Press.

Rolland, J.S. (1988) A conceptual model of chronic and life-threatening illness and its impact on families, in C.S. Chilman, F.M. Cox and E.W. Nunnally (eds.) *Families in Trouble: Knowledge and Practice Perspectives for Professionals in the Human Services.* Newbury Park, CA: Sage.

Rolland, J.S. (1994) *Families, Illness & Disability. An Integrative Treatment Model.* New York: Basic Books.

Rose, L. (2003) *Larry's Way: Another Look at Alzheimer's from the Inside.* New York: iUniverse.

Rossor, M.N., Fox, N.C., Mummery, C.J., et al. (2010) The diagnosis of young onset dementia, *Lancet Neurology*, 9 (8): 793–806.

Sium, A. and Ritskes, E. (2013) Speaking truth to power: Indigenous storytelling as an act of living resistance, *Decolonization: Indigeneity, Education and Society*, 2(1): I–X.

Standing Committee on Indigenous and Northern Affairs (2018) *The Challenges of Delivering Continuing Care in First Nation Communities*, House of Commons. Available at: https://www.ourcommons.ca/Content/Committee/421/INAN/Reports/RP10260656/inanrp17/inanrp17-e.pdf.

Sterin, G. (2002) Essay on a word: a lived experience of Alzheimer's disease, *Dementia*, 1 (1): 7–10.

Sutin, A.R., Stephan, Y., Luchetti, M. (2020) Loneliness and risk of dementia, *Journals of Gerontology*, 75 (7): 1414–22.

Taylor, R. (2007) *Alzheimer's from the Inside Out*. Baltimore, MD: Health Professions Press.

Tindall, L. and Manthorpe, J. (1997) Early onset dementia: a case of ill-timing?, *Journal of Mental Health*, 6 (3): 237–50.

Truswell, D. (2020) Dementia and further common issues affecting several BAME communities, in D. Truswell (ed.) *Supporting People with Dementia in Black, Asian and Minority Ethnic Communities: Key Issues and Strategies for Change*. London: Jessica Kingsley.

Truth and Reconciliation Commission of Canada (TRCC) (2015) *Honouring the Truth, Reconciling for the Future: Summary of the Final Report of the Truth and Reconciliation Commission of Canada*. Winnipeg: Truth and Reconciliation Available at: https://nctr.ca/records/reports/.

UN General Assembly (2008) *United Nations Declaration on the Rights of Indigenous Peoples*. Resolution adopted by the General Assembly, A/RES/61/295. Available at: https://www.un.org/development/desa/indigenouspeoples/declaration-on-%20 the-rights-of-indigenous-peoples.html.

Vernooij-Dassen, M. and Moniz-Cook, E. (2016) Person-centred dementia care: moving beyond caregiving, *Aging and Mental Health*, 20 (7): 667–68.

Walker, J.D., Spiro, G., Loewen, K., et al. (2020) Alzheimer's disease and related dementia in Indigenous populations: a systematic review of risk factors, *Journal of Alzheimer's Disease*, 78 (4): 1439–51.

Walker, J.D., O'Connell, M.E., Pitawanakwat, K., et al. (2021a) Canadian Indigenous Cognitive Assessment (CICA): inter-rater reliability and criterion validity in Anishinaabe communities on Manitoulin Island, Canada, *Alzheimer's and Dementia*, 13: e12213. Available at: https://doi.org/10.1002/dad2.12213.

Walker, J.D., Crowshoe, L., Rowat, J., et al. (2021b) Understanding diagnosis of dementia in Indigenous populations, in *World Alzheimer Report 2021: Journey through the diagnosis of dementia*. London: Alzheimer's Disease International. Available at: https://www.alzint.org/u/World-Alzheimer-Report-2021.pdf.

Williams, T., Dearden, A. and Cameron, I. (2001) From pillar to post: a study of younger people with dementia, *Psychiatric Bulletin*, 25: 384–87.

 **Young onset dementia and employment**

*Louise Ritchie, Laura Lebec
and Rachel Allen*

Overview

Employment is increasingly being recognised as an issue for people with young onset dementia. This chapter aims to outline the experiences of people with young onset dementia in the workplace and the support required to facilitate a positive employment outcome. The chapter will explore the role of employment in maintaining identity and well-being, as well as the other roles people with young onset dementia take in society to maintain purpose in their lives. The chapter concludes with an example of current research that aims to develop an innovative intervention that will support people with young onset dementia with employment and maintaining purposeful activity after diagnosis.

Keywords

Employment, workplace, career, employment support, purposeful activity, identity.

Learning points

- Employment is an integral part of an individual's identity.
- Currently, people with young onset dementia have varied and inconsistent support for employment.
- There is an urgent need to develop person-centred supports for people living with dementia to enable them to negotiate adjustments and make decisions about whether and when to leave work.
- Better awareness of young onset dementia in the workplace may help to improve experiences of employees who develop dementia.
- Career guidance has the potential to provide employment-related support for people with young onset dementia.

Introduction

Many people are still employed when diagnosed with young onset dementia. They may have experienced early symptoms of dementia whilst still in employment, they may have continued working during the diagnostic period, or they may have experienced difficulties in work resulting in them losing employment or taking sick leave. Current research and anecdotal evidence reports varied experiences with employment following a diagnosis of young onset dementia. Regardless of the experience, however, support around employment is essential for people with young onset dementia. Drawing on current research and case studies, this chapter will outline the experiences of people with young onset dementia in employment and the supports required to facilitate positive employment experiences post-diagnosis.

It is important to acknowledge that a positive employment experience does not necessarily mean continuing to work in a job that the person has always done. A positive employment experience could be continuing in a job with appropriate support, but it could also be a well-supported retirement process or being facilitated to explore other options to engage in purposeful activity, such as volunteering, research involvement, advocacy roles and so on (see Chapter 10 for further consideration of meaningful non-employment activities). Whether a person wishes to remain at work or to retire, it is important to recognise that people living with dementia have rights as well as wishes. The Equality Act 2010 gives a person diagnosed while working an entitlement to reasonable adjustments to enable them to remain at work and to protection from discrimination (see Chapter 7 and below for further detail). A person-centred approach is essential when considering employment support, with a focus on what is important to the individual and recognition of the importance of employment to maintaining well-being.

Dementia and employment: understanding the experiences

Over the last 10 years, there has been increasing research interest around the experiences of people with dementia in employment. Qualitative studies have provided insight into the experiences of people who are diagnosed whilst in employment and have helped us to understand the impact of this on their lives. The first symptoms of dementia are often experienced in the workplace and the way this is managed can be crucial for the outcome of the individual. A timely diagnosis is the first step in ensuring a positive employment outcome and limiting the potential financial and social implications of an unplanned workplace exit (Kilty et al., 2023). Our research has established that with appropriate support, people living with dementia can – and do – continue to work after diagnosis (Ritchie et al., 2018). However, the support required can be complex to manage and requires a person- and job-focused approach that addresses what a person can do, rather than what they cannot do (Ritchie et al., 2020).

Employment and identity

It is well established that employment is closely linked to identity, with the benefits of employment reaching far beyond financial remuneration. What a person does for a job, and indeed their career over their life span, can make up a core part of their self-identity and is intrinsically linked to their own well-being. Work roles are found to be integral to the stories of people living with young onset dementia (Chaplin and Davidson, 2016) and our occupational roles are often the most important to us (Bimrose, 2006). Therefore, the intersection of being diagnosed with dementia with an unplanned or unexpected loss of employment after diagnosis has been referred to as a 'double insult' to identity (Robertson and Evans, 2015: 2332).

The first symptoms of dementia are often noticed in the workplace (Ohman et al., 2001; Roach and Drummond, 2014; Ritchie et al., 2018; Evans, 2019). As a result, a person who is developing young onset dementia may experience a shift from knowing they are a competent worker, to making mistakes and feeling unable to explain the reasons for them. This can compromise the person's sense of identity (Ritchie et al., 2018; Andrew et al., 2019).

Along with memory difficulties, symptoms experienced in the workplace include 'tiredness, increased sensitivity in stressful situations, difficulty in reading and writing, and in concentrating and initiating tasks' (Ohman et al., 2001: 37–38), 'feeling irritated, anxious, or fatigued' (Issakainen et al., 2021: 8), and 'loss of ability across many domains' (van Vliet et al., 2017: 1889). Everyday tasks often require more effort (Wawrziczny et al., 2016). The inconsistency (Ritchie et al., 2015), nature (Ohman et al., 2001) and unpredictability (Ashworth, 2020) of symptoms continues to create uncertainty for the individual and can often lead to people taking sick leave or being subjected to disciplinary procedures.

These difficulties and challenges at work can result in a person being perceived as a 'poor worker' by colleagues and others. This causes distress and results in further negative impact on a person's dignity and sense of self (Evans, 2019; Issakainen et al., 2021). Therefore, receiving a timely diagnosis of dementia is an important step to understanding the causes of a change in an employee's work performance and accessing the support required to mitigate negative consequences. People may be reluctant to disclose their diagnosis to employers but it is important to remember that employers have legal obligations towards their employees, including those with a diagnosis of young onset dementia. Employers' obligations give employees the right to raise the issue and expect a non-discriminatory response. Disclosing a diagnosis to an employer should be an opportunity for the person to make sense of what is happening and, ultimately, actively participate in decision-making to ensure a positive employment outcome (Nygard et al., 2023). This may be a decision to continue working, a plan for phased retirement, or a decision to leave the workplace. The important part is that the person has the opportunity to influence their own life, giving them control of the situation, which can profoundly impact their ability to live well (Issakainen et al., 2021).

As our understanding of the experience of dementia at work increases, so does our understanding of how to support a person with dementia with employment issues. We know that it is possible to continue working after diagnosis of dementia (Ritchie et al., 2018) and that people with dementia can continue to make a meaningful contribution to society in a variety of ways. The chapter will next focus on the support required for continuing paid employment, followed by a discussion of the wide and varied roles that people with dementia play in society and the contribution this makes to maintaining well-being and identity.

Supporting employees with dementia: reasonable adjustments

Whilst there is increased awareness that it is possible to continue employment after diagnosis of dementia, there is still a limited amount of information about the types of support that can help a person continue work. In the UK, the Equality Act 2010 prohibits employers discriminating against employees because of age or disability and other protected characteristics and requires employees to make reasonable adjustments to support the individual to access, maintain or return to work. However, research highlights that people who develop dementia whilst in employment do not always receive the 'reasonable adjustments' in the workplace to which they are entitled under the Equality Act (Chaplin and Davidson, 2016) and workplaces are not well equipped to identify and support workers with a cognitive impairment (Evans, 2019). There are a number of reasons for this, including stigma around dementia, not disclosing the diagnosis to employers, and lack of clarity around 'reasonable adjustments'.

Supporting employees with dementia includes developing policies and guidelines for someone experiencing cognitive decline (Cox and Pardasani, 2013) but the question of what reasonable adjustments or accommodations can be made depends on a number of factors, including the job role and the individual work tasks (Karjalainen et al., 2022). Reasonable adjustments need to be agreed in conjunction with the employee and the organisation and should be both person- and situation-specific. It has been suggested that occupational therapists could play an important part in identifying reasonable work adjustments to support the employee to remain in work (McCulloch et al., 2016; Ritchie et al., 2018). Research has sought to define the kind of workplace that is accessible for a person living with a cognitive impairment, as well as better understanding the kinds of accommodations needed for the individual to continue working (Karjalainen et al., 2022). Underpinning this is supportive workplace relationships, including the employee-manager relationship and having supportive colleagues. This allows for open and honest communication of needs and active responses in terms of the individual adjustments required (Karjalainen et al., 2022). Researchers have identified individual adjustments and measures that can be taken to support people with a diagnosis of young onset dementia in the workplace (Ohman et al., 2001; Egdell et al., 2021; Karjalainen et al., 2022). They include:

- modifying work tasks;
- changing roles/responsibilities;
- the use of memory aids;
- offering flexible working;
- remote working;
- re-deployment;
- additional IT support; and
- provision of individual guidance and opportunities to discuss work with one's supervisor.

An exploration of vocational rehabilitation for workers with dementia identifies that workplace support follows a phase of assessing the situation and telling people about the diagnosis and occurs prior to planning a move to a new role or leaving work (Evans et al., 2021).

It is essential that the person with young onset dementia has open and honest conversations about their diagnosis and the impact of their symptoms with their employer (Ritchie et al., 2018) to discuss the adjustments that they will require. Both the UN Convention on the Rights of Persons with Disabilities 2006 and the UK's Equality Act 2010 provide for the right to reasonable adjustments and accommodations at work (Egdell et al., 2018). Additional complexities are added to conversations about diagnosis due to the existing preconceptions some employers hold about dementia, often leading to knee-jerk assumptions about what is best for the employee (Egdell et al., 2021). Many employers base their assumptions about what a person with dementia can do on their own personal experiences and media representations of dementia, with a focus on older people at the later stages of the disease. They often bring this understanding to their position as an employer. A diverse and positive workplace culture supports an environment that enables open and honest conversations to take place. Employees disclosing a diagnosis need to do so knowing they will be supported based on their individual needs rather than on any assumptions employers may have related to dementia.

Although there are few examples of empirical data showing how workplace support happens in practice, the intentions of workplaces when surveyed indicate they would try to respect a person's wishes to work and aim to make that possible (Ritchie et al., 2018; Omote et al., 2020). However, not all workplace interventions in response to disclosing a diagnosis of dementia are helpful. Examples included managers and colleagues observing an employee with dementia covertly (Chaplin and Davidson, 2016) and too much support being provided (Ikeuchi et al., 2022). Excessive workplace support can be disempowering for the person with dementia, in particular when they are not consulted about those changes (Ikeuchi et al., 2022). Employees with young onset dementia should be involved in addressing their own work needs (Issakainen et al., 2021), and this benefits both the employee and employer (Chaplin and Davidson, 2016).

Janet's story: Being supported to continue at work

Janet is a finance officer who was diagnosed with young onset dementia at age 54 in a large organisation. After diagnosis, Janet decided to have an open conversation with her line manager, with the support of her healthcare professional, about the problems she was having in her work. This allowed them to agree a range of adjustments to support Janet to continue working, including assistive software, memory aids and flexible working to support daily tasks. Janet agreed to have regular check-ins with her line manager, which provided opportunities for review. The flexible, inclusive workplace policies that were already in place in her organisation were used to allow her to continue contributing meaningfully to her role, supporting her to maintain normalcy and to continue to provide financial support for her family after diagnosis.

Holistic adjustment of workplaces

While making adjustments on an individual basis may comply with legislation, adjusting existing workplace practice and policies to be inclusive of dementia can ensure the wider inclusion of those living with dementia. Research has started to explore how technology and design interventions could be integrated to provide more effective support (Rodgers, 2021; Shastri et al., 2021). Shastri et al. (2021) identified the untapped potential to develop technologies for supporting people in the workplace, ideally using clear and simple technology, including smart phones that people are already familiar with (see also Chapter 5 on technology). They recognise that, in the work setting, developing cognitively accessible technology could support people to have more agency in how they engage with work.

Rodgers (2021) reports on a series of future work initiatives for people living with dementia where design is used as a disruptive force for good, aiming to allow a person to exercise their right to work and engage in productive, creative and rewarding employment. The disruptive design approach encourages varied solutions to issues by emphasising fun, safe failure and doing things differently. For example, an innovative retail enterprise showcased a variety of creative products, such as ceramics and homeware, co-designed and produced by people with dementia. This research looks to disrupt perceptions, showing that people with a diagnosis of dementia have much to offer society through remaining in the workplace (Rodgers, 2021).

Dementia awareness in the workplace

An important employment support for employees with dementia is dementia awareness training for their colleagues. People with dementia have reported dementia awareness training as one of the most helpful things in enabling them to continue working (Ritchie et al., 2018). However, dementia awareness in the workplace needs to go beyond basic dementia awareness and explore ways to apply understanding of dementia to the workplace context. Training can help colleagues and employers to understand the impact of symptoms on the employee, so they can understand the types of supports a person may need. It also helps to create an open dialogue among colleagues where they can offer support and the employee can discuss their needs.

It is therefore essential that we improve access to dementia awareness training throughout organisations. This will help to challenge preconceptions about the ability of people with dementia to meaningfully contribute to the workforce and improve the experiences of employees in future. Improving knowledge about and attitudes towards dementia in workplaces will help to shift from a deficit-focused perspective to focusing on abilities and meaningful contributions that can be made by employees with dementia (Nygard et al., 2023).

Job loss and financial impacts

While it is possible to continue employment, the reality for many people living with young onset dementia is job loss, through early retirement, dismissal or redundancy. A direct consequence of this is loss of income (Mayrhofer et al., 2021). One study showed that employees with young onset dementia were more likely to leave their jobs sooner than people without young onset dementia (Sakata and Okumura, 2017). In this study the authors found that 14% of participants left their jobs within a year of a diagnosis, which was twice the rate of those without young onset dementia. They conclude that healthcare providers should be providing advice and support to people living with young onset dementia and their families on employment just after the initial diagnosis (Sakata and Okumura, 2017).

Job loss may lead to financial difficulties impacting those with the diagnosis and their families (Tolson et al., 2015; Roach et al., 2016; Bayly et al., 2021). Spouses may have to take up employment, in addition to caring responsibilities, to mitigate the loss of income, which could put a strain on relationships (Kilty et al., 2023). People have further reported losing not just their incomes but also the ability to continue with pension contributions (Mayrhofer et al., 2021). Following job loss, the person may have difficulty finding alternative employment due to their symptoms (Bayly et al., 2021) and it may be difficult to secure government financial assistance if the job loss has been related to performance issues (Roach et al., 2016; Bayly et al., 2021). Leaving work has been reported as being a difficult and emotional decision to make (Tolson et al., 2015). Research further indicates that job loss is associated with a loss of the employee's 'locus of control' (Chaplin and Davidson, 2016: 14). Employees report feeling abandoned by the workplace subsequent to their dismissal (Chaplin and Davidson, 2016). This loss of control can also have a negative impact on the person's mental health (Tolson et al., 2015).

Income losses, depleted savings and unexpected care costs have been described as creating a 'triple effect', creating anxiety around current affordability of life (Mayrhofer et al., 2021), further exacerbated by the current cost of living crisis. The lack of ability to plan for future care needs typically results in anxiety, a sense of disempowerment and stress (Mayrhofer et al., 2021; Kilty et al., 2023). Where people have left their employment or experience difficulties with memory or behaviour prior to receiving a diagnosis of dementia, significant financial strain on households has been reported. People may, for example, find it hard to meet mortgage payments and other household expenses for their dependents (Kilty et al., 2023). The altered financial prospects may result in families having to reduce spending, having difficulty in meeting daily needs, or even selling the family home (Bayly et al., 2021). Receiving a diagnosis of dementia while in the workplace undoubtedly has a serious effect on a person's employment and financial situation, but it is also clear that this has a devastating impact on the wider family unit (Kilty et al., 2023).

Research has shown that people who are diagnosed with dementia whilst in employment need access to specialist advice and information about employment rights, remuneration and pension status (Kilty et al., 2023). Ensuring that a diagnosis is received in good time would help improve the situation, with greater work clarity and supportive employment processes (Kilty et al., 2023). Lack of clarity of processes and procedures around needs assessments, carers' assessments and financial assessments by different organisations resulted in some families having to ask for legal advice and, in some cases, involved lengthy appeal processes (Mayrhofer et al., 2021). These findings highlight a major gap in financial supports for people with young onset dementia (Bayly et al., 2021).

Working beyond diagnosis

Up until this point, this chapter has focused on paid employment and maintaining job roles that people may have done for most of their lives. However, many people with dementia express relief at leaving work due to the stress of trying to cope with symptoms in the work environment (Ritchie et al., 2018). Those who leave work, in whatever situation, often express that they feel that they still have something meaningful to contribute to society. On the other hand, people also feel that if they had had appropriate and timely support whilst still in work, they could have continued. The sense of normalcy and being useful that can be gained from work, is essential to the overall well-being of people with young onset dementia (Kinney et al., 2011; Stamou et al., 2023). It is therefore important, when discussing employment for people with young onset dementia, that we focus on the wide and varied roles people hold in society that could be viewed as a form of work.

Our current research project at the University of the West of Scotland is exploring the potential of career guidance services to support people with young onset dementia. Career guidance practitioners are qualified professionals who provide support and advice to people about their careers. They take a life course approach and can support decision-making around career at any age up to and beyond retirement. Career guidance could make a beneficial contribution at this point in a person's life, by ensuring people with dementia have the option to remain in work, explore the decision-making needed prior to the cessation of work or to explore the other options available to them. Career development interventions, such as guidance interviews and career planning tools, can support the cessation of work, the start of retirement and beyond (Bolger et al., 2023). In our current research project, co-researchers living with dementia are essential to the success of the project. Working in partnership with the researchers and career guidance practitioners, people with young onset dementia are helping us refine the career guidance approach to support people with the condition. As a group, this is underpinned by the concept that living a purposeful life with dementia is required for well-being and that each individual will have different aspirations in terms of what they want to do with their lives, and support should respond to that.

Workplace placement programmes have received some attention over the last decade. These are programmes where people living with young onset dementia, who are no longer able to maintain employment, are provided with opportunities to work alongside employees in other workplaces, instead of attending services such as day care, which may not be appropriate. GOOTH (Get Out Of The House) is an example of a workplace placement programme. In this project, people living with dementia undertook work at a zoo and benefited from socialisation with one another while doing activities they enjoyed (Kinney et al., 2011). Side by Side involved people living with dementia having a 'buddy' at a local hardware store and working with them one day per week (Robertson et al., 2013). These programmes have demonstrated the social benefits of engaging in work, as well as promoting normalcy and routine for individuals. Being in work environments takes the focus away from dementia and focuses again on the skills and abilities of the individual (Kinney et al., 2011; Robertson et al., 2013).

However, while they have promise, programmes like these are not widely available and it is essential that we broaden our view of work for people with young onset dementia to ensure that we maximise the opportunities available to engage in other work-like purposeful activities. People living with young onset dementia are increasingly engaged in research involvement activities, policy influencing and activist roles. From our own research, people living with dementia identify research involvement, working with the Scottish Dementia Working Group and other activities as a form of work. This provides purpose and focus and allows them to maintain confidence by using the skills they have developed over their careers (see Chapter 11 for further discussion of involvement in research).

Alternative activities that could be viewed in a similar way include other caring responsibilities, hobbies (Pipon-Young et al., 2011), campaigning

(Bartlett, 2014), advocacy (Broders and Wiersma, 2022), housekeeping and gardening (Ohman et al., 2001; van Vliet et al., 2017). These types of activities have been found to be important for engagement with the world and provide important opportunities to socialise with others living with young onset dementia (Pipon-Young et al., 2011).

For a person living with young onset dementia, having access to a range of activities and finding a purpose in life after diagnosis is essential to living well. This may be representing people with young onset dementia on high profile political arenas, as some do. Equally, it may be volunteering at a local charity using their electrical expertise to conduct PAT testing to check the safety of electrical items that are being repurposed to families in need, as one participant in a past study did. What is important is that people are supported to realise that they still have skills and abilities that can make a meaningful contribution to society. This could be managed through post-diagnosis services, or we could look to other organisations and services that could provide this support. Such opportunities for meaningful activity are addressed in greater depth in Chapter 10.

Mark's story: Meaningful work-like activity

Mark was diagnosed with young onset dementia at age 60 after experiencing difficulties at his work. He was an electrical engineer and began making small mistakes at work, such as misplacing tools and forgetting to return from his breaks on time. A more serious mistake when Mark left a live electrical panel unsecured and unattended in the busy factory floor resulted in the threat of disciplinary action. Following this, Mark took sick leave from work and the diagnosis process started. When he received his diagnosis, it was recommended by his employer that he take early retirement. Although he stopped paid employment, Mark was keen to maintain his technical skills and find alternative options for work after his diagnosis. He found an opportunity to volunteer for a second-hand furniture charity performing electric testing on small appliances to be donated to families in need. The charity provided a supportive environment, with opportunities for social interaction. Despite leaving his paid employment, Mark found a new opportunity for purposeful activity by continuing to use his skills in a way to make a meaningful contribution to his local community.

Conclusions

It is very common that people with young onset dementia experience employment issues. There is a wide range of challenges that people with young onset dementia will require support with having received their diagnosis. This will include support with identifying appropriate workplace supports, managing workplace relationships, financial and pension advice, and help in identifying opportunities to engage in other purposeful activity after leaving work, for example, volunteering, advocacy and research involvement activities. Although it is encouraging that employment for people with young onset dementia has received increased attention over the last decade, there is still a long way to go in ensuring that there is equity in the support people living with young onset dementia receive with employment. We urgently need increased research, robust policy development, and innovative interdisciplinary interventions to support people with young onset dementia in the workplace. Clear guidance for employers, as well as increased awareness of the meaningful contributions of people with young onset dementia make in society, will help to create positive employment experiences for those diagnosed with young onset dementia in the future.

What does this mean in practice?

If you have received a diagnosis of dementia in the workplace

It is possible for people with dementia to continue working after diagnosis, with appropriate support. In the UK, dementia is considered a disability under the Equality Act 2010, which requires employers to make reasonable adjustments to support employees and to help remain in employment. The following may be helpful when disclosing a diagnosis to an employer:

- Having support from a family member, colleague or trade union representative.
- Disclosing the diagnosis in a way you feel comfortable with, face-to-face, via an email, etc.
- Have a desired outcome from the meeting, for example, a referral to occupational health, specific forms of support.

If you employ someone who has been diagnosed with dementia

People with dementia who have continued working report that the routine and social interactions help to keep them well and preserve their self-confidence. Understanding what the employee is experiencing helps the employer to provide support and make well-informed adjustments to the individual's job description or work environment. Some key points to consider include:

- Dementia awareness training is a very helpful resource for employers and colleagues to support an employee with dementia.
- Dementia is likely to meet the definition of disability defined by the Equality Act 2010.
- Review existing policies and procedures to ensure they are dementia-friendly.

Some examples of 'reasonable adjustments' which have supported people with dementia to continue employment after diagnosis include: flexible working, such as altered shift patterns, reduced hours and working from home; memory aids, such as online calendars, providing written information and instructions; technology, including mobile phones and voice recognition technology; and environmental adaptations to reduce noise and distraction (see Chapter 5 for further information on technologies). If an employee decides to leave work, ensure there is a clear pathway to support this.

If you are working alongside someone with a diagnosis of dementia

If your co-worker has been open about their diagnosis, speak to them about it. They may be happy to explain to you the effect dementia has on their work and how they would prefer to be supported. If you have any worries about your co-worker, ensure there are open and appropriate channels for this to be discussed with management or human resources.

References

Andrew, C., Phillipson, L. and Sheridan, L. (2019) What is the impact of dementia on occupational competence, occupational participation and occupational identity for people who experience onset of symptoms while in paid employment? A scoping review, *Australian Occupational Therapy Journal*, 66 (2): 130–44.

Ashworth, R.M. (2020) Looking ahead to a future with Alzheimer's disease: coping with the unknown, *Ageing and Society*, 40 (8): 1647–68.

Bartlett, R. (2014) Citizenship in action: the lived experiences of citizens with dementia who campaign for social change, *Disability and Society*, 29 (8): 1291–1304.

Bayly, M., O'Connell, M.E., Kortzman, A., et al. (2021) Family carers' narratives of the financial consequences of young onset dementia, *Dementia*, 20 (8): 2708–24.

Bimrose, J. (2006) *The changing context of career practice: Guidance, counselling or coaching?* Centre for Guidance Studies, University of Derby. Available at: https://warwick.ac.uk/fac/soc/ier/people/jbimrose/publications/jb_changing_context_of_career_practice_final_31_8_06.pdf

Bolger, E., Egdell, V. and Ritchie, L. (2023) Dementia in the workplace: implications for career development practice, *British Journal of Guidance and Counselling*, 51 (1): 74–83.

Broders, K. and Wiersma, E. C. (2022) Creating change: the experiences of women living with young onset dementia, *Disability and Society*, 37 (5): 787–808.

Chaplin, R. and Davidson, I. (2016) What are the experiences of people with dementia in employment?, *Dementia*, 15 (2): 147–61.

Cox, C.B. and Pardasani, M. (2013) Alzheimer's in the workplace: a challenge for social work, *Journal of Gerontological Social Work*, 56 (8): 643–56.

Egdell, V., Stavert, J. and McGregor, R. (2018) The legal implications of dementia in the workplace: establishing a cross-disciplinary research agenda, *Ageing and Society*, 38 (11): 2181–96.

Egdell, V., Cook, M., Stavert, J., et al. (2021) Dementia in the workplace: are employers supporting employees living with dementia?, *Aging and Mental Health*, 25 (1): 134–41.

Evans, D. (2019) An exploration of the impact of younger-onset dementia on employment, *Dementia*, 18 (1): 262–81.

Evans, D., Murray, C., Berndt, A., et al. (2021) Supporting people with dementia in employment, in L.-F. Low and K. Laver (eds.) *Dementia Rehabilitation: Evidence-Based Interventions and Clinical Recommendations*. London: Academic Press.

Ikeuchi, S., Omote, S., Tanaka, K., et al. (2022). Work-related experiences of people living with young-onset dementia in Japan, *Health and Social Care in the Community*, 30 (2): 548–57.

Issakainen, M., Mäki-Petäjä-Leinonen, A., Heimonen, S., et al. (2021) Experiences of influencing one's own life when living with working-age dementia, *Ageing and Society*, 43 (8): 1934–53.

Karjalainen, K., Issakainen, M., Ylhäinen, M., et al. (2022) Supporting continued work under the UNCRPD – views of employees living with mild cognitive impairment or early onset dementia, *International Journal of Discrimination and the Law*, 22 (4): 371–85.

Kilty, C., Cahill, S., Foley, T., et al. (2023) Young onset dementia: implications for employment and finances, *Dementia*, 22 (1): 68–84.

Kinney, J.M., Kart, C.S. and Reddecliff, L. (2011) 'That's me, the Goother': evaluation of a program for individuals with early-onset dementia, *Dementia*, 10 (3): 361–77.

Mayrhofer, A.M., Greenwood, N., Smeeton, N., et al. (2021) Understanding the financial impact of a diagnosis of young onset dementia on individuals and families in the United Kingdom: results of an online survey, *Health and Social Care in the Community*, 29 (3): 664–71.

McCulloch, S., Robertson, D. and Kirkpatrick, P. (2016) Sustaining people with dementia or mild cognitive impairment in employment: a systematic review of qualitative evidence, *British Journal of Occupational Therapy*, 79 (11): 682–92.

Nygard, L., Nedlund, A.C., Maki Petaja Leinonen, A. et al. (2023) What happens when people develop dementia whilst working? An exploratory multiple case study, *International Journal of Qualitative Studies on Health and Well-being*, 18 (1): 2176278. Available at: https://doi.org/10.1080/17482631.2023.2176278.

Ohman, A., Nygard, L. and Borell, L. (2001) The vocational situation in cases of memory deficits or younger-onset dementia, *Scandinavian Journal of Caring Sciences*, 15 (1): 34–43.

Omote, S., Ikeuchi, S., Ishiwata, T., et al. (2020). Investigation into the factors relating to the intention of workplaces to retain employees diagnosed with young onset dementia, *Journal of Wellness and Health Care*, 44 (1): 43–52.

Pipon-Young, F.E., Lee, K.M., Jones, F., et al. (2011) I'm not all gone, I can still speak: the experiences of younger people with dementia. An action research study, *Dementia*, 11 (5): 597–616.

Ritchie, L., Banks, P., Danson, M., et al. (2015) Dementia in the workplace: a review, *Journal of Public Mental Health*, 14 (1): 24–34.

Ritchie, L., Tolson, D. and Danson, M. (2018) Dementia in the workplace case study research: understanding the experiences of individuals, colleagues and managers, *Ageing and Society*, 38 (10): 2146–75.

Ritchie, L., Egdell, V., Danson, M., et al. (2020) Dementia, work and employability: using the capability approach to understand the employability potential for people living with dementia, *Work, Employment and Society*, 36 (4): 591–609.

Roach, P. and Drummond, N. (2014) 'It's nice to have something to do': early-onset dementia and maintaining purposeful activity, *Journal of Psychiatric and Mental Health Nursing*, 21 (10): 889–95.

Roach, P., Drummond, N. and Keady, J. (2016) 'Nobody would say that it is Alzheimer's or dementia at this age': family adjustment following a diagnosis of early-onset dementia, *Journal of Aging Studies*, 36: 26–32.

Robertson, J. and Evans, D. (2015) Evaluation of a workplace engagement project for people with younger onset dementia, *Journal of Clinical Nursing*, 24 (15/16): 2331–39.

Robertson, J., Evans, D. and Horsnell, T. (2013) Side by Side: a workplace engagement program for people with younger onset dementia, *Dementia*, 12 (5): 666–74.

Rodgers, P. A. (2021) Designing work with people living with dementia: reflecting on a decade of research, *International Journal of Environmental Research in Public Health*, 18 (22): 11742. Available at: https://doi.org/10.3390/ijerph182211742.

Sakata, N. and Okumura, Y. (2017) Job loss after diagnosis of early-onset dementia: a matched cohort study, *Journal of Alzheimer's Disease*, 60 (4): 1231–35.

Shastri, K., Boger, J., Marashi, S., et al. (2021) Working towards inclusion: creating technology for and with people living with mild cognitive impairment or dementia who are employed, *Dementia*, 21 (2): 556–78.

Stamou, V., Oyebode, J., La Fontaine, J., et al. (2023) Good practice in needs-based post-diagnostic support for people with young onset dementia: findings from the Angela Project, *Ageing and Society*. Available at: https://doi.org/10.1017/S0144686X22001362.

Tolson, D., Ritchie, L., Danson, M., et al. (2015) *Dementia in the workplace: the potential for continued employment post-diagnosis*, University of the West of Scotland. Available at: https://research-portal.uws.ac.uk/en/publications/dementia-in-the-workplace-the-potential-for-continued-employment-.

Van Vliet, D., Persoon, A., Bakker, C., et al. (2017) Feeling useful and engaged in daily life: exploring the experiences of people with young-onset dementia, *International Psychogeriatrics*, 29 (11): 1889–98.

Wawrziczny, E., Pasqier, F., Ducharme, F., et al. (2016) From 'needing to know' to 'needing not to know more': an interpretative phenomenological analysis of couples' experiences with early-onset Alzheimer's disease, *Scandinavian Journal of Caring Sciences*, 30 (4): 695–703.

11 Meaningful activity

Jacqui Hussey and Jan Oyebode

Overview

Having access to age-appropriate, meaningful activities is vital for maintaining a sense of identity, enabling people to maintain their hobbies and express their talents and indeed learn new ones. This chapter will show how sporting, creative and social activities can be offered in a personalised way to people living with young onset dementia. It will also synthesise evidence that shows how effective activity is in reducing isolation, improving well-being and preventing crisis. It will provide specific examples supported, where possible, by empirical research on the types of activity that are beneficial and how they can be delivered. Importantly, it will include feedback from people living with young onset dementia as to the types of activities they wish to access.

Keywords

Age-appropriate, purposeful, choice, risk-positive, empowering, social connection, reduced neuropsychiatric symptoms, reduced anti-psychotic prescribing, well-being.

Learning points

- Younger people living with dementia wish to remain active and engaged. The focus should be on ability, not disability.
- Meaningful activity can improve well-being and results in fewer neuropsychiatric symptoms.
- Adapting services for people living with young onset dementia requires risk-positive approaches.

Introduction

When people first develop the symptoms of young onset dementia, they are likely to be in employment and to be physically active. As memory, communication impairment and/or difficulties in planning and problem-solving emerge, this can make it more challenging to maintain performance at work or to engage in hobbies. By the time of a diagnosis of young onset dementia in the UK, 80% of people have stopped working (London Assembly Health Committee, 2018).

Our needs, hopes and expectations vary according to our different stages of life and most people in their forties, fifties or early sixties expect to be usefully employed and active. Lack of appropriate activities can result in a loss of identity and sense of purpose (Roach and Drummond, 2014), a decline in health, reduced social engagement, and increased risk of psychological and behavioural distress, such as anxiety, depression, agitation and apathy (Bakker et al., 2014).

Whilst cognitive decline may be inevitable in dementia, there is evidence that purposeful activity offers quality of life (QoL) and well-being benefits to both those living with dementia and their families. This is particularly relevant in young onset dementia as differences in clinical manifestation between young and late onset dementia are most prominent with regard to mood disorders and behaviours that may present challenges. It is these aspects (rather than cognitive and functional changes) that are reported to result in more severe consequences for both those diagnosed and their family members (Werner et al., 2009).

Meaningful activity is one of the most frequent unmet needs identified for people living with young onset dementia (Van Vliet et al., 2017). Where people with young onset dementia have opportunities to engage in meaningful physical, cognitive or arts-based activities, these are valued as they reinforce identity and self-esteem (Stamou et al., 2023) and are likely to reduce problems such as restlessness or boredom. One participant in the Angela Project said:

> *I am still full of the person who I used to be, who I am. I am still full of the young-ness, full of energy and enthusiasm … So, what's important for me is something that's compatible with who I am … What's been good for me has been music and situations where people allow me to express myself or recognise what I want to do is relevant.* (Stamou et al., 2023: 13)

Overall, it is important for people living with young onset dementia to have sources of activity that are meaningful and give a sense of accomplishment and contribution to society.

Research evidence

In the health or social care context, activities, hobbies or pastimes that are introduced to improve cognitive or emotional well-being, tend to be conceptualised as 'interventions'. This allows them to be packaged in a reasonably standardised, replicable way that, in turn, means their effectiveness can be tested versus 'treatment as usual'. However, despite the proliferation of interventions, there is a dearth of research looking at their application and benefits in young onset dementia.

Mayrhofer et al. (2018) carried out a systematic review of age-appropriate services for people diagnosed with young onset dementia and identified just 10 peer-reviewed papers which were eligible for inclusion over a 26-year period. Some of these are included later in this chapter. An overview of approaches to promote engagement of individuals with all-age frontotemporal dementia (FTD) by Kortte and Rogalski (2013) showed that activity-based programmes such as painting, collage and theatre improvisation workshops may improve mood and quality of life. They can also create environments which can sublimate socially inappropriate behaviour (that is, they open up ways for people who have potentially problematic behaviour to express themselves in acceptable ways). Individuals with primary progressive aphasia, in particular, appear to benefit from activity-based intervention groups rather than ones based on more verbal interactions (Kortte and Rogalski, 2013).

Anti-psychotic prescribing is thought to be higher in younger onset dementia because these medications are prescribed to lessen the physical challenges associated with agitation. There is possible evidence that regular activity reduces levels of anti-psychotic prescribing. The Younger People with Dementia (YPWD CIO) charity, which provides a weekly programme of activity workshops for people living with young onset dementia, found a low percentage (4.9%) of their attendees were taking anti-psychotic medication (Hussey et al., 2016) compared with a community-based study of 196 people with young onset dementia, of whom 17.3% were prescribed anti-psychotic medication (Koopmans et al., 2014).

To date, most of the research that considers activity-based interventions consists of anecdotal self-reports. There have been very few attempts to quantify outcomes using standard measures, and even fewer that compare the relative benefits of different activities. This represents a significant gap in current knowledge because whilst it is obviously important for people with young onset dementia to have a choice of activities, it is also important to understand the potential impact (and provide hard evidence) of the value of those activities to convince service funders and commissioners to invest in them. There is a clear need for primary intervention studies looking at the impact of meaningful activity. Randomised controlled studies (RCTs), which are viewed as the gold standard, can be hard to conduct in young onset dementia given the rarity of the condition and the varied diagnoses. These factors can make it hard to recruit sufficient numbers of participants for RCTs. However, rigorous qualitative studies and effectively designed single-case series that take individual differences into account could provide useful evidence of efficacy and impact.

Despite the lack of research studies, there is emerging evidence of what younger people living with dementia find useful, which can help to shape services and inform further research.

What activities do people with young onset dementia experience as helpful?

The simple answer is anything an individual finds interesting and relevant. In a quantitative study which looked at why formal services were not being used, people living with young onset dementia and their carers identified five aspects of an ideal service – such a service needs to be unique, flexible, affordable, tailored and meaningful (Cations et al., 2017). These key elements help to support personalised engagement programmes and their accessibility.

Meaningful activity

As noted in Chapter 1, the Angela Project found that services which provide joint working and seek the opinion of people with young onset dementia provide a sense of empowerment, togetherness and of being valued. Maintaining autonomy and 'being myself' through access to age-appropriate services, meaningful activity, relationships, giving/contributing and normalcy were some of the key themes (Stamou et al., 2023).

In the field of dementia generally, a wide range of 'leisure pursuits' have been evaluated for their benefits to those living with dementia (Gray et al., 2023). Many of these can be tailored to age-related factors, such as physical capabilities and generational interests. Meaningful activity can encompass a range of pursuits from household tasks to hobbies, social activities, arts-based activities (such as shared reading, singing, and arts and crafts), volunteering and reminiscence activities (such as sporting memories), through to more physically challenging activities such as gardening, running and cycling (Kinney et al., 2011; Hewitt et al., 2013; Carone et al., 2016; Sansoni et al., 2016). Offering choice is fundamental.

It is not just about being occupied but also about being able to participate in something that is purposeful and rewarding. Focus groups of people with young onset dementia and caregivers in the Netherlands identified a sense of usefulness from having a social role or participating in functional activity, although over time the *pleasure* from activities seemed to supersede a sense of usefulness (Van Vliet et al., 2017). Meaningful activity was also one of 11 themes expressed by people with young onset dementia and their family members in qualitative research by Bannon et al. (2022). Those with young onset dementia wished to stay cognitively challenged, learn new skills and engage in activities that would advance their health and well-being.

Suitable activities vary according to an individual's personality, previous interests and physical health. The suitability of purposeful activity is an important consideration as unsuitable activities may be poorly attended and lack efficacy. Approaches and adaptations need to accommodate a range of cognitive difficulties often experienced in young onset dementia, which can include language and behavioural changes and not just memory loss (see Chapter 3). Activities need to be flexibly adjusted according to changing needs and progression of symptoms.

Age-appropriateness

Traditional services for dementia are designed to meet the needs of older adults and consequently are not relevant and lack appeal to younger adults with dementia who are often physically fitter and identify more with people of their own age. The older age of attendees at mainstream day care services can mean younger people are reluctant to attend (Millenaar et al., 2016). In an Australian study, it was revealed that younger people with dementia were offered activities that were not age-appropriate and, paradoxically, were sometimes unable to access services because they were too young (Cations et al., 2017).

Normality (normalcy)

People should be defined by what they are able or have the potential to do, not by their diagnosis and disability. Enabling people with young onset dementia to continue to live their normal lives supports this positive stance. The Dementia Pathfinders Community Interest Group, a not-for-profit social enterprise which provides 'learning opportunities, resources and services, to enable people with dementia and their families to live with hope, creativity and meaning' (see https://www.dementiapathfinders.org/) sent a clear message that people living with young onset dementia wish to continue with 'normal life' for as long as possible.

> You do not need to put plans on hold or limit your life unduly. Learning to live with dementia includes continuing doing things you enjoy and keeping life as 'normal' as possible. You might need to adapt activities slightly, but life is not over! (Dementia Pathfinders Community Interest Group, 2015)

The Angela Project found that people wish to maintain their identity and 'be seen as adults' (Stamou et al., 2023). One step towards this is to reconsider the use of language that could infantilise or put the individual in the sick role. How often are people 'taken on walks' rather than 'accompanied', 'supervised' as opposed to 'working alongside', or are offered 'painting' when they could be offered 'art classes'? The wish to avoid identity being overtaken by dementia is expressed by a participant in one 2020 study: *'I don't want to be him-with-dementia. I want to live as normal as possible'* (Busted et al., 2020: 4).

Where possible, activities should be offered in community settings, which are often more accessible and provide a sense of normality. The dementia-friendly approach of making appropriate modifications to an existing environment (e.g. by improving signage) can enable access to community venues. A 'dementia-capable' approach that embraces people living with dementia as part of the wider 'disability community' can also be helpful (Lin and Lewis, 2015). Inclusion in the community also helps to educate communities and reduce stigma.

Empowerment

Many people with young onset dementia like to speak about their experiences of living with dementia and express their fears, current needs, ways of coping and their wishes for the future (Busted et al., 2020). Some have found positions on Dementia Boards such as the UK Young Dementia Network steering group and other advisory groups, become members of research advisory groups, lectured at conferences and written books and poetry. Keith Oliver's book *Dear*

Alzheimer's: A Diary of Living with Dementia (2019) and Wendy Mitchell's blog (https://whichmeamitoday.wordpress.com/blog/) and her three books (Mitchell, 2018, 2022, 2023) are shining examples. By sharing their experiences, Keith, Wendy and many other people with young onset dementia have been able to provide valuable insights about their challenges and the strategies they use, and also instil hope for others. Such advocacy and activist roles provide purpose, give identity, and raise self-efficacy and self-esteem.

Empowerment groups such as DEEP (Dementia Engagement and Empowerment Project: https://www.dementiavoices.org.uk/) which comprise, at the time of writing, 80 groups of people living with dementia across the UK, many of them with young onset, promote self-efficacy through raising awareness of dementia and campaigning.

Social engagement

Regular attendance at groups which provide continuity and familiarity fosters identity and belonging (such as belonging to an art group) and helps to promote social relationships and peer support. People start to feel part of a community and have a feeling of 'togetherness' (Johannessen and Möller, 2013; Stamou et al., 2023).

It is recognised that not all people wish to participate in group activities. In the Angela Project, having a buddy who can provide one-to-one support to participate in an activity that is of personal interest was also identified as positive. Examples of activities include walks, going out for coffee, swimming, golf, furniture restoration and attending local community projects. One-to-one support can give people the confidence to join a group, but this depends on individual preference and specific needs. Referring to a buddy with whom he did joint activities, one of the men in the Angela Project said: *'It's just like having a more able version of myself'* (Stamou et al., 2023: 10).

Risk-positive approach

Younger people with dementia report feeling inhibited by the focus on danger and risk conveyed by professionals (Beattie et al., 2004). Over-emphasis on safety and risk neglects the psychological and social well-being of individuals and can reduce quality of life (Clarke and Mantle, 2016). With an emphasis on what people can no longer do, it is unsurprising that caregivers, family supporters and the individuals themselves can struggle to find the right risk balance. The decision to stop driving, for example, may be clear-cut but other aspects are more nuanced. Risk that is positively managed can be life-enhancing.

As an example, the YPWD CIO charity runs regular katakanuing sessions in the Spring and Summer months on the River Thames with an instructor and a member of YPWD staff. The katakanus are six-seater catamarans paddled with single-blade oars. Although this is a group activity, each person's level of ability is taken into account and participants are encouraged to try out paddling or observe the wildlife on the river. The sensory elements of this activity, taking

Table 11.1 Key elements to provide activities

Age-appropriate	Tailored	Meaningful	Normalising	Empowering
Cognitively challenging	Social engaging	Provide peer support	Provide autonomy	Risk-positive

in the sights and sounds of the river, are very important and attendees often reflect on how calming and peaceful the whole experience is.

> *He loves the katakanuing sessions, especially the camaraderie! He likes the feeling of being in nature and watching the birds etc. It's also good exercise for him and lifts his mood. It's also great that he has learned a new skill and feels such a sense of achievement afterwards.* (Family supporter whose husband joins YPWD activities)

The idea of 12 or more people living with young onset dementia katakanuing may seem 'risky' and indeed there are some inherent risks. However, it offers the person living with dementia the chance to spend time on the river working as part of a team and engaging in an activity that is physically challenging, fun and meaningful. Arguably, inactivity and boredom have their own risks, especially for younger people who are often still fit and physically active. Katakanuing channels energy in an observed environment. Scores on the Neuro Psychiatric Inventory (NPI), which measures behavioural and psychological aspects of dementia, have been shown to reduce by half over a 12-month period in people who took part (Hussey et al., 2016).

The key elements to provide beneficial activity, drawn from the research evidence and the experiences described above, are summarised in Table 11.1. Some activities will have a stronger focus on some elements than others and few will address all the elements. However, those that encompass several elements may prove particularly worthwhile.

Delivering meaningful activities

In this section, we provide specific examples of activities which are accessible, have tangible benefits and have been adapted for people living with young onset dementia.

Singing

The rationale

Music can stimulate social interaction, providing a way of relating to others. Singing with others provides a forum where interpersonal interactions can take place that may otherwise be difficult due to impaired verbal ability. It may also be inherently enjoyable and stimulating. Additionally, singing involves the coordinated action of motor, visuospatial and verbal mechanisms in a synergistic way (Sorrell and Sorrell, 2008).

The evidence

Music therapy such as the Alzheimer's Society 'Singing for the Brain' programme has gained recognition (Bannan and Montgomery-Smith, 2008). There is qualitative evidence that group singing can improve health and well-being and have a positive impact (Osman et al., 2016). Choral singing, in particular, has been shown to improve the attention skills of people with Alzheimer's disease (Bannan and Montgomery-Smith, 2008). Choirs have also been shown to have a positive impact on mood, cognitive stimulation, focused attention and social support (Clift et al., 2007), all very relevant to the challenges faced by younger people with dementia.

How it can be delivered

An example is the 'Harmony' choir, supported by YPWD CIO (http://www.ypwd.info), which was established for people living with young onset dementia and their family supporters in Berkshire. Regular members attend weekly on their own if they can, or with family supporters or other carers. All are welcome to stay and join in the singing. The choir is led by a local singer, musician and choir leader, who expressed an interest and passion for working with younger people with dementia and their family supporters. Other members of staff from YPWD CIO and volunteers are also involved.

The choir meets weekly in the same non-clinical setting, a community arts centre. On average, 30–35 people attend and those who start coming along tend to stay. The format seems to work for several reasons: it is familiar and provides routine, there are recognisable faces and a great sense of belonging. This helps to orientate those with dementia, whatever their level of impairment or ability.

Specific aspects of the leader's approach, including visual cues and prompts, help those with young onset dementia with their overall understanding and ability to join in, even if a person's comprehension of language is affected. Helpful techniques include repetition of phrases, visual demonstrations of how to make a more staccato sound, or a scale or progression of notes demonstrated by clever use of the leader's hands. People with mild to more severe impairment appear to benefit. Choir members have a range of diagnoses including Alzheimer's disease, frontotemporal dementia, dementia with Lewy bodies, posterior cortical atrophy and cerebral autosomal dominant arteriopathy with subcortical infarcts and leukoencephalopathy (CADASIL).

Harmony provides a sense of belonging and normalcy, friendship, peer support and fun. The choir also offers cognitive challenges that are sometimes out of the comfort zone: learning new songs, complex rhythms, warm-up exercises and meeting new people. It offers opportunities to perform to audiences including an annual Christmas concert and performances at St George's Chapel at Windsor Castle, which engender a sense of pride. Attendance at different venues helps to reduce stigma and provides empowerment as the audience are paying for their ticket, and the choir makes a wonderful sound which is applauded. Carers feed back that often they, too, see Harmony as their support network – a chance to connect and share experiences with other carers in similar situations.

> *Singing together is a great leveller. Once we are singing, there are no indicators as to who has dementia and who doesn't. We are all choir members for that time together. This is a time when very often happy memories are made and I feel like my old self.* (Member of Harmony who is living with dementia.)

Gardening

The rationale

Gardening provides an opportunity to be outdoors, use physical effort and be in a 'green' and multi-sensory environment. It can be social or solitary according to personal preference. These attributes can engender a feeling of relaxation and a sense of purpose and satisfaction from seeing the 'fruits' of one's labour. Working together in a green space can provide a sense of community, social activity and achievement.

The evidence

A systematic review of the impact of horticulture-based activities for people with dementia living in the community found eight relevant studies and concluded there were positive impacts on engagement, social interactions, and mental and physical well-being (Scott et al., 2022); and a further review and meta-analysis showed it to have significant benefits in reducing agitation and increasing engagement for older people with dementia living in care homes (Lu et al., 2020). However, it cannot be assumed these findings are transferable to people living with young onset dementia, due to differences in life stage and nature of dementia.

Only one study has been published that is specific to young onset dementia. In 2013, Hewitt and colleagues evaluated the impact of a structured gardening programme of 2 hours per week over 46 weeks. It showed that structured gardening could maintain or improve well-being and mood in the presence of cognitive deterioration. Self-identity, purposeful activity and feeling useful were common themes identified by participants (Hewitt et al., 2013). Clearly more research is needed to establish the physical, cognitive and QoL benefits in younger people.

How it can be delivered

A flexible and tailored approach based upon positive reinforcement was adopted throughout Hewitt's structured gardening research programme. The group comprised people with Alzheimer's disease, mixed Alzheimer/vascular dementia, posterior cortical atrophy and dementia with Lewy bodies. Tasks could be pitched at different levels. Some required complex planning and sequencing, whereas others were tailored to provide 'hand over hand' help for someone with posterior cortical atrophy. 'Examples of tasks included digging and planning a bed with spring flowering bulbs or a one-step task such as sweeping leaves or sensory activities' (Hewitt et al., 2013: 357). Participants were given options to help maintain autonomy and a specific routine was adopted each week that included a group meeting at the start to plan but also have the opportunity to socialise, followed by an hour of gardening. A communication book was completed after each session that included written reminders of the activity and photos.

University College London provides guidance on how community gardens can support people living with dementia (Griffin et al., 2022).

Physical activity

The rationale

There are clear benefits of exercise for people of any age. Beyond the health advantages for individuals living with young onset dementia, physical exercise can help maintain motor skills, sequencing and provide socialisation and enjoyment. However, opportunities to be physically active, which many in their forties, fifties or sixties take for granted, can be denied to younger people living with dementia. This can be for multiple reasons: prejudice and assumptions about risk; lack of trained people to support activities; and personalised support plans which do not prioritise physical care in dementia. Support workers, for instance, who have been trained to deliver care may not have the confidence or opportunity to support someone to play golf.

The evidence

Qualitative research into the experience of a weekly community-based sports group for men with young onset dementia established by Notts County Football in the Community (NCFC) revealed four main themes. Two of these reflected the negative consequences of having young onset dementia and the lack of age-appropriate services but, importantly, two reflected positive gains from the sports activities, including enjoyment and positive anticipation from being part of a group, and attending a 'dementia-free' environment (Carone et al., 2016).

Sport for Confidence is an organisation through which allied health professionals deliver sport sessions in leisure centres. People living with young onset dementia were each allocated a sports coach and offered a choice of sporting activities such as hockey, boccia (a ball-based sport for those with high levels of support needs) or swimming. Research with 60 attendees showed participants developed increased fitness levels, flexibility, cognition and self-esteem. They benefited from social interaction and took part in more conversation

(Tilki et al., 2022). More empirical research is needed in this field to ascertain how long cognitive and physical improvements last and to assess the impact for family supporters.

How it can be delivered

Sports and physical activities need to be individually chosen and tailored and offer choice to take part on a 1:1 basis or in a group. The Notts County football and Sport for Confidence projects demonstrate the benefits of partnership working to deliver community-based physical activity. For those who are unable to physically take part in their sport of interest, sports reminiscence may be an alternative; for example, Sporting Memories (https://www.sportingmemories.uk) is a social enterprise which offers reminiscence groups for people over the age of 50 living with dementia. The groups focus on a wide range of sports, and they also offer resources, including a kitbag for people to use at home and a resource pack for use in care homes.

Art-based activities

The rationale

As dementia progresses, individuals may have reduced ability or opportunity to initiate or access creative hobbies they once enjoyed. With facilitation, either through a supporter or groups, milieux such as art and crafts, drama, film and reading can still be explored. The benefit of these activities is deemed to arise from a person-centred approach that highlights competencies and minimises deficits. This in turn supports well-being. Art and drama in particular are multisensory, and can enhance QoL through creativity and expression. This can be helpful particularly for younger people with language-based dementias, such as primary progressive aphasia (PPA) and semantic dementia, who may have impaired verbal communication. Such activities can promote choice and independence.

The evidence

Morhardt et al. (2019) developed, delivered and evaluated an arts-based group programme for people living with PPA of mixed ages from 55 to 82 years (mean 67). Their programme involved elements of education and support as well as activities. The activities, including art, collage and theatre improvisation, were chosen for being creative but also non-verbal. The sessions were delivered twice a month over 6 months to nine people living with PPA and eight carers. The people living with PPA in particular appreciated the creative activity element.

Theatre work alone has not been evaluated as an activity for people living with young onset dementia, although an ongoing study is looking into the use of an approach called Neuro Dramatic Play as the basis for supporting relationships and bonds for people living with young onset dementia and their family and close friends (Holmwood et al., in press).

There is also emerging evidence of the benefits of shared reading for older people with dementia, though the approach is just starting to be transferred to younger people (described below). The Reader is a national charity which runs groups where stories and poems are read out loud by attendees, evoking discussion and reactions to the literature. The 'Get into Reading' programme, which involved reading together in a facilitated group, was introduced to 61 participants in a care home, in-patient or day centre setting over an 18-week period. A reduction in behavioural and psychological distress was observed, measured by a reduction in NPI-Q scores (Kaufer et al., 2000), with improvements in mood, agitation and concentration. It was also observed that participants' verbal communication improved, and was more purposeful and less disconnected (Billington et al., 2013). A further study by The Reader charity showed improvement in QoL scores (The Reader Organisation, 2014).

How it can be delivered

Shared reading groups are delivered by YPWD CIO. Groups for 6–8 younger people living with dementia run for six consecutive weeks with a parallel course for family supporters. The same short story, book chapter or poem are read with both people with young onset dementia and their carers so they can jointly discuss the material at home afterwards. This also offers the person with dementia the same opportunity to generate discussion and have a voice as much as the carer. The stories are read a few sentences at a time and then discussion encouraged. This way people can retain information more easily through 'chunking' of information and can offer opinion in the here and now. Participants show support for each other and camaraderie. They also concentrate and actively listen and have confidence to provide opinion and to disagree. There is often carryover of the benefits in between the group sessions. One carer attending a group with his wife commented:

> *My wife hadn't read for 2 years but the next day got a book off the shelf for us to read together.* (Family supporter whose wife attends a reading group)

Shared reading accommodates individuals with different subtypes of dementia, including frontotemporal dementia and posterior cortical atrophy (PCA). People only read aloud if they wish to. It has been observed that people develop increased confidence across the sessions. Adaptations can be made, such as changing the font and presenting fewer and shorter lines of text on a page to reduce 'visual crowding' for an individual with PCA (Yong et al., 2015). One person with significant expressive speech problems had the confidence to read aloud by the end of 6 weeks.

More generally, Arts 4 Dementia, a UK charity (https://arts4dementia.org.uk/home/), has a rich programme of workshops and advertises artistic events in community settings such as dementia-friendly film screenings and opera. It

Table 11.2   Suggested activities for younger people living with dementia

Sports	Arts-based	Other
Badminton	Art	Cooking
Cycling (adapted bikes are available)	Choir	Equine therapy
Football	Crafts	Furniture restoration
Golf	Drama	Gardening
Indoor wall climbing	Photography	Involvement in research
Running	Shared reading	Public speaking
Table tennis		Reminiscence
Walking		Volunteering

also offers training. Although not specifically directed at younger people with dementia, many people with young onset dementia are involved and can sign up to their wide range of creative activities.

Table 11.2 shows a summary of suggested activities for people living with young onset dementia, based on experience at YPWD CIO.

Conclusions

In this chapter, we have looked at the role of meaningful activity in maintaining functioning and well-being for people living with young onset dementia. We argue that it is important that people in mid-life, who are often physically fit and who expect to be busy and contributing to society, have opportunities to engage in creative, sporting and other pastimes and hobbies to maintain their personal identity, health and quality of life. We have summarised key elements that are essential for person-centred choice of activities, have given detailed examples where available of how to provide different types of activity, and have summarised the rather scant research on their impact. Although there is little research on the impact of activity, there is a clear need to further explore the perceived benefits reported by people living with young onset dementia to inform future service adaptations and design. There is also a need for those living with young onset dementia, wherever they live, to have access to a choice of appropriate activities.

So what does this mean in practice?

If you are diagnosed with young onset dementia, what should your approach be to developing meaningful activity?

See if you can still pursue hobbies and roles you enjoy by adapting the way you connect with them. Be open to new pursuits – many people discover their creative side after a diagnosis of young onset dementia. Consider a wide range of opportunities to find what you might want to try: physical, art-based or social activities, volunteering or taking part in advisory, advocacy or research groups.

If you are a family member or friend of someone living with young onset dementia, how should you support them in developing meaningful activity?

Look for some things you can do together and others you can each pursue. Doing something enjoyable together can bring new energy to a relationship. Having time apart can be nurturing for both of you.

If you are a professional or support worker, to assist people in maintaining or developing meaningful activity

Try to focus on people's individual interests and adapt activities to make them achievable. Maintain a risk-positive approach so that people with young onset dementia can still have adventure and excitement. Look for opportunities for people with young onset dementia to take part in activities in ordinary community settings.

If you have a role in providing leisure, arts or sports activities

Participation in activities with people of a similar age helps to foster peer support and social connection – could you set up some specific young onset dementia sessions? Activities provided in community settings are attractive because they offer a sense of normality – are there places you could go out to together? Affordability is key – consider ways to reduce cost. Offering choice and taster sessions may help people to engage.

References

Bakker, C., de Vugt, M.E., Van Vliet D., et al. (2014) The relationship between unmet care needs in young-onset dementia and the course of neuropsychiatric symptoms: a two-year follow-up study, *International Psychogeriatrics*, 26 (12): 1991–2000.

Bannan, N. and Montgomery-Smith, C. (2008) 'Singing for the brain': reflections on the human capacity for music arising from a pilot study of group singing with Alzheimer's patients, *Journal of the Royal Society for the Promotion of Health*, 128 (2): 73–78.

Bannon, S.M., Reichman, M.R., Wang, K., et al. (2022) A qualitative meta-synthesis of common and unique preferences for supportive services among persons with young onset dementia and their caregivers, *Dementia*, 21 (2): 519–39.

Beattie, A., Daker-White, G., Gilliard, J., et al. (2004) 'How can they tell?': a qualitative study of the views of younger people about their dementia and dementia care services, *Health and Social Care in the Community*, 12 (4): 359–68.

Billington, J., Carroll, J., Davis, P., et al. (2013) A literature based intervention for older adults living with dementia, *Perspectives in Public Health*, 133 (3): 165–73.

Busted, L.M., Nielsen, D.S. and Birkelund, R. (2020) 'Sometimes it feels like thinking in syrup': the experience of losing sense of self in those with young onset dementia, *International Journal of Qualitative Studies on Health and Well-Being*, 15 (1): 1734277. Available at: https://doi.org/10.1080/17482631.2020.1734277.

Carone, L., Tischler, V. and Dening, T. (2016) Football and dementia: a qualitative investigation of a community based sports group for men with early onset dementia, *Dementia*, 15 (6): 1358–76.

Cations, M., Withall, A., Horsfall, R., et al. (2017) Why aren't people with young onset dementia and their supporters using formal services? Results from the INSPIRED study, *PLoS One*, 12 (7): e0180935. Available at: https://doi.org/10.1371/journal.pone.0180935.

Clarke, C. and Mantle, R. (2016) Using risk management to promote person-centred dementia care, *Nursing Standard*, 30 (28): 41–46.

Clift, S., Hancox, G., Morrison, I., et al. (2007) Choral singing and psychological well-being: findings from English choirs in a cross-national survey using the WHOQOL-BREF, *International Symposium on Performance Science*, AEC.

Gray, K., Russell, C. and Twigg, J. (2023) *Leisure and Everyday Life with Dementia*. London: Open University Press.

Griffin, L., Ashton, J., Roche, M., et al. (2022) *Supporting people with dementia: A guide for community gardens*. London: University College London. Available at: https://www.ucl.ac.uk/bartlett/development/sites/bartlett_development/files/dementia_community_garden_guide_griffin.pdf.

Hewitt, P., Watts, C., Hussey, J., et al. (2013) Does a structured gardening programme improve well-being in young-onset dementia? A preliminary study, *British Journal of Occupational Therapy*, 76 (8): 355–61.

Holmwood, C., Ward, A. and Collard-Stokes, G. (in press) Dementia, younger onset dementia and the Arts, *Healthcare Counselling and Psychotherapy Journal*.

Hussey, J., Draper, C., Blanchette, C., et al. (2016) Younger people: an innovative partnership, *Journal of Dementia Care*, 24 (6): 20–22.

Johannessen, A. and Möller, A. (2013) Experiences of persons with early-onset dementia in everyday life: a qualitative study, *Dementia*, 12 (4): 410–24.

Kaufer, D.I., Cummings, J.L., Ketchel, P., et al. (2000) Validation of the NPI-Q, a brief clinical form of the Neuropsychiatric Inventory, *Journal of Neuropsychiatry and Clinical Neurosciences*, 12 (2): 233–39.

Kinney, J.M., Kart, C.S. and Reddecliff, L. (2011) 'That's me, the Goother': evaluation of a program for individuals with early-onset dementia, *Dementia*, 10 (3): 361–77.

Koopmans, R.T., Reinders, R., van Vliet, D., et al. (2014) Prevalence and correlates of psychotropic drug use in community-dwelling people with young-onset dementia: the NeedYD-study, *International Psychogeriatrics*, 26 (12): 1983–89.

Kortte, K.B. and Rogalski, E.J. (2013) Behavioural interventions for enhancing life participation in behavioural variant frontotemporal dementia and primary progressive aphasia, *International Review of Psychiatry*, 25 (2): 237–45.

Lin, S. and Lewis, F. (2015) Dementia friendly, dementia capable, and dementia positive: concepts to prepare for the future, *The Gerontologist*, 55 (2): 237–44.

London Assembly Health Committee (2018) *Young-onset dementia*. Available at: https://www.london.gov.uk/sites/default/files/yodfinal.pdf (accessed 21 May 2023).

Lu, L.C., Lan, S.H., Hsieh, Y.P., et al. (2020) Horticultural therapy in patients with dementia: a systematic review and meta-analysis, *American Journal of Alzheimer's Disease and Other Dementias*, 35: 1533317519883498. Available at: https://doi.org/10.1177/1533317519883498.

Mayrhofer, A., Mathie, E., McKeown, J., et al. (2018) Age-appropriate services for people diagnosed with young onset dementia (YOD): a systematic review, *Aging and Mental Health*, 22 (8): 933–42.

Millenaar, J.K., Bakker, C., Koopmans, R.T., et al. (2016) The care needs and experiences with the use of services of people with young-onset dementia and their caregivers: a systematic review, *International Journal of Geriatric Psychiatry*, 31 (12): 1261–76.

Mitchell, W. (2018) *Somebody I Used to Know*. London: Bloomsbury.

Mitchell, W. (2022) *What I Wish People Knew about Dementia: From Someone Who Knows*. London: Bloomsbury.

Mitchell, W. (2023) *One Last Thing: How to Live with the End in Mind*. London: Bloomsbury.

Morhardt, D.J., O'Hara, M.C., Zachrich, K., et al. (2019) Development of a psycho-educational support program for individuals with primary progressive aphasia and their care-partners, *Dementia*, 18 (4): 1310–27.

Oliver, K. (2019) *Dear Alzheimer's: A Diary of Living with Dementia*. London: Jessica Kingsley.

Osman, S., Tischler, V. and Schneider J. (2016) 'Singing for the brain': a qualitative study exploring the health and well-being benefits of singing for people with dementia and their carers, *Dementia*, 15 (6): 1326–39.

Roach, P. and Drummond, N. (2014) 'It's nice to have something to do': early-onset dementia and maintaining purposeful activity, *Journal of Psychiatric and Mental Health Nursing*, 21 (10): 889–95.

Sansoni, J., Duncan, C., Grootemaat, P., et al. (2016) Young onset dementia: a review of the literature to inform service development, *American Journal of Alzheimer's Disease and Other Dementias*, 31 (8): 693–705.

Scott, T.L., Jao, Y.L., Tulloch, K., et al. (2022) Well-being benefits of horticulture-based activities for community dwelling people with dementia: a systematic review, *International Journal of Environmental Research and Public Health*, 19 (17): 10523. Available at: https://doi.org/10.3390/ijerph191710523.

Sorrell, J.A. and Sorrell, J.M. (2008), Music as a healing art for older adults, *Journal of Psychosocial Nursing and Mental Health Services*, 46 (3): 21–24.

Stamou, V., Oyebode, J., La Fontaine, J., et al. (2023) Good practice in needs-based post-diagnostic support for people with young onset dementia: findings from the Angela Project, *Ageing and Society*. Available at: https://doi.org/10.1017/S0144686 X22001362.

The Reader Organisation (TRO) (2014) *Read to care: An investigation into the quality-of-life benefits of shared reading groups for people living with dementia*. Available at: https://www.thereader.org.uk/wp-content/uploads/2022/11/Read-to-Care-2014-Final. pdf.

Tilki, M., Curran, C., Burton, L., et al. (2022) Sport for confidence: a collaborative programme of physical activity, sport and exercise for people with young onset dementia, *Working with Older People*, 27 (2): 128–36.

Van Vliet, D., Persoon, A., Bakker, C., et al. (2017) Feeling useful and engaged in daily life: exploring the experiences of people with young-onset dementia, *International Psychogeriatrics*, 29 (11): 1889–98.

Werner, P., Stein-Shvachman, I. and Korczyn, A.D. (2009) Early onset dementia: clinical and social aspects, *International Psychogeriatrics*, 21 (4): 631–36.

Yong, K., Rajdev, K., Shakespeare, T.J., et al. (2015) Facilitating text reading in posterior cortical atrophy, *Neurology*, 85 (4): 339–48.

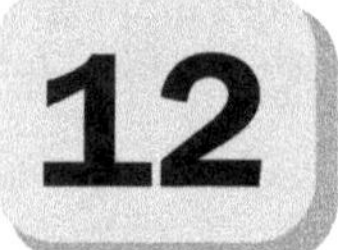

12 Involving people with young onset dementia in research

*Jacqueline Parkes, Laura Cole
and Natasha Bayes*

Overview

When a person retires prematurely from work due to a younger onset dementia, a role as an expert-by-experience in research can provide a sense of purpose, maintain social connections, preserve a sense of identity, and enhance self-confidence and self-esteem. This chapter will describe why people with dementia want to be involved in research, and why younger people are particularly motivated to engage in dementia research studies and projects. Lessons learned from a recently completed project to set up a national Public and Patient Involvement and Engagement Research Network of people living with young onset dementia and other related literature, will be presented to help others to consider why involving people with young onset dementia is beneficial for the development of future young onset dementia research and the ongoing well-being of persons living with the diagnosis.

Keywords

Young onset dementia, research, public and patient involvement and engagement, occupational purpose, identity.

Learning points

- Understand the importance of involving people with young onset dementia in research for the design and development of dementia research studies.
- Recognise the importance and value of being involved in research for the well-being of the person with young onset dementia, to enhance feelings of worth, self-esteem and purpose.

- Evaluate the different ways to involve people with young onset dementia in research and decide on the most appropriate approach for different types of research designs.
- Create and design future research with the involvement, engagement and participation of people living with young onset dementia.

The involvement of people with young onset dementia in research

Due to the progressive degenerative changes in the brain which cause a decline in cognitive functioning, academic researchers have historically tended to exclude people with young onset dementia from active participation in research, assuming them to be incapable of understanding, and therefore unable to offer anything of great value to the research process (Rivett, 2017). In turn, this can reinforce societal perceptions that receiving a dementia diagnosis means that the person is no longer able to make a meaningful contribution to society. As Cantley et al. argued, 'the challenge of involving people with dementia is in essence the challenge of addressing their social inclusion' (2005: 3). However, increasingly over the past decade, people living with dementia have stated loudly and clearly that they should have the right to be actively and meaningfully involved in research and evaluation studies (DAA, 2018). Those who fund dementia care research have heard this and many funders now expect meaningful Public Patient Involvement and Engagement Representatives (PPIE) to be included in all projects (Biggane et al., 2019).

In general, people often have an innate desire to participate in meaningful activities. Some people with a young onset dementia may be in a position to fulfil this wish by taking part in research and evaluation projects as a PPIE representative. The inclusion of such experts-by-experience as PPIE representatives ensures those living with a health condition or using a service have a voice in the development and conduct of research studies, above and beyond being participants. It is one way people living with young onset dementia can continue to contribute to society, while deriving personal benefit in the form of cognitive stimulation and improved self-confidence and self-worth. People with dementia have a variety of reasons for wanting to contribute to research projects. Participating in research enables them to describe their encounters, voice their concerns, challenge the system and, perhaps, improve the delivery of future dementia care and support. Involvement in PPIE work can leave people with dementia feeling valued and still able to contribute to society at a time in their lives when they are experiencing significant cognitive, physical and social changes.

In the Angela Project, two people with young onset dementia represented the young onset dementia community. Their feedback during the project

PPIE Forum meetings was that they knew of a number of people with young onset dementia who would welcome the opportunity to become actively and meaningfully involved in research studies and projects, if they were effectively supported to engage in the process (Oliver et al., 2020). Their motivation for getting involved was to help design and develop research proposals and funding applications that were truly informed by the people affected by dementia. They were keen to enhance the knowledge of clinicians, policy-makers and academics about the unique challenges that people under the age of 65 experience when diagnosed with dementia. They also wanted to suggest ideas for future research projects that could improve the future diagnostic and post-diagnostic experiences of other people with young onset dementia. Being involved in research as an equal and valued partner on the project team could also leave them feeling a sense of continued worth to society.

The involvement and engagement of people with dementia in research and evaluation projects provides a unique perspective on the effects of the disease process both on themselves and their family and friends. Sharing their lived and often complex experiences of the effects of the disease, their journey to diagnosis, and the level of post-diagnostic support they have received can significantly illuminate the strengths and challenges of the health and social care system. Their insights, comments and feedback can help researchers to craft project proposals and funding applications for activities that could ultimately influence health and social care providers, clinical commissioners and policy-makers to review and improve care provision.

People with young onset dementia *can* be involved in research

As far back as 2005, Cantley et al. drew attention to a broad range of participatory approaches that can be employed to effectively capture the knowledge and experiences of people with dementia in research and evaluation studies, including both individual and group consultation (Cantley et al., 2005).

As research participants, people with young onset dementia may give first-hand accounts of their experiences during an interview or by completing a questionnaire. A more collective approach to acquiring several 'voices' during data collection may involve organising focus groups or a consultation event. Multiple views can also be accessed via existing Forums or social sup port groups. However, beyond this, people who have undergone appropriate training in research methods, such as the one developed by Parkes et al. (2014), can also assist with co-designing and producing research studies (Parkes et al., 2022). In the Angela Project, the PPIE members were actively involved throughout all stages of the study, helping to design the project logo, the survey questionnaires, interview schedules, participant information leaflets, and contributing to publications.

The 'Balanced Participation Model' was specifically designed to support the active engagement of people in the early stages of dementia to design and deliver their own research projects (Schack Thoft et al., 2018). Building on 'Partners in Projects' (Parkes et al., 2014), combined with the 'Authentic Partnerships Model' (Dupuis et al., 2011), Schack Thoft and colleagues proved that with appropriate training and robust support, people with dementia could be both participants and co-researchers in their own projects. They can also assist academic researchers to co-design research projects (Dupuis et al., 2011) or even design and lead their own studies as principal investigators (Schack Thoft et al., 2018). Indeed, in the UK, 26 small-scale research projects have been led by groups of people with dementia engaged on the Dementia Enquirers Programme (2018–23; Litherland and Hare, 2024).

Developing a PPIE Network Model for younger people with dementia

In 2019, a University of Northampton (UK) project team secured funding from the Wellcome Public Engagement Fund for a 2-year project to establish the 'Dementia Experts for Involvement Network-Young Dementia' (DEfIN-YD). The aim was to develop a PPIE Research Network across England specifically for people with young onset dementia who would be interested in shaping future research into different aspects of the condition. Having strong links with the national Young Dementia Network and building on the Angela Project PPIE Forum findings (Parkes et al., 2022), Parkes recognised the need to grow and develop a body of people with young onset dementia who could identify specific young onset dementia research priorities and help co-design and produce young onset dementia-focused studies. Consequently, the research team invited people with young onset dementia, who were willing and able to participate, and to potentially lead research, evaluation and audit projects.

The vision was that the creation of a PPIE Research Network where the 'voices' of people with young onset dementia could be heard would provide a vehicle whereby knowledge about young onset dementia research could be shared, future project ideas could be identified and developed, and group members could contribute their expertise to young onset dementia research, evaluation and audit projects across the UK and beyond.

Informed directly by feedback from a DEfIN-YD Advisory Steering Committee member, the DEfIN-YD project team developed the project aims and protocol, and organised three regionally located PPIE groups in England. Each regional group undertook a series of five workshops, led by facilitators and supported by the project team. Having completed the workshops, the group members, facilitators and project team participated in individual interviews and focus groups to ascertain why members had got involved in DEfIN-YD, what their experiences had been of being involved, and what the team could have done differently to maximise involvement, satisfaction and sustain future engagement. Ultimately, the project focus was to explore:

- whether the groups attracted a strong and representative membership;
- whether the workshops were structured, organised and facilitated in a supportive way;
- what the perceived purpose of each group was; and
- if the delivery of the groups could be sustained beyond the life of the project.

The intention was to develop a national network of uniquely placed individuals who, given appropriate support and training, could either develop their own research or be available to other researchers to improve societal understanding, at all levels, about the experience of living with young onset dementia.

In the remainder of this chapter, we draw out some of our experiences in running the DEfIN-YD Project that may be of value to researchers who wish to run similar groups or involve people with young onset dementia in the planning, design and development of research. We also give an account of the feedback from people with young onset dementia who took part in the project evaluation. This gives valuable insights into the benefits people with young onset dementia may gain from being partners in research and may inspire others to get involved in research too.

Designing and delivering the Dementia Experts for Involvement-Young Dementia (DEfIN-YD) Project

Initially planned to be in-person, due to the COVID-19 pandemic, the DEfIN-YD Project officially launched via a virtual online Conference Day event. Twenty-one people were recruited to form three regional PPIE groups (North, Midlands, South of England). Each was associated with a university that was directly involved in the project. The group members were recruited via the Young Dementia Network, Dementia UK, the Alzheimer's Society, the Dementia Engagement and Empowerment Project (DEEP) Network, as well as local NHS services. Members came from urban and rural settings, and had a variety of diagnoses. They were at different stages of their dementia journey but all had been diagnosed with dementia before the age of 65 years. They included both men and women and represented a variety of socioeconomic and cultural backgrounds.

Care was taken to ensure members were adequately informed and supported to join the project. Each member received an information pack (electronic and hard copy) that included a project information sheet and consent form (original and easy-read formats), some stationery, and an 'I want to speak please' card (www.dementiavoices.org.uk) that could be easily shown when on video-calls to facilitate participation. One of the project team spoke with members via an online video application to explain the project, answer any questions, and establish if members were able to give their informed consent to participate in the evaluation of the project, recording verbal consent. These procedures reflect the Gold Standards for Ethical Research set out by The Dementia Enquirers (2023).

Group members participated, alongside the project team members (Jacqueline Parkes, Laura Cole, Natasha Bayes and Anna Crawford), in a series of five 90-minute independently facilitated online workshops in each of the regions. Some members attended the meetings alone and others were supported by advocates, usually family members. The first workshop, delivered by a member of the research team (Parkes), provided all the group members and the independent facilitators with training in research methods and processes. Subsequent workshops then explored:

- the reasons why someone with young onset dementia might want to get involved in research;
- how they could actively and meaningfully participate in project work;
- group ideas for future young onset dementia projects; and
- how the regional groups might be sustained beyond the life of the project.

When all five of the workshops had been completed in each region, the 15 group members with young onset dementia who were still participating in the project completed online individual interviews, which were recorded, transcribed verbatim and analysed thematically (described below) (Braun and Clarke, 2006). Finally, during an end of project event, all DEfIN-YD members – the project team, advisory steering group members and independent facilitators – came together in person to hear the findings and recommendations of the evaluation, consider the future of the young onset dementia PPIE Research Network and celebrate the project's success.

Why people living with younger onset dementia joined the DEfIN-YD Project

During the online interviews, the participants explained whether they had any previous knowledge or experience of being involved in research-related studies or project work; described what taking part had meant for them; and provided guidance on whether future DEfIN-YD meetings should be on an online platform or in-person.

The main reason why DEFIN-YD members wanted to get involved in research and evaluation was to improve the experience of living with dementia for themselves as well as others, both now and in the future. The primary motivation was to help shape future young onset dementia research. The group members still wanted to be useful to society, despite having ceased paid work (see Chapter 10). They wanted to feel valued and to have a sense of purpose and achievement; and they wanted to belong to a team where they would bene-fit from peer support, camaraderie, and greater knowledge and understanding of their condition.

The core motivations revolved around wanting to raise awareness and edu-cate others so that people with a diagnosis could be better understood and supported. One member of the research network described how he was keen to raise awareness of young onset dementia, while still having the cognitive ability to make a contribution:

> *My reasons for any research project never changes ... I know I am on a time bound fuse now. And no matter what goes on, whether it be research into services, research into medication, research into non-clinical interventions, whatever it might be, it is not going to be any use to me whatsoever. But the reason I do all this training and university and all that sort of thing is to get that awareness into the next generation in the hope that what will come from that will be a better world for those coming through with dementia. So that's why I will join any project.*

There was a sense from the DEfIN-YD project members that there are cur-rently a limited number of studies ongoing that focus purely on young onset dementia, and this should be significantly expanded. The suggestion was also made that involvement and engagement opportunities are currently poorly communicated or advertised; and that many people with young onset dementia may not be engaging in projects because they do not know how to get involved. A PPIE member explained how he was very keen to get more academic and practitioner researchers, as well as people with young onset dementia, involved in young onset dementia research:

> *Well myself I'm an eager and prolific participant in research studies, I have been since the day of my diagnosis. And I wanted to encourage other people like me to step forward to help those recruiting and to understand how best to address the needs of potential candidates.*

Another reason offered by members for why people with young onset dementia do not currently engage with research included a lack of familiarity with online platforms:

> *People are keen [to engage in research] but they don't know how. So I give them the Join Dementia Research website details, they go on there and it's just, it's so unfriendly that a lot of them just fall at the first hurdle and don't register. That's the only trouble, I think, is to make the process easy, welcom-ing, inclusive and rewarding.*

Other explanations included people not feeling academic enough to engage in research, some studies having limited or restrictive inclusion criteria, and there being fewer research opportunities in the North compared to the

South of England. Some members also suggested that many people with young onset dementia still have extensive life commitments, such as caring responsibilities for dependent family members, which prevent them from participating in PPIE activities. Sadly, there were also those individuals with a diagnosis who felt that they would be perceived to be too unwell with their dementia to make a valid contribution to study design or implementation.

Many of the DEfIN-YD members had already been involved in a range of research, evaluation, audit and educational projects. They found that being involved gave them a sense of identity and purpose, as described by a PPIE member's spouse:

> The reasons for taking part in the first place were a desire to be useful really. I think she really desires a purpose and that's been the worst thing about having dementia for her. She wanted to be involved with something that was going to be useful and had a purpose.

For many members, the experience of being involved in research made them feel validated and useful:

> And I know that my lived experienced helped to provide useful insights into some aspects of the research process. I felt valued and for me that's very important because not being able to work anymore, you know, not feeling sorry for myself. But, you know, one of the things about being at work is every now and then you feel good about something that you've done, don't you. It's a good feeling, that's what I like most about work ... achieving something, and I felt I was achieving something at those [DEfIN-YD] meetings. So, from a quite selfish perspective, I got something out of it. But I could also see that I was playing a small part in shaping things at every meeting. And that's great, that's how you learn a lot.

Generally, the feedback offered during the participant interviews clearly indicated that most group members had really enjoyed the experience of attending the DEfIN-YD workshops. They felt they had 'learnt a lot' from each other, the facilitators and the research team, and they also felt that they had been listened to and respected for their contributions. However, some members also disclosed that there were some elements of the organisation and delivery of the workshops which they felt would help to maximise everyone's input equally. We will highlight these in turn.

Lessons learnt from organising and delivering the DEfIN-YD workshops

All the members who attended the five workshops of the DEfIN-YD Project unanimously agreed that they wanted to continue with a young onset dementia PPIE Research Network in the future. They felt that their opinions were respected and their suggestions for improving the group meetings were listened and responded to. Future recommendations for the DEfIN-YD Project to consider, which would also be relevant to others who wished to consider setting up something similar, were:

- to encourage people with young onset dementia from different social, economic and cultural backgrounds to get involved;
- to attract members from a wide range of geographical locations and living arrangements, such as people with young onset dementia living alone;
- to have a clear purpose and focus for each group meeting, with co-designed expectations, ground rules and communication processes;
- to involve anyone with a diagnosis of dementia aged 65 years or younger who wished to join the groups;
- to continue to include members with a young onset dementia diagnosis to attend the groups past the age of 65 years, as long as they have capacity to clearly consent to their involvement;
- to optimise the size of the groups, with a minimum of eight and a maximum of 10 people;
- to have strong facilitation from a researcher or an academic with experience of working with people with young onset dementia;
- to have administrative support for the groups, carried out by someone with knowledge and understanding of the abilities and capabilities of people with young onset dementia; and
- recompense members for their involvement and engagement in the groups, acknowledging that some members may wish to donate their payment to a charity of their choice due to the potential impact on the benefits they receive.

Conclusions

Without a doubt, all people with a young onset dementia should be given an opportunity to participate as a PPIE representative in research and evaluation studies and projects, should they wish to take part. They have a lot to offer, in terms of their existing strengths and capabilities from having recently left work, alongside their unique insight of living with young onset dementia, with its impact on multiple aspects of their lives. Participating in projects such as DEfIN-YD can also provide a sense of purpose, and help retain personal identity and a feeling of being of value to society.

Why should people with young onset dementia be encouraged and supported to become research active? People with young onset dementia can inform and influence policy-makers, clinicians and commissioners who assess and care for people with young onset dementia, and research leaders and project designers who create the knowledge and evidence base for young onset dementia research. Through this route, people living with young onset dementia can make a difference to the care and support both they and others in similar circumstances receive once diagnosed with a dementia. At the same time, being involved in research may improve feelings of self-worth and enhance wellbeing. For far too long people with young onset dementia have been excluded from involvement activities, but the DEfIN-YD Project has clearly shown that if opportunities are widely advertised and people are aware of them, given the right support, training and guidance, people with young onset dementia are able to actively and meaningfully contribute to society by becoming a PPIE Representative.

So what does this mean in practice?

If you are living with young onset dementia or supporting someone with young onset dementia

If you are not sure whether to get involved in young onset dementia research, ask your peers if anyone has been involved in research and chat with them about their experiences to see if you then feel inspired to get involved. To help you decide, read accounts from people living with young onset dementia who have been involved in research, such as Keith Oliver's paper referred to above, dip into Litherland and Hare (2024), or have a look at websites such as The Dementia Enquirers (https://dementiaenquirers.org.uk/).

If you would like to get involved in young onset dementia research and are in the UK, have a look at the Young Dementia Network website (https://www.youngdementianetwork.org/get-involved/current-research-studies/) to see current young onset dementia research studies that are looking for people with the condition or family members to participate and consider signing up to Join Dementia Research. Wherever you live, you can ask your consultant or a dementia care worker if they know of studies or local universities you could become involved with.

If you are a young onset dementia researcher

Inform yourself about participatory approaches to research, for example by reading Litherland and Hare (2024) to see accounts of co-production, and read the Gold Standards for Ethical Research set out by The Dementia Enquirers (2023) to inform your thinking.

You could also consider setting up a PPIE group of people living with young onset dementia and their supporters who can meet regularly and get to know your university (or other base) and your work. You could find out from this group what support people living with young onset dementia or their supporters need from you to make an effective contribution, in terms of preliminary discussion, advance information and support during meetings.

Consult people living with young onset dementia and their supporters about *your* research ideas and about *their* research ideas before you start writing your proposal. Work with people living with young onset dementia and their supporters to put together a feasible PPIE strategy so that they are involved in various aspects of your study, including design, delivery, analysis and dissemination of findings.

If you sit on funding panels or review bids for research funding

Inform yourself about participatory approaches to research, for example by reading Litherland and Hare (2024) to see accounts of co-production, and read the Gold Standards for Ethical Research set out by The Dementia Enquirers (2023) to inform your thinking. When you review bids, check bids to see how strong the PPIE strategy and representation are. Do not hesitate to suggest ways these can be strengthened.

References

Biggane, A.M., Olsen, M. and Williamson, P.R. (2019) PPI in research: a reflection from early stage researchers, *Research Involvement and Engagement*, 5: 35. Available at: https://doi.org/10.1186/s40900-019-0170-2.

Braun, V. and Clarke, V. (2006) Using thematic analysis in psychology, *Qualitative Research in Psychology*, 3 (2): 77–101.

Cantley, C., Woodhouse, J. and Smith, M. (2005) *Listen to us: Involving people with dementia in planning and developing services*. Newcastle: Dementia North and Northumbria University. Available at: http://www.mentalhealthpromotion.net/resources/listen-to-us.pdf.

Dementia Action Alliance (DAA) (2018) *National Dementia Declaration*. Available at: www.dementiaaction.org.uk/assets/0000/1157/National_Dementia_Declaration_for_England.pdf (accessed 1 December 2023).

Dementia Enquirers (2023) *The Dementia Enquirers gold standards for ethical research*. Available at: https://www.dementiavoices.org.uk/wp-content/uploads/2020/07/The-DEEP-Ethics-Gold-Standards-for-Dementia-Research.pdf (accessed 1 December 2023).

Dupuis, S.L., Gillies, J., Carson, J., et al. (2011) Moving beyond patient and client approaches: mobilizing 'authentic partnerships' in dementia care, support and services, *Dementia*, 11(4): 427–52.

Litherland, R. and Hare, P. (2024) *People with Dementia at the Heart of Research: Co-Producing Research through The Dementia Enquirers Model*. London: Jessica Kingsley

Oliver, K., O'Malley, M., Parkes, J.H., et al. (2020) Living with young onset dementia and actively shaping dementia research: The Angela Project (special edition), *Dementia*, 19 (1): 41–48.

Parkes, J.H., Pyer, M., Wray, P., et al. (2014) Partners in projects: preparing for public involvement in health and social care research, *Health Policy*, 117 (3): 399–408.

Parkes, J., O'Malley, M., Stamou, V., et al. (2022) Lessons learnt from delivering the public and patient involvement forums within a younger onset dementia project, *Dementia*, 21 (7): 1–14.
Rivett, E. (2017) Research involving people with dementia: a literature review, *Working with Older People*, 21 (2): 107–14.
Schack Thoft, D., Pyer, M., Horsbol, A., et al. (2018) The balanced participation model: sharing opportunities for giving people with early-stage dementia a voice in research, *Dementia*, 19 (7): 2294–2313.

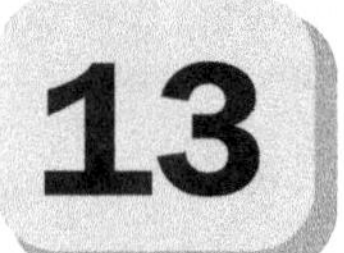

Maintaining identity over time when living with young onset dementia

Aud Johannessen and Kirsten Thorsen

Overview

The self is a central and unique aspect of the human personality, character-ised by the individual's organised and lasting experiences of their own identity. There is at least some evidence for persistence of self in all the mild, moder-ate and severe stages of dementia, although many studies record some degree of deterioration in aspects of self or identity. Most people with dementia can speak for themselves about their experience of living with the disease. This chapter focuses on how younger people with dementia experience changes of identity over time, including changes of identity in the early stage, general issues managing stigma at early stages, changes in identity in the moderate and late stages, and supporting environments. In addition, we address how living in an accepting, considerate and supportive environment may validate the new personhood, when the person with young onset dementia is experiencing more cognitive impairment and disability as their dementia progresses.

Keywords

Alzheimer's disease, young onset dementia, individuality, personhood.

Learning points

- People with young onset dementia can provide their own subjective accounts of their experiences.
- People with dementia should be listened to and included in planning for person-centred public health services.
- Living in an accepting, considerate and supportive environment validates personhood.

Introduction

The self is a central and unique aspect of the human personality, characterised by the individual's organised and lasting experiences of their own identity (in Norwegian this is referred to as the person's *leksikon*). The self is a central concept in recent psychological theories of personality, where it is emphasised, among other things, that people at all times try to act in accordance with their own self-image.

A review of studies on self in dementia found all of them suggested that there is some evidence for persistence of self in the mild, moderate and severe stages of dementia, although many studies find some degree of deterioration in aspects of self or identity (Caddell and Clare, 2010, Trindade et al., 2020). It is also the case that to find out about self in dementia it is possible to talk directly with those living with dementia. Studies underpin that most people with dementia can provide their own subjective account of their experiences of living with the disease (Johannessen et al., 2019; Trindade et al., 2020). A study by Baptista et al. (2019) showed that there is a difference between young onset dementia and late onset dementia when it comes to awareness. The young onset group in their study had higher levels of disease awareness than the late onset group, even though they had greater impairment in functionality. People with young onset dementia, therefore, may be in a relatively strong position to give their own insights, even as their dementia advances.

In this chapter, we will illustrate the main points with reference to a longitudinal study conducted in Norway. The first part of our longitudinal study lasted for over 2 years, interviewing people living with young onset dementia every 6 months. The study focused on how identity was experienced by people with young onset dementia, as they faced the prospect of living with a disease, for which there is no curative treatment, from mid-life onwards (Johannessen et al., 2018). We found that people with young onset dementia experience that their dementia impacts on their ability to look after themselves, and that the awareness of this has a marked effect on everyday life. The study revealed that people with young onset dementia can express how they experience life with progressing dementia, even at later stages when they are greatly handicapped by cognitive problems, such as with short-term memory and loss of vocabulary. This is also apparent in books written by people with dementia themselves (de Baggio, 2002, 2003; Taylor, 2007), as well as in reports and recorded stories (Rose, 2003, Voris et al., 2009).

In our longitudinal study, we continued to conduct further interviews every 6 months over a period of 3 years with one of the participants (Thorsen et al., 2020). Despite her considerable cognitive impairment, she had a large vocabulary to describe feelings and changes in her cognitive capacity and her social interactions, and she described how these domains are interwoven (Thorsen et al., 2018). Even if many words disappear for people as dementia worsens, much rich vocabulary can be preserved for a long time, and people with dementia can give very valuable narratives of 'Alzheimer's from the inside' (Rose, 2003).

The first interviews with participants in our study were conducted about 6 months after a diagnosis was made, at which point they still had quite fluent verbal abilities (Johannessen et al., 2018). Each person had their own socio-lect (language used by particular social groups) and dialect. Each person also had a unique personal tone, what Greenwood (Power, 2014: 78) calls a 'word palette'. This forms the basis of each person's communications when dementia sets in. Power (2014: 79) has emphasized how the words, signs, body language, mimicry and metaphors used by each person carry their own meaning. There-fore, those who know the person well are in a good position to understand and communicate if and when dementia interferes with straightforward verbal communication.

Due to communication difficulties, some researchers and clinicians resort to talking to family members rather than directly to people living with demen-tia. However, studies have shown that information about the quality of life of people with dementia by proxy (family members, healthcare personnel) devi-ate from the person's own experiences (Sands et al., 2004; Arons et al., 2013). Hence, in our study, we focused on speaking with people living with young onset dementia themselves rather than taking any accounts from family mem-bers, even when dementia had become more advanced. The citations in this chapter come from conversations with two of our research participants, Anne and Arne (both pseudonyms). Anne participated in seven and Arne in ten inter-views (Thorsen et al., 2020).

Changes of identity over time

The main overriding theme in the participants' stories about living with young onset dementia is changes of identity over time (Johannessen et al., 2018; Thorsen et al., 2018, 2020). The participants' narratives revolved around:

- how to preserve their identity over time;
- how to continue to experience a lust for life and vitality; and
- how to participate in human interactions that validate and support identity.

The most significant aspects of the participants' experiences of how young onset dementia was influencing them over time were the initial signs, coping efforts, concealing the diagnosis, social withdrawal, existential anxiety and strivings to revive the self. The overriding experience was that living with young onset dementia was aggravating and uncomfortable (Johannessen et al., 2018; Thorsen et al., 2018, 2020).

Existential challenges for human beings concern issues such as:

- managing our mortality and fear of death;
- existential loneliness vs. being part of a community;
- facing meaninglessness vs. finding meaning;

- living with freedom vs. responsibility; and
- fear of life.

Our participants faced these issues as the condition worsened, but their main concern was to preserve and protect their identity (Johannessen et al., 2018; Thorsen et al., 2018, 2020). This resonates with Kitwood's assertion that maintaining identity – that is, 'to know who one is, in cognition and in feeling' (Kitwood, 1997: 43) – is a fundamental need in life with dementia.

The study revealed how individuals reacted to handle this challenge. People with young onset dementia experienced and reflected on the changes brought by the disease. They had adequate insight for a long time, and tried to master and control their life as the disease progressed. Participants adapted and preserved a feeling of living quite a good life by using various coping strategies. Interactions with health personnel were integrated into participants' stories. High quality public support was important to assist them in sustaining quality of life and vitality (Johannessen et al., 2019). In particular, personalised care, from 'support contacts', was valued. A support contact in Norway is a local authority key worker or someone who provides personally tailored care like a 'befriender'. Our findings suggest that this sort of service should be more widely available to assist people with young onset dementia to preserve their identity through living a normal everyday life as far as possible (Johannessen and Thorsen, 2018). The insight from this finding emphasises that the voices of people with dementia should be listened to and included in planning public health services.

Identity in the initial stages

In the initial stages, we found that the increasing cognitive difficulties were mainly seen as creating everyday problems. Those with young onset dementia tried to cope with these through different practical means, such as taking notes and using post-its (Johannessen et al., 2018, 2019). Gradually, cognitive problems interfered more and more annoyingly with both their daily life and with social relationships. These two areas of managing day-to-day life and social interaction were closely related. Power (2014) has also pointed out that there is a close tie between identity and social connectedness and, of course, Kitwood placed great emphasis on interpersonal interaction, which he felt was crucial to support sense of self in dementia (Kitwood, 1997).

Anne's experiences

Our stories showed that people can have very different experiences after diagnosis of young onset dementia. Not all have experiences like Anne's, but we use her account here as an example. Anne (a pseudonym) is divorced. For more than 30 years she worked as a director of a commercial firm and was engaged, busy and hardworking. This is the core of her identity.

> *Then I had, for a long time, recognised that something was wrong. Now I am about to become crazy! Forgetting, remembering, suddenly being scared about things I have always done without any problems, like taking the train to the airport. Ah! It is a nightmare. So, I went to the doctor.*

Anne's account shows that she was busy with typical mid-life activity at this point. A lot of tests were performed, and at the next visit the doctor abruptly informed her that she had got the diagnosis of Alzheimer's dementia. She described that the message came like 'a BOMB'! Even though she suspected that something was wrong, she had never thought of dementia:

> *I thought it was something that could be fixed, so it became a little ... [...] When I did not know anything, I could just burst into anger, from frustration to getting furious. I, who never used to be angry. Now I have turned the anger towards myself.*

As shown, getting the diagnosis of young onset dementia was a very severe blow to her everyday life and her activities, a total break in her life course and life plans, and a blow to her identity. The impact of the diagnosis on her identity is made worse by her directing her anger in on herself.

At the next interview, Anne reported that her dementia contact had suggested that she should join a coffee-group with others living with dementia. She went along once, but it seemed to make her fearful: '*Then I just went down. It was just too much for me. I was miserable for many days afterwards.*'

The social occasion and seeing all the people with more severe dementia than her own, made her think that she would have a grim future with dementia and made her break down. The meeting demonstrated to her that her identity would be further eroded over time. As a result, she withdrew from being connected with this group and her days felt empty and depressing, and her existence meaningless.

> *Often, when I get up in the morning, I just return to bed. This is the worst, to get my days to pass on, to get finished one day after another. I can't read any longer, I was a passionate reader. I just watch very simple programmes on TV. Films are outside my reach. Tried listening to books on CD, and they read too fast. I feel so stupid!*

Anne said she postponed everything to tomorrow. She avoided meeting people, and social occasions got more and more difficult.

It is so hard to communicate. I use so much energy. And I feel I must use a lot of energy just to sit silent!

The future seemed very frightening.

I have got a sort of panic. I do not know. I have written down what I want to and do not want, the day I no longer can decide for myself. It rotates in my head.

We will return to Anne's story later in the chapter.

General issues around managing stigma during early dementia

To preserve normal relationships as far as possible, our participants avoided presenting themselves to the outside world as carrying the diagnosis of dementia (Johannessen et al., 2018). They wanted to escape the stigma of the disease and the very negative images it evokes. They felt that disclosing the diagnosis would aggravate the situation, for others as well as for themselves.

The stigma of dementia is well documented by research (Behuniak, 2011) and by reports from people with dementia (Aquilina and Hughes, 2006; Taylor, 2007). People with a diagnosis describe how others immediately change the way they communicate and behave towards them when they learn of the diagnosis (Simpson and Simpson, 1999). Metaphors often used about people with dementia, like 'half-empty', 'fading away', 'no longer there' or 'the living dead', underline the dehumanisation of those with the condition (Behuniak, 2011). In addition, the biomedical model characterises the reactions of the person diagnosed with dementia as symptoms of the disease (Power, 2014). Van Gorp and Vercruysse (2012) analysed how TV and news media seem to reinforce the public perception of dementia as a highly dreaded disease in western society. People with dementia become 'the demented other' (Sabat et al., 2011). To avoid becoming 'the other', the participants in Sabat and colleagues' (2011) study preferred to present themselves as 'a person with a memory problem', a more usual and accepted issue than dementia.

Despite this, most of the participants in a study by Aminzadeh et al. (2007) seemed remarkably able to cope with the disease for a long time and to live a satisfying life, after the initial shock of the diagnosis. In the early phases of our study (Johannessen et al., 2018), most participants found their strategies for handling their life situation enabled them to live a satisfying and good life. Participants emphasised that they focused on the positive side of life. If they were able to live 'the normal life' they were used to, feel valued and be connected to others in a life that was meaningful to them, most of these people living with young onset dementia found that their quality of life was rather good.

Identity in the moderate and late stages

Continuity vs. flexibility

Several of our participants were still satisfied with life right up to the last interview we conducted in the 2-year longitudinal study (Johannessen et al., 2018). Living their familiar life, as they had done before the diagnosis, functioned as protection against serious depression. Arntzen et al. (2016) also found something similar, demonstrating that identity can be better retained in moderate to late dementia when:

- everyday life takes place in a routine that is well known, and
- where people, neighbourhood and community, physical structures and material things are recognisable and support established habits.

We also found that forced changes to their familiar lifestyle had an impact on sense of self, more so than the immediate symptoms of young onset dementia itself (Johannessen et al., 2018). The participants focused on the impact of undesired changes in everyday life, like losing their job and their social and familial network, and moving to a new flat or to a nursing home. Such autobiographical disruptions are more severe for people with young onset dementia than for those with late onset dementia, since those with late onset are generally already retired, drawing a pension and adjusting to disabilities associated with ageing.

The continuity theory of ageing of Atchley (1989) underlines the importance of *outer* and *inner* continuity (i.e. subjective experiences of the outer world and the inner self). It suggests that a feeling of continuity can be preserved even when the circumstances of life change. This theory holds that, in making adaptive choices, middle-aged and older adults attempt to preserve and maintain the existing internal and external structures that give them a sense of continuity. They accomplish this by using well-established strategies tied to their past experiences of themselves and their social world. Changes are therefore linked to the person's perceived past, producing a sense of continuity in inner psychological characteristics, as well as in social behaviour and in social circumstances. Continuity is thus a grand adaptive strategy that is promoted by both individual preference and social approval.

The theory of continuity may explain why familiarity fosters a sense of security. It can be especially reassuring for those living with young onset dementia to have the sense of 'normalcy' this brings, and our study demonstrated that feeling safe is important when dementia progresses. However, wishing for continuity can also become dysfunctional; that is, aiming to continue life as it has always been can cause difficulties when old habits and ways of handling tasks no longer function well in the face of increasing cognitive impairment. In this situation, flexibility is needed. Anne expressed flexibility, as she moved into a nursing home and then started to adapt to her move, in this way:

> *Here in this nursing home, life is good. People are kind and it is safe. Still, inside me it goes up and down. I am a bit calmer, but I can become emotional, cry and be angry.* (Anne, living with dementia)

Family and friends' reactions to change

In our study (Johannessen et al., 2018), some participants reported that clinging onto continuity was an issue for spouses, partners and families. Some family members hung on tightly to the idea of the person with young onset dementia as they used to be and were not able to accept, tolerate and adapt to the changes in the person that young onset dementia entailed. In these situations, the person living with young onset dementia felt a lack of understanding from others and, consequently, might then withdraw and become isolated. Anne described the changes in her social relations and the gap between her experiences and their perceptions of her:

> *I have realised that to live with this [the dementia] is a hell, both for me and for others. It is no fun. People do not see it, but I feel it. So, I isolate myself more and more.* (Anne)

Studies have documented the great burden family members can experience in caring for people with advanced dementia. Family carers themselves find that family and friends often pull away from social contact, resulting in the carers themselves becoming isolated. Mirroring the experience of the person living with young onset dementia, they may then lose their own autonomy and personal life world (Johannessen et al., 2017; Helvik et al., 2024).

There seems to be a tendency in research literature to overlook the conflicts and problems people with young onset dementia may experience in family care. Support is not always given with warmth, love, support and concern. Anne's story illustrates how the 'new person with young onset dementia' that she became was no longer recognisable, acceptable or tolerated by those nearest to her, particularly her partner and family. The 'gap' between the former well-functioning person and the new, more cognitively challenged person is especially great when younger people are diagnosed with dementia (Thorsen et al., 2018). Young onset dementia is unusual, unexpected and difficult to understand. Our study (Johannessen et al., 2018) showed how people with young onset dementia often found that social relationships with friends and partners became so complicated and destructive to their existential self that those diagnosed preferred to break the contact. This resulted in them becoming more isolated and getting less identity support, catching them in a negative spiral.

Living alone

The study showed that living alone was not seen as a great disadvantage among single people, in contrast to other research highlighting the importance of social support for quality of life, assistance and avoidance of depression (WHO/ADI, 2012; Johannessen et al., 2018). Our participants included three women who were divorced from their husbands. They explicitly expressed that living alone was an advantage. To manage alone was their preferred way of life. At later stages, however, the three participants were no longer able to sustain existence on their own. This posed a new challenge to their sense of identity, because they then needed help with basic activities of daily life and could not necessarily access adequate community support services.

Supportive environments

Living in an accepting, considerate and supportive environment may validate the 'new person with young onset dementia', when the former cognitively intact person is gradually being changed by their dementia and needs much more daily support. Here we include extracts from our continuing interviews with Anne, demonstrating how she thrived after moving into supported living. This is a positive example of the value of moving to a supportive environment. We do not wish to imply, however, that everyone would thrive in supported living. There might be other ways forward for some, like moving in with family or employing a live-in carer.

In our later interviews with Anne, we heard that her dementia contact had suggested that she move to a flat in a complex with supported living for people of all ages with varied disabilities. She accepted this suggestion because she had become so afraid of being in her own flat and had become anxious being on her own.

At the sixth interview, she had moved into supported living, and her mood and tone had changed completely. She talked eagerly about how she was decorating her new flat, with encouraging assistance from her mother and her support contact. She was enjoying shopping for furniture, curtains and new gadgets. She expressed that the new environment would show her as a modern woman, valuing beauty and presenting her as able to decorate a new home, a central part of her female identity. Some of the new appliances – washing machine, dishwasher, TV – were impossible challenges, and written instructions were of no use. However, she got assistance, as needed, from personnel in the building.

She talked about outings with friends to cinemas, concerts and cafés. She had made plans to travel with her daughter: 'We have so many plans. We would like to go to Africa.' Her everyday life was bringing her joy, and she viewed her future as holding hope and anticipation of pleasure. The researcher remarked that she seemed to be thriving and doing better than before. She answered:

> *Yes, I am more satisfied. I am! I was more anxious in my former flat. Now I feel much safer. I have landed in a way. There are so many who ask, 'Don't you miss your former flat?' I say, 'Not for a minute!'* (Anne)

Anne praised the kind and considerate personnel at the complex. She summarised the changes: '*Yes. I thrive better and better and better. I really do, although I sense that I have deteriorated. Then I get very annoyed.*' She persisted in avoiding people from the dementia team as they cause her to feel much worse. She stated, '*All my life, I have said yes. Now I will end that. Learn to say no!*' Bidding farewell to the researcher, she remarked, '*I think it was a very good thing that I moved while I was as well as I am. Then I can get new habits and adapt to everything.*'

The final interview with Anne focused mostly on everyday events, joys and minor practical problems. In her new social environment, with people around, she looked forward to being alone:

> *It is very important to have time for myself. I am never bored with my own company. I think it is wonderful! Eat when I want, sleep when I want, go walking when I want, and not when I don't want.* (Anne)

Her depression and anxiety and bouts of panic had vanished. But even in her life at this point, filled with pleasures and plans, a continuing stream in her existential experience was the awareness of her deterioration due to the disease:

> *I am tired of being ill. I am fed up. I can get furious because I have heard that it takes 5 to 12 years. Then I think, when 12 years have passed, maybe I will be relieved of all this. Finished. I am not afraid of dying. I have planned. When I am leaving, everything shall be in order!* (Anne)

Overall, we can see in Anne's account how she greatly valued the acceptance, support and validation she got in her new living arrangements.

Another participant, Arne, who also moved into a care home, had a contrasting experience and was less content. He found his days empty and did not feel existentially confirmed in his new surroundings. Possibly the female-dominated environment was alien to him. He mentioned that he had much time on his own: '*I do not thrive with everyone here. We have little in common.*' However, he later formed a close friendship with a female resident who shared his interest in nature and travelling. They have a chat every day. He stated: '*She is a light in my day. She means rather much to me.*'

Having a sense of himself as an active man, he explained that every day he thinks that he has to be more active, cycling or cross-country skiing, but he says he is lacking the means to do it, like a car. However, overall he says:

> *I see no reason for complaining of life in the nursing home, the personnel are kind and considerate, and the food is good. I am very comfortable. Do not have to make any decisions. Long live laziness.* (Arne, living with dementia)

In these accounts, we see the security and support people with young onset dementia can feel from staff who at their best strengthen the person and their identity. After a period of floundering in the community, without enough support, people with young onset dementia may experience that they manage better again, as they did in their former life. The account illustrates the great importance of dedicated and accepting staff in good supported living and nursing homes.

Supporting identity and personhood – summary and recommendations

Hearing people living with young onset dementia

To achieve the World Health Organisation's (WHO) policy goals as expressed in 'Towards a Dementia-Inclusive Society' (WHO, 2021) and care for the needs of people with dementia, society must include those diagnosed more thoroughly, ask appropriate questions of the relevant people, and listen to their stories and answers. A society that hears people with dementia and supports their involvement in community and social life is a core aspect of a dementia-friendly and person-centred culture.

To achieve the WHO's goals, further research should focus on the voices of people with dementia, including young onset dementia. A lack of research regarding people with young onset dementia will negatively affect the level of knowledge required to meet the WHO and governmental goals of developing dementia-friendly societies (Alteren et al., 2023). Our study underpins that having an independent safe life with societal inclusion, both in private homes as well as in neighbourhoods and public spaces, is important for people with young onset dementia (Alteren et al., 2023). Our findings underline the importance of supporting personhood for well-being among those living with young onset dementia, in line with the theory of dementia care presented by Kitwood and Bredin (1992).

Focus on preservation of identity

Power (2014) has written about dementia 'beyond disease' and how to contribute to well-being in dementia. He encapsulates key principles for enabling people with advanced dementia to live well in one phrase: 'Preserve identity, celebrate personhood and create meaning in the moment for people with dementia' (Power, 2014: 42).

Many strategies for preserving identity focus on life in the past – the individual's life history. But, in the dementia process, memories are often eroded, starting with more recent memories but then moving back to more remote ones. Therefore, remembering and referring to the past becomes increasingly difficult and less meaningful. Studies have also shown how social interaction may become too demanding. They have revealed that people living with young onset dementia might prefer to sit and see others, knowing that they are there, rather than making the effort needed to join in fast-paced conversations. Even though not acting or participating, a person's inner life may be fine, relaxed and rich. Just being and being safe may come to be more comforting to the self than acting and talking. In advanced dementia, acting and talking may always seem to expose shortcomings or failings. Protecting well-being, rather than being active, becomes all-important when dementia is severe (Thorsen et al., 2018, Trindade et al., 2022).

Meaningful personal support

In our study, care staff such as community nurses were not mentioned by the participants as significant supporters. They seemed to belong to a taken-for-granted background of everyday life. Although the people with young onset dementia received the necessary health and social care, these care staff were not experienced as central to the participants' existential life. The staff were viewed as giving tolerable support, sometimes being nice, sometimes a nuisance, sometimes even scaring the participants when they did not recognise who had come to their home. In contrast, the participants emphasised with warmth the 'support contacts', who were valued for their personalised and adapted contact. They were 'like a friend' or a befriender (see also Johannessen et al., 2016; Johannessen and Thorsen, 2018).

In common with a number of other countries, including the UK, the Norwegian Government's 'Dementia Plan 2020' recommends that people with dementia and their caregivers should have a contact person in the health system – a person who should know the individual and coordinate and plan their assistance throughout the disease process. The individual should get varied support, outlined in an individualised care plan (Norwegian Ministry of Health and Care Services, 2020).

In contrast to this ideal, care in the community and in nursing homes is too often based on standardised systems regulated by working schedules. The diagnosis of dementia places the person within the biomedical model, transforming the person into a patient. Norway, like many other western countries, has many and shifting part-time health workers (Statistics Norway, 2011), implying that people living with young onset dementia meet many care staff, who are therefore difficult to distinguish and remember.

Different concepts have been introduced to try and change biomedical and non-person-centred cultures of care. These include person-centred care (Kitwood and Bredin, 1992; Edvardsson et al., 2008; Kitwood and Brooker, 2019), person-directed care (Fox et al., 2005), relationship-centred care (Suchman, 2006) and authentic partnerships in care (Dupuis et al., 2012). Our study underpins that it is vital that public care is transformed to be person-orientated, to support the identity of the person with young onset dementia. However, to achieve transformation, the influences of the cultural, organisational and economic contexts must be taken into account (McCormack et al., 2002). To transform caring systems, it is crucial to direct strategies both at the culture and the physical/organisational structure, to give people with young onset dementia a better life (McCormack and McCance, 2006).

Learning from those with advanced dementia

Our study highlights that the stage of the dementia influences the narratives people living with young onset dementia give, and the progressive disease restricts their dialogue over time. Yet people with quite severe young onset dementia were still able to tell us about their experiences. In this chapter, we have drawn heavily on the narrative of Anne, who was divorced and living alone. People living with a partner or who still have children or young people in the household will have other experiences. People with young onset dementia might also be from other cultures or have different diagnoses. Still, we found that the variations in our sample of persons with young onset dementia offered new insights (Johannessen et al., 2018).

Even though our sample was small, the themes have broader validity. Qualitative research findings cannot be generalised in a statistical sense but the results can be transferred to other contexts of individuals living with young onset dementia. They may contribute to a better understanding of how to contribute to the development and organisation of services for people with young onset dementia in a way that supports identity, especially as dementia advances.

Ethical research

Finally, a point about research methodology. Here, we want to emphasise the need for applied dementia care researchers to apply an ethical, person-centred and relational approach to their studies. A narrative longitudinal study depends on trust and a positive relationship between the interviewer and the participant (Thorsen and Johannessen, 2020). We analysed our own interview processes with attention to the concept of 'responsive identity support'. This is the idea that participants – for example, people living with young onset dementia – should be seen, confirmed and supported to preserve their self and dignity as they take part in research interviews (Johannessen et al., 2019). In examining our interview dialogues, we located examples of how the interviews supported the identity and self-esteem of the participants through sensitive interaction that validated interviewees' points and indicated they had been heard, using person-centred communication. We conclude that dialogue with responsive identity support is a fruitful research method in young onset dementia research (Thorsen and Johannessen, 2020).

Conclusions

People with dementia can tell their subjective stories about living with young onset dementia over time. The most significant aspects of their experiences over time were: the initial signs, coping efforts, concealing the diagnosis, social withdrawal, existential anxiety, and strivings to revive the self. The voices of people with dementia, not only around the time of diagnosis but also over time, should be listened to and included in planning for person-centred health and care services, because their experiences can be very different after diagnosis and later on.

People with young onset dementia highlight that the diagnosis provokes key existential concerns. To be aware of this, and that stigma still exists, can give us glimpses of how we can contribute so that people with young onset dementia can live 'the normal life' they were used to, feel valued and be connected to others in a life that is meaningful to them. A society that hears people with dementia and supports their involvement in community and social life is an important aspect of a dementia-friendly and person-centred culture. Living in an accepting, considerate and supportive environment may validate the new 'person living with young onset dementia', when the formerly cognitively competent person is gradually changing due to their dementia.

So what does this mean in practice?

If you are living with young onset dementia

Despite your diagnosis and premature retirement, you can support your identity by continuing to do things that make you who you are. Consider which activities and relationships are central to who you are. Think about whether and how you can keep these as part of your life. Discuss with others any support you need to do so and who could offer this. Think about replacements for things you can no longer do, so that these aspects of your life are not lost altogether. Try and find that one person from services, such as a 'side-by-side' worker or 'personal assistant', who can understand, support and guide as time goes on.

If and when your cognitive impairment gets worse, you may find it most comfortable to live 'in the moment', sometimes observing rather than being more involved. Think about what would help you do this. What would you most like to watch? What sounds or music do you find relaxing? How can you recreate the atmosphere you like best, whether it is a calm green setting, being with, or being able to see, photos of precious people and places, or having a cat on your lap.

If you are a family member or friend of someone with young onset dementia

You can support the person's identity early on by finding ways to help them to keep as much independence as possible and continue aspects of life that are important to them. Are there barriers that stop the person being able to go out that you could overcome so that the person you support feels safe and included?

As someone who knows your friend/family member well, you probably know what brings them pleasure, relaxation and enjoyment. When the dementia is more severe, think about what could provide these things and how this can be made available.

If you are a professional supporting people with young onset dementia

People with young onset dementia often have high levels of awareness, including as cognitive difficulties get worse over time. So be sure to ask people with young onset dementia who you support for their opinions on how to retain their quality of life. Ensure care is person-centred, taking the individual's culture, values and personal likes and dislikes into account.

If you are a researcher

Think about the impact your data collection could have on the identity and self-esteem of those who take part. Look for methods and ways of involvement that will support not undermine identity and well-being.

If you are involved in policy

Keep the goal of making communities inclusive in mind and think about how to create safe, welcoming public spaces in neighbourhoods, so that people with young onset dementia are not excluded. Remember the value placed by people living with young onset dementia on having a consistent 'key worker' over time and set up systems that foster this as a core part of service support.

References

Alteren, J., Johannessen, A., Lyberg, A.M., et al. (2023) Giving voice to people with dementia and perspectives regarding a dementia-friendly society: a synthesis of qualitative studies, *Journal of Multidisciplinary Healthcare*, 16: 851–61.

Aminzadeh, F., Byszewski, A., Molnar, F.J., et al. (2007) Emotional impact of dementia diagnosis: exploring persons with dementia and caregivers' perspectives, *Aging and Mental Health*, 11 (3): 281–90.

Aquilina, C. and Hughes, J. (2006) The return of living dead: agency lost and found?, in J. Hughes, S. Louw and S. Sabat (eds.) *Dementia: Mind, Meaning, and the Person.* Oxford: Oxford University Press.

Arntzen, C., Holthe, T. and Jentoft, R. (2016) Tracing the successful incorporation of assistive technology into everyday life for younger people with dementia and family carers, *Dementia*, 15 (4): 646–62.

Arons, A.M., Krabbe, P.F., Schölzel-Dorenbos, C.J., et al. (2013) Quality of life in dementia: a study on proxy bias, *BMC Medical Research Methodology*, 13: 110. Available at: https://doi.org/10.1186/1471-2288-13-110.

Atchley, R.C. (1989) A continuity theory of normal aging, *The Gerontologist*, 29 (2): 183–90.

Baptista, M.A.T., Santos, R.L., Kimura, N., et al. (2019) Differences in awareness of disease between young-onset and late-onset dementia, *Alzheimer's Disease and Associated Disorders*, 33 (2): 129–35.

Behuniak, S. (2011) The living dead? The construction of people with Alzheimer's disease as zombies, *Ageing and Society*, 31 (1): 70–92.

Caddell, L.S. and Clare, L. (2010) The impact of dementia on self and identity: a systematic review, *Clinical Psychology Review*, 30 (1): 113–26.

De Baggio, T. (2002) *Losing My Mind: An Intimate Look at Life with Alzheimer's Disease.* New York: Free Press.

De Baggio, T. (2003) *When it Gets Darker: An Enlightened Reflection on Life with Alzheimer's.* New York: Free Press.

Dupuis, S.L., Whyte, C., Carson, J., et al. (2012) Just dance with me: an authentic partnership approach to understanding leisure in the dementia context, *World Leisure Journal*, 54 (3): 240–54.

Edvardsson, D., Winblad, B. and Sandman, P.O. (2008) Person-centred care of people with severe Alzheimer's disease: current status and ways forward, *Lancet Neurology*, 7 (4): 362–67.

Fox, N., Norton, L., Angelelli, J., et al. (2005) *Well-Being: Beyond Quality of Life.* Rochester, NY: The Eden Alternative.

Helvik, A.S., Hvidsten, L., Engedal, K., et al. (2024) Living with young-onset dementia in the family: a mixed method study, *Aging and Mental Health*, 28 (2): 254–61.

Johannessen, A. and Thorsen, K. (2018) Personsentrert omsorg i praksis: Fire perspektiver på støttekontakttjenesten i demensomsorgen-en case studie design, *Nordisk tidsskrift for helseforskning*, 14: 2. Available at: https://doi.org/10.7557/14.4323.

Johannessen, A., Engedal, K. and Thorsen, K. (2016) Family carers of people with young-onset dementia: their experiences with the supporter service, *Geriatrics*, 1 (4): 28. Available at: https://doi.org/10.3390/geriatrics1040028.

Johannessen, A., Helvik, A.S., Engedal, K., et al. (2017) Experiences and needs of spouses of persons with young-onset frontotemporal lobe dementia during the progression of the disease, *Scandinavian Journal of Caring Sciences*, 31 (4): 779–88.

Johannessen, A., Engedal, K., Haugen, P.K., et al. (2018) 'To be, or not to be': experiencing deterioration among people with young-onset dementia living alone, *International Journal of Qualitative Studies on Health and Well-being*, 13 (1): 1490620. Available at: https://doi.org/10.1080/17482631.2018.1490620.

Johannessen, A., Engedal, K., Haugen, P. K. et al. (2019) Coping with transitions in life: a four-year longitudinal narrative study of single younger people with dementia, *Journal of Multidisciplinary Health*, 12: 479-492.

Kitwood, T. (1997) *Dementia Reconsidered: The Person Comes First.* Buckingham: Open University Press.

Kitwood, T. and Bredin, K. (1992) Towards a theory of dementia care: personhood and well-being, *Ageing and Society*, 12: 269–87.

Kitwood, T. and Brooker, D. (eds.) (2019) *Dementia Reconsidered, Revisited: The Person Still Comes First.* London: Open University Press.

McCormack, B. and McCance, T.V. (2006) Development of a framework for person-centred nursing, *Journal of Advanced Nursing*, 56 (5): 472–79.

McCormack, B., Kitson, A., Harvey, G., et al. (2002) Getting evidence into practice: the meaning of 'context', *Journal of Advanced Nursing*, 38 (1): 94–104.

Norwegian Ministry of Health and Care Services (2020) *Dementia Plan 2020.* Oslo. Available at: https://extranet.who.int/mindbank/item/6403.

Power, G. (2014) *Dementia beyond Drugs: Enhancing Wellbeing*, Baltimore, MD: Health Professions Press.

Rose, L. (2003) *Larry's Way: Another Look at Alzheimer's from the Inside*. New York: iUniverse Inc.

Sabat, S.R., Johnson, A., Swarbrick, C., et al. (2011) The 'demented other' or simply 'a person'? Extending the philosophical discourse of Naue and Kroll through the situated self, *Nursing Philosophy*, 12 (4): 282–92, discussion 293–96.

Sands, L.P., Ferreira, P., Stewart, A.L., et al. (2004) What explains differences between dementia patients' and their caregivers' ratings of patients' quality of life?, *American Journal of Geriatric Psychiatry*, 12 (3): 272–80.

Simpson, R. and Simpson, A. (1999) *Through the Wilderness of Alzheimer's: A Guide in Two Voices*. Minneapolis, MN: Fortress Press.

Statistics Norway (2011) *Stort omfang av deltidsarbeid [Much part-time work among health personnel]*. Samfunnsspeilet, 2. Available at: https://www.ssb.no/en/arbeid-og-lonn/statistikker/regsys/aar/2016-05-27.

Suchman, A.L. (2006) A new theoretical foundation for relationship-centered care: complex responsive processes of relating, *Journal of General Internal Medicine*, 21 (suppl. 1): S40–44.

Taylor, R. (2007) *Alzheimer's from the Inside Out*. Baltimore, MD: Health Professions Press.

Thorsen, K. and Johannessen, A. (2020) Lydhör identitetsstötte i samtaler med personer med demens: En studie av intervjuer i en femårig narrativ forlöpsstudie, *Nordisk tidsskrift for helseforskning*, 16: 2. Available at: https://doi.org/10.7557/14.5345.

Thorsen, K., Dourado, M.C.N. and Johannessen, A. (2018) Developing dementia: the existential experience of the quality of life with young-onset dementia – a longitudinal case study, *Dementia*, 19 (3): 878–93.

Thorsen, K., Dourado, M.C.N. and Johannessen, A. (2020) Awareness of dementia and coping to preserve quality of life: a five-year longitudinal narrative study, *International Journal of Qualitative Studies on Health and Well-being*, 15 (1): 1798711. Available at: https://doi.org/10.1080/17482631.2020.1798711.

Trindade, P.G.E., Santos, R.L., Johannessen, A., et al. (2020) Awareness of functional Status: people with Alzheimer's disease abilities to self-report impairment in activities of daily living, *Journal of Alzheimer's Disease Reports*, 4 (1): 405–15.

Trindade, P.G.E., Johannessen, A., Baptista, M.A.T., et al. (2022) 'I do not enjoy too much being with people, it takes me a long time to interact': a qualitative analysis of awareness of relationships in people with dementia, *Aging and Mental Health*, 27 (6): 1120–26.

Van Gorp, B. and Vercruysse, T. (2012) Frames and counter-frames giving meaning to dementia: a framing analysis of media content, *Social Science and Medicine*, 74: 1274–81.

Voris, E., Shabahangi, N. and Fox, P. (2009) *Conversation with Ed: Waiting for Forgetfulness. Why Are We So Afraid of Alzheimer's Disease?* San Fransisco, CA: Elders Academy Press.

World Health Organisation (WHO) (2021) *Towards a dementia-inclusive society: WHO toolkit for dementia-friendly initiatives*. Available at: https://www.who.int/publications/i/item/9789240031531.

World Health Organization and Alzheimer's Disease International (WHO/ADI) (2012) *Dementia: A public health priority*. Available at: https://www.who.int/publications/i/item/dementia-a-public-health-priority.

14

The impact of young onset dementia on the identity and well-being of family carers

Christian Bakker and Marjolein de Vugt

Overview

Family carers of people with young onset dementia face unique challenges and experiences compared with carers of older adults with dementia. As mentioned in earlier chapters of this book, young onset dementia is often difficult to diagnose, which can be frustrating for family carers who may have been noticing, and coping with, changes in their family member's behaviour or cognition for a long time. Delayed diagnosis results in a delay in the initiation of appropriate help and support, adding to any anxiety, worries or burden already experienced (Millenaar et al., 2016a). The impact of young onset dementia on family supporters can be particularly pronounced due to the unexpected nature of the condition and the rapid decline in cognitive function or significant changes in behaviour that can occur. Caring for a relative with young onset dementia can also have a profound impact on family carers' identity and well-being. This chapter explores how young onset dementia impacts family carers' identity and well-being, drawing on research from the scientific literature. The chapter also includes discussion of supportive strategies and psychosocial interventions available for mitigating the impact of young onset dementia on carers' well-being.

Keywords

Young onset dementia, role change, family-based support, supportive strategies, healthcare and social services.

Learning points

- Providing family care for a person with young-onset dementia impacts family members' roles, relationships and sense of identity at the individual level, but also the family as a whole.

- It is crucial that health and social care professionals acknowledge and address the emotional distress, social isolation and financial strain experienced by family members of persons with young onset dementia in order to support the overall well-being of those family members.
- Supportive strategies for young onset dementia carers that include tailored information about young onset dementia, access to peer support networks, counselling services and respite care can be beneficial.
- The introduction of a specialised key contact person, such as a case manager, can facilitate adaptation of support to the changing needs of the family along the course of the disease.
- Experiences of family carers of a person living with young onset dementia differ, for example between a partner who takes most responsibility and children or other family members who also step up to provide care. However, as family members share common challenges, a system-focused approach can create mutual understanding, improve communication and strengthen family relationships.

Changes in roles and family dynamics

Following a diagnosis of young onset dementia, family members may experience shifts in their identity because of their caregiving role (Chirico et al., 2022). Spouses or partners, for example, may, over time, experience a shift from being a partner to being a carer. This can be a difficult adjustment, as the dynamics of the relationship change. The partner may need to provide hands-on care, such as helping with personal hygiene or managing behaviour, which can be emotionally challenging. Partners may also need to take on additional household responsibilities, such as cooking and cleaning, which can be time-consuming and physically demanding (Millenaar et al., 2017). As partners often have to combine these tasks with work, parenting and societal roles, this can add to the burden already felt (Massimo et al., 2013). As a person's dementia progresses, partners often find they are no longer able to discuss their experiences or worries with the person with dementia, for instance regarding parenting issues. The experience of this shift from partner to carer can also be amplified by changes in intimacy or a sense of loss of reciprocity in the relationship. Depending on the diagnosis or stage of dementia, the person with dementia may have difficulty showing empathy, reflecting on how the dementia may affect other family members or reflecting on their own abilities to provide support. Such changes are often gradual, except for conditions such as frontotemporal dementia. If these changes occur gradually, this allows couples to adjust. However, many partners find it difficult to continue their caregiving role as reciprocity diminishes (Lockeridge and Simpson, 2013).

In young onset dementia, it is most often the partner who acts as the primary carer, with about 80% of primary carers being spouses or partners

(Stamou et al., 2021). About 50% of these carers are men and 50% women, giving quite an even gender split. This contrasts with late onset dementia where a larger proportion of carers are female, most often wives, daughters or daughters-in-law. However, children may have similar experiences to partners regarding changes in their role as they lose a parent figure and have to adapt to a caregiving role. Their ability to do so depends on their pre-existing relationship with their parents and family dynamics, as well as their coping abilities. It is also influenced by whether they are still living at home and their willingness to undertake caregiving tasks. Decisions about whether to perform care duties impact on future plans, such as moving out or taking a break from studies, and can have a pronounced impact on children's lives (Millenaar et al., 2014).

Family members not only have to adapt to the changes caused by the dementia at the individual level, but also at the family level. For instance, expectations regarding the caregiving situation and perspectives of individual family members need to be managed. Parents often feel that they ought to shield their children from a caregiving role as they believe that the children should be able to grow up without having to worry too much about such things. At the same time, children are often worried about their healthy parent, when aware of all the challenges that parent is faced with. Children are often more focused on the needs of their parents than they are on their own needs, with the risk of parentification in which the parent-child role becomes reversed (Millenaar et al., 2014). Organising care together as a family can have positive effects for all family members by increasing cohesion, strengthening interaction and communication, and creating a sense of companionship (Bruinsma et al., 2022a). The challenge for (young) adult children is to find space for their own development according to their own needs. Young adults may cope with this through detachment, for example by avoiding difficult situations at home and participating more in activities outside the family. This can provide protection in stressful times when they are not able to take control of the situation (Johannessen et al., 2016). The impact on children and young people is addressed further in Chapter 15, which focuses on family relationships, and Chapter 16, which focuses on the well-being of children.

Overall, the experiences of spouses/partners and children or young people caring for a parent with young onset dementia will differ based on their relationship to the person with dementia. Some challenges experienced may be best addressed through one-to-one support. On the other hand, different family members share many common challenges that can be addressed in a system-focused approach that involves all close family members. This can create mutual understanding, improve communication and strengthen family relationships.

Impact on mental and physical health

Family members may experience a range of emotions, such as grief, anger and guilt, as they try to cope with the impact of the condition on the person with dementia and themselves. These emotions can be particularly difficult to manage when caring for a relative with young onset dementia, as the person's cognitive decline may be more rapid and unpredictable (Day et al., 2022). Family members may also experience frustration and helplessness as they struggle to communicate with their relative, who may become increasingly confused or agitated.

Research has shown that family members caring for a person with young onset dementia may experience higher levels of emotional distress than those caring for a person with later-onset dementia. Kimura et al. (2021) reported that spouses caring for a partner with young onset dementia appear to experience higher levels of burden and depression than those caring for a partner with late-onset dementia. Research has also shown that, although caring for a person with dementia in general impacts on the health-related quality of life of carers, the impact of this reduction in quality of life on the ability to perform care and other responsibilities appears more pronounced among younger carers (Millenaar et al., 2016b). Providing hands-on care may also result in physical strain. If carers have less time to engage in physical activity or attend to their own healthcare needs due to care responsibilities, this may result in negative health outcomes. On the other hand, their resilience and adaptability may be higher than that of elderly carers, because they are more likely to be healthy and still physically fit.

However, in general, the impact of caring for someone with dementia on the mental well-being of carers is clear. They may feel that they are one step behind all the time in adjusting to the changes that occur. Family members may also struggle with how to involve the person with dementia in care decisions and as the dementia advances, this becomes more difficult or even impossible. As we have seen in earlier chapters, retaining control over their own care is important for people with young onset dementia, probably more so than in late-onset dementia. Making care decisions for the person with dementia is often stressful for family members. In particular, decisions regarding transitions in care, such as initiating day care or a move into a residential or nursing home, often results in feelings of guilt. As one partner stated during a support group: '*I feel so guilty. I am still young, I should be able to care for him, but I am exhausted, I can't go on any longer.*'

Loss is a significant theme in family carers' descriptions of caring over time. Most carers report experiencing continuing loss with each phase of the disease. One daughter, talking about her father with young onset dementia, described this process: '*There is not much left, although physically he is still here, I feel that I have already lost him.*' Putting things in your own life on hold (e.g. work, social and sporting events, hobbies) in order to provide care can also result in feelings of loss and increase the subjective burden. Being able to hold on to such activities is an important aspect of self-care. Family members who feel that they can continue with these activities tend to experience lower levels of distress than family members who are not able to do so. Changes in intimacy can cause a sense of loss as the person with young onset dementia may no longer be able to show affection or provide comfort to family members. Partners may find it difficult to be intimate with the person with young onset dementia, often because of changes in the person's behaviour, self-care or incontinence. However, some partners feel that the quality of their relationship has improved despite the dementia because of an increased focus on each other and on joint activities that are still possible (Bruinsma et al., 2020).

Family members often find it difficult to keep the family going when the role of the person with young onset dementia within the family diminishes over time. This is especially the case when the person moves into a care home and after their death. During the period of caregiving, family members often feel guilty that their relative is no longer able to join in family outings. However, family events and activities are essential for carers to retain a balance between caregiving and connectedness of family members. Family members are often very much aware during the course of the disease of the fact that at some point they will have to find a way to continue their lives without their relative. As one partner described it:

I knew we would lose him at some point; still his death came as a surprise. I feel that I did not take the time to grieve before, because I was too busy managing everything.

Social isolation

Research shows that caring for a person with young onset dementia can result in social isolation. Family members may experience social isolation as a result of their caregiving responsibilities. They may need to reduce their working hours or leave their job to provide care, which can impact their social connections. They may find it difficult to maintain their social relationships because caring for a relative with young onset dementia can be time-consuming and emotionally draining. Many family members also experience that people around them don't understand what it means to care for a person with dementia. As one partner stated: '*They tell me that he still looks fine. It hurts when they question me sending him to day care, suggesting this is too soon for him.*' They also find that as time passes, family and friends visit less often. One partner said: '*I know that her behaviour has changed a lot due to the dementia. I think they do not know how to talk to her and simply stay away.*' This may apply in particular to conditions such as frontotemporal dementia, which have pronounced behavioural changes as one of the core symptoms (Bruinsma et al., 2022b). In this focus group study, participants expressed that they experienced little understanding and support from family, relatives and friends who felt that the carer was exaggerating the condition of the person with young onset dementia (Bruinsma et al., 2022b). Such reactions influence the quality of the relationship with others and can amplify the feeling of being socially isolated.

As caring for a person with young onset dementia can be a lengthy process, it is important that carers feel supported and understood by others.

Decades of research have shown that social support is very important for the well-being of carers and serves as a protective factor in a stressful process. Received support, satisfaction with support, and social networks can moderate the relationship between the objective and subjective burden in carers (Xu et al., 2021). This means that the presence and quality of social connections can influence how caregivers perceive and experience the challenges of caregiving.

Use of formal care alongside informal, family care can increase benefits for the carer by providing respite, helping them persevere and facilitating access to resources such as peer support, although formal care use is generally limited in young onset dementia. The reluctance to use formal care services is related to the stigma of dementia, lack of perceived need and limited availability of specific services tailored to the needs of persons with young onset dementia (Cations et al., 2017). Because of these barriers, carers often do not seek formal care until impairment is very severe and formal care becomes inevitable (Bakker et al., 2013). Access to tailored care and support that fit the needs of carers at the early stages of the disease trajectory can improve timely acceptance of care, with important implications for the quality of life of the carer as well as their relative with young onset dementia.

Financial strain

Young onset dementia has a financial impact on families. First of all, the person with young onset dementia will often have to stop working early in the course of the disease, which results in a loss of income despite any compensation that may be available (see Chapter 9 for a discussion of employment and young onset dementia). Family members may also experience financial strain because of their caregiving responsibilities. They may need to pay for care services or equipment, reduce their working hours or leave their job to provide care, or pay for the person's medical expenses. This can impact their financial stability and create additional stress. In a study by Kandiah and colleagues (2016), family carers of individuals with young onset dementia experienced higher levels of financial burden than those caring for individuals with late onset dementia. The financial burden was highest in families caring for a person with frontotemporal dementia.

The financial impact of dementia in young families is especially high because of their younger life stage, in which they may still have a mortgage, have to pay tuition fees for the education of children and may have other financial responsibilities. Family members may also experience negative effects on their career, such as reduced career opportunities or promotions resulting in overall lower earnings or reduced pension. Additionally, people with young onset dementia may not have access to certain benefits or these benefits may be very low (see Chapter 6 for further in-depth discussion of financial considerations). This underlines that dementia has a profound impact on the lives of families over time.

Supportive strategies

In order to mitigate the impact of young onset dementia on family carers' identity and well-being, it is important for family members to seek support and to prioritise their own self-care. Support can come from a range of sources, including health and social care professionals, support groups, ehealth support and respite care services. These services can provide family carers with the resources and information they need to manage their relative's condition and to take care of their own needs. Prioritising self-care can include activities such as exercise and meditation, as well as spending time with friends and family. It is important for family members to recognise that caring for a person with young onset dementia will have a significant impact on their own lives. Finding a balance between taking care of the person with dementia versus taking care of themselves is critical but challenging.

Information and education

Timely support starts directly after the diagnosis is established. Higher quality of the way the diagnosis is disclosed is important for better adjustment and less negative emotional impact on carers (Woods et al., 2019; see also Chapter 3). Information must be tailored to individual characteristics and needs, taking into account expectations and experiences in the pre-diagnostic period. This applies broadly to dementia of all ages but in young onset dementia this may be more challenging (O'Malley et al., 2021). For example, atypical presentations occur more often at a young age and these might be more difficult to explain and understand. Access to additional resources and high quality information, such as brochures, books or web-based information on young onset dementia, can help to improve the understanding and acceptance of the diagnosis.

Acceptance of the diagnosis is an important factor that influences the acknowledgement of needs and openness to additional care and support. In the European RHAPSODY-project, a multimedia online programme was developed specifically for young onset dementia carers (Metcalfe et al., 2019). The programme covered a range of topics, including causes and treatments, common difficulties and suggested strategies, and where to access further care and support. A pilot of the programme showed promising results in participants regarding acceptability, programme satisfaction and carer well-being. In an additional study in the Netherlands, the programme was tailored to the Dutch context and integrated into the online platform of the Dutch Alzheimer Society. The evaluation showed that carers appreciated finding trustworthy, tailored information on young onset dementia in one place, including young onset dementia subtype-specific information (Daemen et al., 2022). A daughter of a person with Alzheimer's dementia stated:

> *As a carer, there is always the question, 'Where do I find all the information?' You can't see the forest for the trees. After looking into this programme, this is the place where I would recommend people visit.*

Self-management and ehealth

Carers have to cope with many problems and stressors in daily life. Due to the progressive nature of dementia, the needs of the person with young onset dementia change, challenging the knowledge and skills of the carer who is trying to manage their caregiving role. Self-management support for carers can, on the one hand, help to increase carer confidence to address the needs of the person with dementia, while on the other, identify their own needs and wishes. Self-management can also contribute to strengthening the carer-care recipient relationship. This can help carers to take charge of the changes in their life and increase self-efficacy, lower carer stress and improve their well-being.

The blended care 'Partner in Balance' intervention was found to be an effective and feasible self-management tool for family carers of persons with dementia (Boots et al., 2018). It is referred to as 'blended' owing to its combination of coaching from a professional and online materials. It proved to be an especially good fit for carers of persons with young onset dementia as they liked the online accessibility that offered support at their own convenient place and time. In light of this feedback, the programme was further developed to fit the specific needs of this younger carer group (for example, by using thematic modules and appropriate video vignettes). A feasibility study showed that the programme was positively evaluated and carers expressed feeling more confident to cope with future challenges after participating in the intervention (Bruinsma et al., 2021a).

Based on these positive results, a further version was developed with tailored content for carers of people with frontotemporal dementia (Bruinsma et al., 2021b). This group felt recognised by the tailored programme, since the majority of available support for carers of people with young onset dementia has been designed with Alzheimer's disease in mind (Bruinsma et al., 2021a). These developments were in Dutch and in the context of the Netherlands, but an English version is currently being developed.

Peer support

Carer support can be more impactful when offered by individuals who are undergoing similar circumstances and facing comparable experiences. This form of support, commonly known as peer support, aids in normalising experiences and cultivating effective coping strategies (Carter et al., 2020). Carers of young family members with frontotemporal dementia (FTD) emphasised the significance of peer support groups in fostering a sense of acknowledgement and understanding. They found it challenging when receiving tailored guidance from healthcare professionals regarding coping strategies for emotional and behavioural changes in individuals with FTD. Consequently, carers felt unseen and misunderstood by healthcare providers, which led them to delay seeking care and support services. Peer support played a vital role in making carers feel heard and helping alleviate feelings of isolation (Bruinsma et al., 2022b). Research on peer support for (young) children is scant, but experiences with initiatives such as 'Breinspoken' (a summer camp and supporting online digital platform for children with a parent with young onset dementia) and support groups for children in the Netherlands are promising (see the links in the appendix to this chapter).

Peer support can be provided through face-to-face support groups or online platforms, both of which have proved beneficial for carers. A recent co-design study, involving people living with young onset dementia and their carers, stressed that the lack of awareness about other families living with young onset dementia in their local area was a significant obstacle to establishing peer support networks (Mayrhofer et al., 2020). Online peer support, in particular, holds potential not only as a cost-effective method of delivery but also as a means of reaching affected families even in remote areas.

Counselling and psychotherapy

Counselling and psychotherapy are valuable forms of support that can be offered to both persons living with young onset dementia and their carers. These interventions involve regular sessions between an individual, dyad or the family as a whole and a therapist. Commonly used approaches are cognitive behavioural therapy, supportive counselling, acceptance and commitment therapy, and mindfulness-based interventions. Psychotherapy can enhance acceptance of the situation and reduce the negative impact of caregiving on the psychological health of carers of people with dementia (Cheng et al., 2020; Cheston, 2022). A family-oriented approach regarding counselling and psychotherapy may be valuable in young onset dementia, especially given evidence for more intact self-awareness in early than in late onset dementia (see recommendations section below and Chapter 15) (van Vliet et al., 2013; Baptista et al., 2019). However, specific evidence regarding counselling and psychotherapy for family carers of people with young onset dementia is lacking, compared with the broader population of carers for individuals with late onset dementia. More studies are needed to explore psychotherapeutic interventions and counselling strategies specifically targeting carers of young individuals with dementia.

Care coordination

A key contact person, such as a case manager, is crucial to support family carers in accessing appropriate care and support when needed. This person acts as a central point of contact who can gather and disseminate relevant information about the person with dementia, family members, their needs and available resources. They maintain continuity of care by monitoring the changing needs of the person with dementia and other family members, and overseeing and coordinating the different aspects of care during the care trajectory. This will support the family to regain and/or retain a sense of balance in living with dementia throughout the caregiving trajectory. The case manager's knowledge about the specific problems and needs in young onset dementia will facilitate access to tailored support and age-appropriate services for this population.

For example, in the Netherlands, dedicated training programmes are available at the national level to equip healthcare professionals such as case managers and nurses with the skills necessary to provide optimal support in young onset dementia (Bakker et al., 2021).

Respite services

As stated earlier, carers of individuals with young onset dementia often face challenges in balancing their own needs with caregiving responsibilities. These challenges are further amplified by additional obligations such as employment and parenthood. As a result, carers often struggle to find time for themselves and report high levels of unmet needs. Feelings of loyalty, self-sacrifice and obligation may contribute to resistance to seeking support from respite care services (Bressan et al., 2020). A study focusing on this issue in young onset dementia revealed that carers with more unmet psychological needs, including the need for respite care, are at higher risk of limitations in social functioning, as well as feelings of depression and anxiety (Bakker et al., 2014).

Respite care, particularly in the form of day care, is a common type of support that can have positive outcomes for both carers and the person with dementia. In the broader population of dementia carers, the utilisation of day care services has been associated with a decrease in carer burden and other stress-related factors. These benefits are particularly pronounced when carer support is integrated into the day care programme (Vandepitte et al., 2016). However, respite services for persons living with young onset dementia should be age-appropriate, increasing the likelihood that these services can accommodate their particular needs and that family members perceive a good fit as well. Acknowledging and addressing the need for respite care is crucial in supporting carers' overall well-being and mental health.

Recommendations for an integrative, family-based approach

Existing support systems and interventions often fail to consider the dynamics and complexities of family relationships when caring for a person with young onset dementia. They tend to focus on the primary carer, neglecting the experiences and needs of other family members. There is a lack of insight into how young onset dementia impacts the entire family unit, including their internal dynamics and relationships. The few studies to adopt a family-based approach have revealed that poorer family relationships and higher levels of stress are associated with less positive adaptation to dementia. These challenges can manifest as ineffective communication, a lack of connectedness among family members, and difficulties in coping with the impact of dementia on their lives (Hutchinson et al., 2020). A family-based study of frontotemporal dementia (FTD) demonstrated individual differences in involvement, coping strategies and bereavement experiences due to the dynamic interplay between symptoms and family life (Bruinsma et al., 2022a). Another study

(La Fontaine et al., 2022) which followed seven families with a member with behavioural variant FTD (bvFTD) over approximately 2 years, found there was an interplay between the family relationships in the way bvFTD impacted on these relationships and families' understanding of the condition. The authors concluded that to support families of those with bvFTD, we need to provide 'tailored, relational-focused and specialised information concerning the experience of living with bvFTD' (La Fontaine et al., 2022: 1).

Recognising the importance of involving the entire family in education about dementia and support can significantly influence their future functioning and interactions. Obtaining comprehensive knowledge about the family's background, history and beliefs early on is crucial. This information helps to create a sense of mutual understanding among family members and reduces the risk of a family crisis. Facilitating open communication can greatly assist families in navigating the challenges of shared decision-making and organising care for a relative with dementia. By adopting a family-centred approach, support services can better address the holistic needs of the entire family unit, promote healthier family dynamics, and enhance their ability to cope with the demanding task of caring for a person with dementia at a young age. This topic is addressed further in Chapter 15 on sustaining family relationships.

Conclusions

In conclusion, the impact of young onset dementia extends beyond the individual with the condition and affects the well-being and identity of family carers. In the case of young onset dementia, the main carer is usually the partner/spouse and most research has therefore focused on spouse/partner carers but there is also an impact on the well-being of parents, children, young people and siblings who take on caregiving roles. Emotional distress, social isolation and financial strain are the common challenges they face. It is crucial for health and social care professionals to acknowledge and address these impacts in order to support the overall well-being of family members.

Implementing supportive strategies tailored to the needs of carers can be beneficial. Providing tailored information about young onset dementia, access to peer support networks, counselling services and respite care can help alleviate some of the burden they experience. The presence of specialised key contact persons, such as case managers, is essential in facilitating access to age-appropriate services and support that adapts to changing needs during the course of the disease. Taking a family-centred approach is vital in providing comprehensive support. By recognising the holistic needs of the entire family unit, support services can promote healthier family dynamics and enhance carers' ability to cope with the challenges of caring for a relative with young onset dementia. This approach aims to improve the overall well-being and resilience of family members as they navigate the complexities of young onset dementia caregiving.

References

Bakker, C., De Vugt, M.E., Van Vliet, D., et al. (2013) The use of formal and informal care in early onset dementia: results from the NeedYD study, *American Journal of Geriatric Psychiatry*, 21 (1): 37–45.

Bakker, C., De Vugt, M.E., Van Vliet, D., et al. (2014) Unmet needs and health-related quality of life in young-onset dementia, *American Journal of Geriatric Psychiatry*, 22 (11): 1121–30.

Bakker, C., Verboom, M. and Koopmans, R. (2021) Reimagining postdiagnostic care and support in young-onset dementia, *Journal of the American Medical Directors Association*, 23 (2): 261–65.

Baptista, M.A.T., Santos, R.L., Kimura, N., et al. (2019) Differences in awareness of disease between young-onset and late-onset dementia, *Alzheimer Disease and Associated Disorders*, 33 (2): 129–35.

Boots, L.M., De Vugt, M.E., Kempen, G.I., et al. (2018) Effectiveness of a blended care Self-management program for caregivers of people with early-stage dementia (Partner in Balance): randomized controlled trial, *Journal of Medical Internet Research*, 20: e10017. Available at: https://doi.org/10.2196/10017.

Bressan, V., Visintini, C. and Palese, A. (2020) What do family caregivers of people with dementia need? A mixed-method systematic review, *Health and Social Care in the Community*, 28 (6): 1942–60.

Bruinsma, J., Peetoom, K., Millenaar, J., et al. (2020) The quality of the relationship perceived by spouses of people with young-onset dementia, *International Psychogeriatrics*. Available at: https://doi.org/10.1017/S1041610220000332.

Bruinsma, J., Peetoom, K., Bakker, C., et al. (2021a) Tailoring and evaluating the web-based 'Partner in Balance' intervention for family caregivers of persons with young-onset dementia, *Internet Interventions*, 25: 100390. Available at: https://doi.org/10.1016/j.invent.2021.100390.

Bruinsma, J., Peetoom, K., Boots, L., et al. (2021b) Tailoring the web-based 'Partner in Balance' intervention to support spouses of persons with frontotemporal dementia, *Internet Interventions*, 26: 100442. Available at: https://doi.org/10.1016/j.invent.2021.100442.

Bruinsma, J., Peetoom, K., Verhey, F., et al. (2022a) Behind closed doors: a case study exploring the lived experiences of a family of a person with the behavioral variant of frontotemporal dementia, *Dementia*, 21 (8): 2569–83.

Bruinsma, J., Peetoom, K., Bakker, C., et al. (2022b) 'They simply do not understand': a focus group study exploring the lived experiences of family caregivers of people with frontotemporal dementia, *Aging and Mental Health*, 26 (2): 277–85.

Carter, G., Monaghan, C. and Santin, O. (2020) What is known from the existing literature about peer support interventions for carers of individuals living with dementia: a scoping review, *Health and Social Care in the Community*, 28 (4): 1134–51.

Cations, M., Withall, A., Horsfall, R., et al. (2017) Why aren't people with young onset dementia and their supporters using formal services? Results from the INSPIRED study, *PLoS One*, 12 (7): e0180935. Available at: https://doi.org/10.1371/journal.pone.0180935.

Cheng, S.T., Li, K.K., Losada, A., et al. (2020) The effectiveness of nonpharmacological interventions for informal dementia caregivers: an updated systematic review and meta-analysis, *Psychology and Aging*, 35 (1): 55–77.

Cheston, R. (2022) *Dementia and Psychotherapy Reconsidered*. London: Open University Press.

Chirico, I., Ottoboni, G., Linarello, S., et al. (2022) Family experience of young-onset dementia: the perspectives of spouses and children, *Aging and Mental Health*, 26 (11): 2243–51.

Daemen, M., Bruinsma, J., Bakker, C., et al. (2022) A cross-sectional evaluation of the Dutch RHAPSODY program: online information and support for caregivers of persons with young-onset dementia, *Internet Interventions*, 28: 100530. Available at: https://doi.org/10.1016/j.invent.2022.100530.

Day, S., Roberts, S., Launder, N.H., et al. (2022) Age of symptom onset and longitudinal course of sporadic Alzheimer's disease, frontotemporal dementia, and vascular dementia: a systematic review and meta-analysis, *Journal of Alzheimer's Disease*, 85 (4): 1819–33.

Hutchinson, K., Roberts, C., Roach, P., et al. and (2020) Co-creation of a family-focused service model living with younger onset dementia, *Dementia*, 19 (4): 1029–50.

Johannessen, A., Engedal, K. and Thorsen, K. (2016) Coping efforts and resilience among adult children who grew up with a parent with young-onset dementia: a qualitative follow-up study, *International Journal of Qualitative Studies on Health and Well-being*, 11: 30535. Available at: https://doi.org/10.3402/qhw.v11.30535.

Kandiah, N., Wang, V., Lin, X., et al. (2016) Cost related to dementia in the young and the impact of etiological subtype on cost, *Journal of Alzheimer's Disease*, 49 (2): 277–85.

Kimura, N.R.S., Simoes, J.P., Santos, R.L., et al. (2021) Young- and late-onset dementia: a comparative study of quality of life, burden, and depressive symptoms in caregivers, *Journal of Geriatric Psychiatry and Neurology*, 34 (5): 434–44.

La Fontaine, J., Larkin, M. and Oyebode, J.R. (2022) Intergenerational family relationships and the impact of behavioural variant frontotemporal dementia (bvFTD): a qualitative longitudinal study, *Ageing and Society*. Available at: https://doi.org/10.1017/S0144686X22001088.

Lockeridge, S. and Simpson, J. (2013) The experience of caring for a partner with young onset dementia: how younger carers cope, *Dementia*, 12 (5): 635–51.

Massimo, L., Evans, L.K. and Benner, P. (2013) Caring for loved ones with frontotemporal degeneration: the lived experiences of spouses, *Geriatric Nursing*, 34 (4): 302–6.

Mayrhofer, A.M., Mathie, E., Mckeown, J., et al. (2020) Young onset dementia: public involvement in co-designing community-based support, *Dementia*, 19 (4): 1051–66.

Metcalfe, A., Jones, B., Mayer, J., et al. (2019) Online information and support for carers of people with young-onset dementia: a multi-site randomised controlled pilot study, *International Journal of Geriatric Psychiatry*, 34 (10): 1455–64.

Millenaar, J.K., Van Vliet, D., Bakker, C., et al. (2014) The experiences and needs of children living with a parent with young onset dementia: results from the NeedYD study, *International Psychogeriatrics*, 26 (12): 2001–10.

Millenaar, J.K., Bakker, C., Koopmans, R.T., et al. (2016a) The care needs and experiences with the use of services of people with young-onset dementia and their caregivers: a systematic review, *International Journal of Geriatric Psychiatry*, 31 (12): 1261–76.

Millenaar, J.K., De Vugt, M.E., Bakker, C., et al. (2016b) The impact of young onset dementia on informal caregivers compared with late onset dementia: results from the NeedYD study, *American Journal of Geriatric Psychiatry*, 24 (6): 467–74.

Millenaar, J., Hvidsten, L., De Vugt, M.E., et al. (2017) Determinants of quality of life in young onset dementia: results from a European multicenter assessment, *Aging and Mental Health*, 21 (1): 24–30.

O'Malley, M., Parkes, J., Campbell, J., et al. (2021) Receiving a diagnosis of young onset dementia: evidence-based statements to inform best practice, *Dementia*, 20 (5): 1745–71.

Stamou, V., La Fontaine, J., Gage, H., et al. (2021) Services for people with young onset dementia: the 'Angela' Project national UK survey of service use and satisfaction, *International Journal of Geriatric Psychiatry*, 36 (3): 411–22.

Vandepitte, S., Van Den Noortgate, N., Putman, K., et al. (2016) Effectiveness of respite care in supporting informal caregivers of persons with dementia: a systematic review, *International Journal of Geriatric Psychiatry*, 31 (12): 1277–88.

Van Vliet, D., De Vugt, M.E., Kohler, S., et al. (2013) Awareness and its association with affective symptoms in young-onset and late-onset Alzheimer disease: a prospective study, *Alzheimer Disease and Associated Disorders*, 27 (3): 265–71.

Woods, B., Arosio, F., Diaz, A., et al. (2019) Timely diagnosis of dementia? Family carers' experiences in 5 European countries. *International Journal of Geriatric Psychiatry*, 34 (1): 114–21.

Xu, L., Liu, Y., He, H., et al. (2021) Caregiving intensity and caregiver burden among caregivers of people with dementia: the moderating roles of social support, *Archives of Gerontology and Geriatrics*, 94: 104334. Available at: https://doi.org/10.1016/j.archger.2020.104334.

Appendix

For more information about the Breinspoken initiative of summer camps and online information to support children and young people who have a parent with dementia, see the following web pages. All are in Dutch but Google Translate or similar can give you a reasonable translation.

For a news item about the camps, see: https://www.omroepzeeland.nl/nieuws/15796379/yade-10-heeft-een-vader-met-alzheimer-en-ziet-op-kamp-dat-ze-niet-de-enige-is

For an article about the digital platform, see: https://nos.nl/artikel/2497365-alzheimercentrum-lanceert-website-voor-kinderen-van-jonge-ouders-met-dementie

For the digital platform: see https://breinspoken.nl

Reflections on Part 2

The second part of the book has focused on identity. The first chapter took a broad view concentrating on the importance of culturally safe dementia care to support the identity of people from minoritised ethnicities. The chapter centres around two issues: the need for care appropriate to a person's ethnic identity and the importance of culturally safe care.

The former issue is quite widely recognised. We know we should take into account distinctive cultural values, religious needs, family roles, music and food preferences, and the appropriateness of reminiscence materials when providing personally tailored support. There is much more that could be done better in this regard but there is at least some awareness of this. There is very little relevant research focused specifically on young onset dementia but there is a small body of more general dementia research (Botsford and Dening, 2015; Parveen and Oyebode, 2018; Alzheimer's Europe, 2020). Readers may also be interested in Ronald Amanze's account of his life and experiences as a London child of Jamaican immigrants who now has a diagnosis of young onset vascular dementia (Amanze, 2023).

Most strikingly, Chapter 9 demonstrates that history and our own lived experience fundamentally influence the trust people from minoritised ethnic groups have in mainstream authorities and services. The chapter authors, Pam Roach and Jennifer Walker, show how and why trust has been badly damaged among Indigenous people in Canada. This has a major impact on whether people feel able to approach health and social care services. Keith Oliver, series editor, who knows Australia well, makes a point about wider relevance: 'whilst it related to the Indigenous Canadian population, often I was thinking of Indigenous communities in Australia and the United States of America'. Indeed, as noted by the authors, the issues apply equally to minoritised ethnic immigrant groups in the UK and other European countries. In many cases, established minority ethnic groups are first, second or later generations of immigrants from former colonies. Historical experiences of trauma and disenfranchisement, as well contemporary experiences of racism, are salient for these groups. Like Indigenous Canadians, people from minoritised ethnicities in the UK, USA and Europe also suffer health disparities, tend to underuse dementia care services, and may also be on the receiving end of invalid cognitive assessments. These parallels stress the relevance of this chapter to every diverse society. Roach and Walker's stance is echoed in contemporary work on trauma-informed care (Office for Health Improvement and Disparities, 2022) and in the 'critical dementia' field (Zubair, 2023).

The three central chapters of Part 2 focused on aspects of meaningful activity: employment, hobbies and pastimes, and becoming active in research.

The chapters speak for themselves. They show the value of thinking of young onset dementia within a framework of disability and rights (Cahill, 2018). They highlight needs for further research, including into how employers can better support people with young onset dementia who are working. We also need more evidence of benefits from age-appropriate personalised activities that can be used to justify the commissioning of services that foster and support recreational and creative activities.

Maintaining identity over time as young onset dementia progresses was addressed by Aud Johannessen and Kirsten Thorsen in Chapter 13. Their work is important in reminding us that even in the presence of quite severe cognitive impairment, people with young onset dementia have and express their unique selfhood. This was a fundamental tenet of Kitwood's work. This chapter shows how vital it is to provide considerate and accepting supportive care. However, this is a very neglected area of research.

Of course, advanced dementia is not the end of the story but, just as we were unable to commission a chapter on minority ethnic issues focused on UK research, we were equally unable to commission a chapter focused on end-of-life care for young onset dementia, due to neglect of the area. A single recent study of palliative care for people with young onset dementia in nursing homes in the Netherlands noted that swallowing difficulties were the most common dementia-related health problem and that agitation was common (Maters et al., 2024). This is a start, but we need much more research about how to support people living with young onset dementia in the advanced stages and at end-of-life.

The final chapter moved away from the identity of people living with young onset dementia to consider family carers' identity, with an emphasis on the main carer, usually a spouse or partner. Again, a comment from our series editors highlighted gaps in research. It was suggested that information should be included on the needs of friends performing the caregiver role, the complexities of second or third marriages, and any differences or similarities between the experiences of people in same-sex relationships compared with those in mixed relationships. On none of these is there young onset dementia-related research.

Issues of connection and relationship are addressed in Part 3 of our book but essentially, as social beings, connection and identity are intertwined. Chapter 14, focused primarily on the identity of family carers, provides a good complement to the chapters on family relationships and impact of young onset dementia on children and young people that form two of the three chapters in Part 3, before the final chapter on the significant area of peer support.

References

Alzheimer's Europe (2020) *Intercultural dementia care: A guide to raise awareness amongst health and social care workers.* Available at: https://www.researchgate. net/publication/347423967_Intercultural_dementia_care_-_A_guide_to_raise_ awareness_amongst_health_and_social_care_workers (accessed 4 June 2024).

Amanze, R. (2023) Small quantities at a time, in R. Ward and L.J. Sandberg (eds.) *Critical Dementia Studies: An Introduction*. London: Routledge.

Botsford, J. and Dening, K.H. (2015) *Dementia, Culture and Ethnicity*. London: Jessica Kingsley.

Cahill, S. (2018) *Dementia and Human Rights*. Bristol: Policy Press.

Maters, J., van der Steen, J.T., de Vugt, M.E., et al. (2024) Palliative care in nursing home residents with young-onset dementia: professional and family caregiver perspectives, *Journal of Alzheimer's Disease*, 97 (2): 573–86.

Office for Health Improvement and Disparities (2022) *Guidance: Working definition of trauma-informed practice*. Available at: https://www.gov.uk/government/publications/working-definition-of-trauma-informed-practice/working-definition-of-trauma-informed-practice (accessed 6 June 2024).

Parveen, S. and Oyebode, J.R. (2018) Dementia and minority ethnic carers, *Better Health Briefing*, 46 (12). Available at: https://raceequalityfoundation.org.uk/wp-content/uploads/2022/10/REF-Better-Health-463.pdf.

Zubair, M. (2023) Reframing 'ethnicity' in dementia research: reflections on current whiteness of research and the need for an anti-racist approach, in R. Ward and L.J. Sandberg (eds.) *Critical Dementia Studies: An Introduction*. London: Routledge.

Part 3

Being Connected

People with young onset dementia and their family members need to feel connected with those around them. This can include support or services:

- to help maintain family relationships;
- for children and young people to be properly acknowledged, supported and connected; and
- to enable people with young onset dementia to feel part of their wider community and networks.

15 Maintaining positive relationships in families affected by young onset dementia

Vasileios Stamou

Overview

Togetherness is at the core of human relationships, including family relationships. Family needs, relationships and dynamics change over time. Additional challenges may result from external influences, such as the unexpected diagnosis of a condition. These can induce significant strain and place family relationships at risk of breakdown. Dementia at midlife influences family roles and dynamics, and disrupts the sense of togetherness in the family. Spousal and parent-child relationships are severely affected and require specialist support to address distinct relational needs of younger people with dementia and their families. Research has provided insights into the shortcomings of services and recent advances have enabled a better understanding of 'what works' in services that help families to stay together and maintain their family bonds and relationships. Continuous age-appropriate, family-centred care through multi-specialist teams and professionals seems to be of particular value from the point of diagnosis onwards, to maintain meaningful family relationships and the sense of togetherness in families affected by young onset dementia.

Keywords

Family-centred, age-appropriate, meaningful relationships, togetherness, relational needs, relational challenges, younger people with dementia, spouse, dyad, parent, child,

Learning points

- Meaningful relationships can be maintained in families affected by young onset dementia, though not without significant challenges.

- Relational challenges in dyad and parent-child relationships can be overcome through age-appropriate, relationship-centred psychosocial interventions.
- A family-centred approach could address individual and collective needs within the family, through an ongoing alliance with a multi-specialist team of professionals.

Introduction

Tom Kitwood's flower of needs for people affected by dementia represents the 'gold standard' of person-centred dementia care. Love is at the core of the model, synthesised from and manifested through different needs, including attachment (Baldwin and Capstick, 2007). Like most theoretical models associated with human needs and well-being, Kitwood's model can be considered as universal in concept, but adjustable in terms of how it may apply to different individuals and families affected by dementia. For instance, the need for meaningful attachment through positive relationships and togetherness in the family may be met in different ways at distinct life stages in the context of unique family circumstances.

Young onset dementia occurs in the distinct stage of midlife and affects the whole family, including young children of those living with the diagnosis (Roach and Keady, 2008). As noted in Chapter 14, it can influence roles, bonds and dynamics within couple and parent-child relationships, as well as the sense of togetherness in the whole family (Chirico et al., 2022). This chapter focuses on relationships in particular, and will examine:

- how family relationships are affected by young onset dementia;
- the relational needs of those affected by the condition; and
- individual or family-oriented forms of support that can be employed by services to foster meaningful relationships and enhance the sense of togetherness in families living with young onset dementia.

Dyad/spousal relationship

During the journey to diagnosis

The relationship between the person with dementia and their spouse or partner (hereafter referred to as the 'dyad relationship') can be significantly affected by young onset dementia (Holdsworth and McCabe, 2018). Challenges in dyad relationships begin from the onset of symptoms, the spouse/partner struggling to understand the changes in behaviour, mood or daily functioning of the person with dementia (Holdsworth and McCabe, 2018), which can result in conflicts and place the relationship under significant pressure or at risk of breakdown (Draper and Withall, 2016; Chirico et al., 2022). The dyad struggles to get along and the spouse/partner may blame the person with young onset dementia (Lai et al., 2023), often assuming that they do not care or love them anymore (Holdsworth and McCabe, 2018). Delays in receiving a diagnosis can increase confusion and pressure and further reduce the quality of the relationship (Kilty et al., 2019).

By contrast, the understanding enabled by the diagnosis can come as a relief and even renew the relationship (Draper and Withall, 2016). The spouse/partner can become more understanding of challenging or unexpected behaviours, knowing that these are due to dementia and not to how their loved one feels for them (Thorsen and Johannessen, 2023). Indeed, for some spouses/partners the diagnosis may signal the end of uncertainty and the beginning of new life plans with dementia for the dyad (Lai et al., 2023). For others, however, diagnosis can come as a shock, as it can instil a sense of loss of the relationship and uncertainty about the future (Kilty et al., 2019). This seems to be slightly more prominent in couples who may be in denial or tend to downplay the cognitive deterioration of the person with the diagnosis (Lockeridge and Simpson, 2013). This fear-driven denial can lead to delays in accessing support and increase conflicts within the relationship if continued (Millenaar et al., 2016).

Irrespective of the initial relief or shock in response to diagnosis, couples may benefit from early dyadic interventions delivered by professionals with specialist knowledge of young onset dementia. Early interventions can focus on:

- Addressing the negative impact of receiving a diagnosis – focusing on coping with challenging emotions resulting from diagnosis could help to alleviate emotional strain and feelings of fear or loss (Grunberg et al., 2022).
- Enabling the couple to maintain and build on their sense of togetherness – focusing on enhancing communication within the dyad may help to maintain a sense of reciprocity within the relationship during the challenging period of receiving the diagnosis (Grunberg et al., 2022).

The overall approach of professionals should focus on reinforcing the dyad to approach present and future challenges together, which is key to maintaining a positive relationship. Thus, it is essential to promote collaborative communication and a teamwork approach within the dyad, to prevent emotional distancing, negative communication and any conflict that may result from avoidance (Bannon et al., 2021).

The dyad relationship after diagnosis

As the condition progresses, spouses/partners, irrespective of gender, may experience a shift in the relationship in terms of emotional connection and the sense of reciprocity within the dyad. Spouses/partners may often feel that the person with dementia is:

- becoming a different person who does not have feelings for them anymore, due to gradually withdrawing from communication (Thorsen and Johannessen, 2023); and/or
- gradually 'drifting away', along with the sense of love and partnership within the relationship (Kilty et al., 2019; Thorsen and Johannessen, 2023).

It becomes evident that the dyad's sense of togetherness can be severely affected as young onset dementia progresses, due to emergent feelings of loneliness, isolation or grief, reduced reciprocity and sexual intimacy, and emotional distancing (Holdsworth and McCabe, 2018). Without needs-appropriate support, the dyad relationship may become at risk of changing from a romantic relationship to a symbiotic nurse-patient one (Millenaar et al., 2016; Kilty et al., 2019; Chirico et al., 2022).

Not everything, however, is dark and gloomy. There is a bright side, since changes in the relationship dynamics can also be experienced as positive and renew the dyad relationship. The cognitive decline of the person with dementia may loosen restraint and allow them to express their love and affection more openly than previously. Spouses/partners can find satisfaction in expressing their love towards the person with dementia in the form of care (Flynn and Mulcahy, 2013) and experience sustained emotional satisfaction in the relationship (Bruinsma et al., 2020). Dyads may have the opportunity to spend more time together (Wawrziczny et al., 2016) and feel more relaxed due to the unexpected liberation from work stressors. Unique moments, such as a romantic walk together or a loved activity, are still possible on a daily basis (Bergman et al., 2016). Indeed, research has shown that couples affected by dementia can experience love and high levels of emotional intimacy (de Vugt et al., 2003; Riedijk et al., 2008; Massimo et al., 2013).

Whether the situation results in breakdown of the dyad relationship or the transformation to a new closeness, as described above, may depend on the quality of the relationship prior to the onset of symptoms and, most importantly, on the timely provision of specialist support. Different forms of support could favour maintaining a positive relationship over a breakdown. For instance:

- Early and regular assessment of relational needs can be a key differentiating factor in identifying the couple's unique needs and determining the appropriate type of support.
- Emergent challenges with communication could be addressed through specialist speech and language therapy, which younger couples perceive as relationship counselling due to the positive impact it has on their relationship (Stamou et al., 2021).
- Regular support from a clinical psychologist with specialist knowledge of young onset dementia could address emergent feelings of loss or grief (Draper and Withall, 2016) and contribute to reconstituting the relationship.

- Relationship counselling or couples therapy with a young onset dementia specialist could assist with maintaining important aspects of the relationship, such as emotional reciprocity, intimacy and sexual activity (Cheston, 2022; Chirico et al., 2022).
- Relational interventions could also enable dyads to understand how to plan and spend quality time together (e.g. arranging date nights, or not being together all the time) and enhance the quality of highly valued interactions (Bannon et al., 2022).
- Social outings, trips and excursions organised by young onset dementia groups may offer the opportunity for meaningful social interaction with other younger couples in a relaxed, safe environment (Stamou et al., 2021) and enhance or renew the sense of togetherness within the dyad relationship.

The dyad relationship can also be affected by changes in working roles and responsibilities. The caring tasks of the spouse/partner can increase to make up for tasks the person with dementia is no longer able to carry out, such as for driving or household tasks (Chirico et al., 2022). The spouse/partner may often have to make family decisions alone, while also working and providing care for dependent members of the family, such as young children or parents (Millenaar et al., 2016). In contrast, the person with young onset dementia may perceive their role in the relationship to be undermined by over-protective behaviours of the spouse/partner (Wawrziczny et al., 2016) and feel cut-out from family decisions (Harris, 2004). Such feelings can add tensions and elicit feelings of frustration, which may remain hidden and exacerbate relational challenges.

Different forms of support can address these challenges and minimise their impact:

- External support, such as in-home or respite care, can address the multiple roles taken up by the spouse/partner and allow space and time for self-care and personally meaningful activities, which can help to maintain the quality of the relationship.
- Admiral Nurses could offer the listening ear of a specialist who understands the relational challenges of dementia at a young age and provide meaningful information and advice on how these can best be addressed (O'Malley et al., 2021).
- Locally delivered community-based psychosocial interventions can enable the person with dementia and their spouse/partner to better understand their relational challenges, and receive information and advice from other couples affected by the condition on ways to cope and adapt to living with young onset dementia (Brooker et al., 2017, 2018).
- Specialist support with advance care planning could enhance the sense of partnership within the dyad and enable younger people with dementia to have a voice in important decisions made by the couple. Research has shown that advance care planning in young onset dementia requires a holistic and relational approach focusing on active communication and partnership between family members (Van Rickstal et al., 2022).

> **Box 15.1: Key recommendations for maintaining the dyad relationship**
>
> - Interventions should focus on enabling couples to maintain and build on their sense of togetherness throughout their experience with young onset dementia; this could be facilitated by paying early, then regular, attention to individual and joint needs to identify appropriate types of support.
> - Interventions focusing on relationships, such as relationship counselling, could address emergent relational needs. These could help the dyad to maintain emotional reciprocity and sexual intimacy, and continue spending quality time together in a balanced, meaningful way.
> - Dyad interventions focusing on communication, such as through speech and language therapists or clinical psychologists, can enable dyads to have more constructive ways of talking with each other and maintain a sense of togetherness.
> - Social activities where both partners meet up with others who understand the challenges of living with young onset dementia can enhance the sense of togetherness within the dyad.
> - Strategies to cope with emergent feelings of loss or grief may be particularly useful; these could be addressed in the context of individual counselling with a young onset dementia specialist for each member of the dyad.
> - In-home and respite care can enable the spouse/partner to engage in self-care and personally meaningful activities, which can help the dyad to maintain the quality of their relationship.
> - Advance care planning employing a relational approach could enhance collaborative communication and the sense of teamwork within the dyad.

Finally, couples affected by young onset dementia often have to abandon long-term life plans due to the progressive nature of the condition (Chirico et al., 2022). Couples have reported a preference to focus on the here-and-now and live one day at a time in a meaningful way (Roach et al., 2014; Grunberg et al., 2022). Mindfulness-based interventions can facilitate achieving this goal (Grunberg et al., 2022) and may provide the opportunity for a renewed sense of fulfilment in the dyad's everyday life. Key recommendations for maintaining the dyad relationship are summarised in Box 15.1.

The relationship between children and parents living with dementia

Changes at the point of diagnosis

Just like dyad relationships, parent-child relationships can be influenced by young onset dementia as early as the onset of symptoms. Initially, children may find it difficult to understand the changes in their parent's behaviour or come to terms with a dementia diagnosis at a young age. The confusion and lack of understanding can lead to feelings of anger, frustration or embarrassment towards the parent with dementia, and conflicts within their relationship (Poole and Patterson, 2022; Grundberg et al., 2023), which may require time and external interventions to be re-established (Chirico et al., 2022). It is therefore imperative that a sustainable age-appropriate support network of specialists is in place from the point of diagnosis onwards, to help children accept the diagnosis, address children's relational needs, and prevent early detachment or drifting away from the family (Allen et al., 2009; Chirico et al., 2022).

Indeed, without support to understand the condition, its impact and how to cope, children may feel that they live in a confusing state of limbo (Chirico et al., 2022) and tend to distance themselves from the parent with dementia physically and emotionally, in an effort to protect themselves (Wiggins et al., 2023). At this stage, the distancing may partly result from fear and confusion around the condition and the changes it may bring, rather than the actual impact of dementia. Different interventions can facilitate identifying and addressing children's relational needs:

- An early collaboration of different specialists with both parents and children can be established to understand unique family circumstances and living situations (e.g. family size, number and age of children in the family, quality of parent-child relationship before the onset of symptoms, availability of health and social care services in the area), and identify the nature, type and level of relational support required for each child (Barca et al., 2014; Groennestad and Malmedal, 2022).
- The provision of age-appropriate advice and information in a safe environment could alleviate children's confusion about dementia and reduce the fear of changes it may bring in family relationships. For instance, young children can receive information and advice in the context of informal activities offered in play-based scenarios and non-threatening environments (Stamou et al., 2023).
- Early one-to-one counselling could offer children a safe space to talk to allow addressing more complex or challenging emotions within the parent-child relationship, normalising dementia, and acquiring coping strategies that help to maintain a healthy attachment to the parent.

Taken together, these interventions may reduce the initial emotional strain, prevent early emotional detachment, and facilitate maintaining a positive relationship with the parent (Stamou et al., 2023).

The initial shock of the diagnosis may be followed by feelings of grief, due to a sense of loss of the parent at a young age and children's perception that they will no longer be able to share any experiences or future with them (Poole and Patterson, 2022). As such, children may experience loneliness, even when with friends and family, and keep their feelings hidden (Gelman and Rhames, 2020; Grundberg et al., 2023). At this stage, children could benefit from specialist emotional support by empathic and compassionate professionals (Stamou et al., 2023), to address complex emotions, ongoing relational challenges, and misconceptions about irreparable strain in the parent-child relationship.

Relational challenges after diagnosis

As dementia progresses, changes in the behaviour or personality of the parent with young onset dementia may make it more difficult for children to feel close and relate to their parent in a meaningful way (Aslett et al., 2019). Both younger and adult children may experience a sense of premature loss of their parent (Svanberg et al., 2010) and the relationship fading away (Groennestad and Malmedal, 2022; Poole and Patterson, 2022), as they may no longer feel able to turn to their parent for emotional affection, support or advice (Allen et al., 2009). As in earlier stages of the condition, children may feel an urge to detach themselves, physically and/or emotionally, from the family, due to the reduced physical and emotional availability of both parents (one parent due to dementia and the other one due to caregiving) (Svanberg et al., 2010).

Specialist support could prevent children's detachment and enable a transition towards a meaningful relationship with the parent living with dementia. Individual counselling from a health or social care specialist (Barca et al., 2014) could gradually:

- promote acceptance of the relational changes brought about by the condition;
- address emergent feelings of grief (Svanberg et al., 2010; Groennestad and Malmedal, 2022); and
- enable the development of a newly formed parent-child relationship, of which dementia can be a part (Svanberg et al., 2010), without any unintended negative feelings towards the parent (Svanberg et al., 2010; Cartwright et al., 2021).

Children value the time they spent with their parent with dementia before diagnosis (Allen et al., 2009). Previously cherished activities, such as trips or holidays, may be possible through social trips and outings organised by professionals facilitating age-appropriate social groups for families affected by young onset dementia. Such activities could enable younger people with dementia and children to spend quality time together and realise that a sense of togetherness within their relationship is still possible. They could also enable meeting other children of families living with young onset dementia, which might help to normalise the condition and alleviate unintended negative feelings towards the parent (see Chapter 16 on the well-being and identity of children and young people).

Children often contribute to caring for the parent with young onset dementia, but reversed caregiving roles at an early age can be hard to accept (Chirico et al., 2022). At first, children may miss their old relationship with the parent and feel hurt or ignored (Barca et al., 2014; Cartwright et al., 2021). At this stage, individual counselling or talking therapy could enable meeting important relational needs, such as reappraising the relationship with the parent in the context of living with dementia, focusing on what is possible here and now, and normalising caregiving (Allen et al., 2009; Svanberg et al., 2010; Aslett et al., 2019; Cartwright et al., 2021). It could also facilitate expressing and addressing challenging emotions, alleviating feelings of loss or fear of attachment, and renewing the relationship with the parent.

Of interest, children have reported caregiving bringing them closer to the parent with dementia (Hall and Sikes, 2018; Grundberg et al., 2023) and eliciting an elevated sense of purpose, accomplishment, self-worth, self-esteem and resilience (Chirico et al., 2022; Poole and Patterson, 2022; Wiggins et al., 2023). The positive impact of caregiving on the parent-child relationship may be hindered by difficulties in communicating with the parent with dementia (Chirico et al., 2022). Specialist interventions could help children adjust their communication style when interacting with the parent with young onset dementia, so that they can spend and enjoy more time with them (Svanberg et al., 2010). Joint speech and language/communication therapy for parent-child pairs could facilitate maintaining positive communication and relationships.

Children being the primary caregiver can act as a barrier to renewing the relationship with the parent with dementia (Grundberg et al., 2023). Without additional support to achieve a balance with other aspects of their lives, children may experience caregiving in a negative manner and gradually withdraw from the relationship with their parent. They may feel hopeless or trapped (Grundberg et al., 2023) and seek detachment as a way out (Grundberg et al., 2023). Additional in-home care in the context of collective caregiving within the family could address these needs and enable children to maintain a meaningful relationship with the parent with dementia.

Children may also not know how to provide care, which could hinder their capacity to renew the relationship with the parent in the context of caregiving. Balanced meaningful education on the condition and how to provide care at a young age could enable children to transform the relationship with their parent through caregiving. Information should be provided in a non-medical age-appropriate manner by empathic and compassionate professionals. The level and nature of information to be revealed should be assessed in advance on a case-by-case basis, as some children may find certain information empowering whereas others may find it confusing or even frightening (Groennestad and Malmedal, 2022).

Finally, the progressive nature of dementia requires continuously adapting to changing circumstances (Cartwright et al., 2021). For children to maintain a positive relationship with the parent, regular assessments of relational needs and access to relevant psychosocial interventions are required. Key recommendations maintaining the relationship between children and young people and parents, when one parent has young onset dementia are summarised in Box 15.2.

Box 15.2: Key recommendations for maintaining the relationship between children and young people and parents, when one parent has young onset dementia

- Age-appropriate one-to-one counselling can address challenging emotions, such as grief or anger, and prevent children's detachment from the family.
- Age-appropriate activities can help children to understand the changes brought about by diagnosis, normalise dementia, and maintain a healthy attachment to the parent living with the condition.

- The parent-child relationship may be renewed in the context of dementia and caregiving, with the help of individual counselling, interventions addressing communication difficulties, and additional in-home care.
- Regular assessments of parent-child relational needs and access to relevant psychosocial interventions may facilitate maintaining positive parent-child relationships.
- Parent-child quality time can be offered through age-specific social activities for families affected by young onset dementia.

Maintaining togetherness as a family

Just as in all social units undergoing major changes, the coherence of families affected by young onset dementia can be challenged by the diagnosis. Family functioning can affect and be affected by the way dementia is experienced in the family (Roach et al., 2014). This means that family-centred support should consider each family's unique course of development (Roach et al., 2014) and the individual and collective needs within the family (Chirico et al., 2022) after diagnosis.

As with dyad relationships, how family relationships are affected will depend on the nature and quality of pre-existing relationships (Bellass, 2016; Aslett et al., 2019). The type of family should also be considered. Relationships in blended families have additional layers of complexity. This means those in blended or step families may be especially vulnerable to distress and breakdown in relationships (Zeleznikow and Zeleznikow, 2015). In troubled relationships, young onset dementia may provide the ground for the expression of pre-existing tensions, whereas in families that have remained close and supportive to each other, it can enhance the pre-existing family bonds and bring the family closer (Bellass, 2016). It is therefore important that professionals understand the changing family needs and dynamics within which support will be provided.

Families may benefit from confronting dementia together as a unit (Roach et al., 2014). Two factors could play a key role in this process:

- the development of an alliance with a team of specialists who will be responsible for assessing needs and providing care throughout the experience with dementia, including a link worker (Stamou et al., 2022); and

- open and honest communication and cooperation between all family members, to sustain family bonds and coherence (Groennestad and Malmedal, 2022) and enable the family to provide care to the person with dementia through different roles of each family member.

For instance, children value honesty from their parents (Svanberg et al., 2010; Chirico et al., 2022), as this helps them to maintain a personal relationship with them and understand dementia better. Parents, on the other hand, may be hiding important information from the children to protect them. When children start noticing the impact of caregiving on the parent providing care, they may choose to hide their emotions and needs to avoid adding to that parent's concerns. As a result, the parent may think that children are coping well and may not be affected by the diagnosis (Gelman and Rhames, 2020). This can gradually drive members of the family apart, as children may stop confiding in their parents, and the quality of their relationship may eventually decline (Gelman and Rhames, 2020).

Professionals can emphasise the importance of openness and honesty during early discussions with the family at the stage of diagnosis. Openness may not only improve communication within the family but also allow professionals to better understand the needs of all family members and signpost to appropriate support in a timely manner (Gelman and Rhames, 2020). The latter may often require professionals to read between the lines, as some family members may initially be reluctant to share their true story, emotions or needs (Roach et al., 2014). Professionals need to relay a clear message that family members are entitled to experience negative feelings and emotions, even those which they may consider inadmissible (Gelman and Rhames, 2020). Individual counselling could facilitate addressing these needs (Roach et al., 2014) and enhance open communication within the family and with the professionals providing care.

As described earlier, children often contribute to caring for the parent with young onset dementia. Under the right conditions, this can be a gratifying experience and enable children to establish themselves as important members of the family and redefine their relationship with both parents (Poole and Patterson, 2022). For example, children may feel proud and increasingly mature for caring for their parent with young onset dementia, helping the parent who provides care by contributing to caregiving, and reciprocating support for the family (Svanberg et al., 2010; Grundberg et al., 2023). Indeed, the contribution of children to caregiving may be valuable for parents as they may need that additional support (Gelman and Rhames, 2020). However, depending on their age and emotional capacity, some children may be more ready than others to contribute to caregiving or take part in making important decisions as a family (Gelman and Rhames, 2020). Professionals could engage in active discussions with all family members to identify age-appropriate ways for children's involvement in caregiving and key decision-making processes, if deemed appropriate.

Children may also be concerned about the impact of dementia on the health of the parent who provides care (Chirico et al., 2022; Grundberg et al., 2023). Excessive worrying may prevent children from maintaining a positive relationship with the parents (Allen et al., 2009). External practical support (e.g. in-home and/or respite care) could help to alleviate this stress and allow relationships to be sustained or enhanced within a less demanding familial environment. The same applies for counselling or one-to-one emotional support, which could facilitate addressing emotional challenges experienced by different family members and allow parent-child relationships to be maintained (Allen et al., 2009).

External support should enable children to make important transitions without worrying about the parents. As much as caregiving may be an important aspect of their family lives, children should not be deprived of making important life decisions, such as moving away from home or going to college or university (Gelman and Rhames, 2020), even if this takes them away from caregiving. Age-appropriate in-home or respite care and emotional support should be available to the whole family, to facilitate the transition. Making these important transitions may improve and enhance children's relationship with the parents (Johannessen et al., 2016), as the opposite could result in future feelings of regret and blaming the parents for lost opportunities.

Family members value working as a team (Svanberg et al., 2010; Barca et al., 2014), as this can prevent isolation and enhance family bonds in the context of changing relationships resulting from a young onset dementia diagnosis (Allen et al., 2009). For instance, when siblings gain support from each other this has been reported to bring the family closer (Cabote et al., 2015), as it may increase their sense of solidarity and of facing issues together. However, conflicts may arise from disagreements between family members regarding the management of the condition (Chirico et al., 2022; Poole and Patterson, 2022). Younger people with dementia wish to be actively included in conversations with their children, particularly regarding issues related to the impact of young onset dementia and how this can be addressed in the family (Bannon et al., 2022). Thus, the balance between a positive and negative family experience of young onset dementia can be, at times, thin.

Professionals can actively engage the whole family in planning their current and future care. Flexible advance care planning could enable the family to make informed decisions on different aspects of care (e.g. practical, social, psychological, medical) based on what matters most to the family as a whole (Van Rickstal et al., 2022). The focus should be placed on the process through an active dialogue between all family members (Van Rickstal et al., 2022), and the voices of all those affected should be represented, particularly the voices of younger people with dementia. This approach could facilitate resolving potential disagreements, assigning clear roles, preventing feelings of exclusion, and enhancing family bonds and the family's sense of coherence. Care planning through family consensus can also instil a sense of security within which families can live one day at a time with less fear or stress, enjoy the good moments, and cope well with the difficult ones.

The progressive nature of dementia has a continuous impact on family needs and dynamics over time (Roach et al., 2014). One of the most challenging transitions that families have to face takes place if the person with young onset dementia needs to move into a care home facility (Barca et al., 2014; Chirico et al., 2022). The family is responsible for making a critical decision on the timing of the transition and the type of facility that would best meet the person's needs. Family discussions with knowledgeable young onset dementia professionals need to take place at early stages of the condition to ensure that the wishes and preferences of the person with young onset dementia are considered when making this decision. Before the transition takes place, family members should be provided with the opportunity to visit different facilities and interact with the staff, so that they feel reassured regarding the quality and age-appropriate nature of the care offered (Chirico et al., 2022; Groennes-tad and Malmedal, 2022). Nevertheless, the time for the decision comes with mixed emotions of high intensity. Family members may feel some sense of relief that the person with dementia will be in the hands of specialists, as they cannot continue providing effective informal care. At the same time, family members experience deep sorrow for being separated from a loved member of the family (Svanberg et al., 2010; Cabote et al., 2015; Chirico et al., 2022; Poole and Patterson, 2022).

To assist with this, families may benefit from specialist support from knowl-edgeable professionals who can help them to make the decision at the best time. Professionals should provide ample time for family members to reflect and gradually accept the necessity to make the decision if needed. They should also inform the family about the available options, the advantages and disadvan-tages of each option, and provide reassurance when the decision is finally made.

It is equally important that the care team remains in touch with the family after the person with the diagnosis moves into a care home, to prevent feel-ings of abandonment. At this stage, family needs may change and the family members may require practical and emotional support. For instance, anxiety regarding the quality of care provided to the person with dementia, and feel-ings of guilt or grief are quite common (Barca et al., 2014; Chirico et al., 2022). These can be addressed through individual and family counselling, so that the family stays together and does not fall apart (Hayo, 2015). It is also important to enable the family to stay connected with the person with dementia through regular visits and to provide continuous well-informed reassurance regarding the quality of care provided. A summary of key recommendations to address whole-family relationships is given in Box 15.3.

Box 15.3: Key recommendations to address whole-family relationships together

- An ongoing alliance with a multi-specialist team may enable families to confront dementia as a unit.
- Changing individual and collective needs in the family require regular assessments and signposting to age-appropriate support.
- Professionals can actively engage the whole family in planning current and future care, including formal care, through flexible advance care planning.
- Practical and emotional support should be available during important tran-sitions, to maintain the family's sense of togetherness.
- Children's contribution to caregiving may enhance family coherence under the right circumstances.
- Family support should not be interrupted when the person with dementia moves into formal care; family needs should be reassessed, and individual and family counselling should become available.

So what does this mean in practice?

If you are a person diagnosed with young onset dementia

Think about your relationship with your spouse/partner and other members of your family. You may initially feel the urge to withdraw or to deny that you are facing challenges. You may feel others in your family do not understand you or neglect you and you may find it difficult to communicate with them.

There is support that could help you address these challenges and help you to maintain or improve your family relationships. For this to happen, it is important that your voice is heard, so that others understand your relational needs.

- You might want to consider speaking to a young onset dementia specialist who provides individual counselling. A counsellor will take time to understand how you feel and can provide you with advice and support with your family relationships.
- Specialists, such as clinical psychologists and speech and language therapists, may be able to help you and your spouse/partner and family talk more easily with each other. They may also be able to help you to continue feeling close to your spouse/partner and help you maintain good relationships with your children.
- Young onset dementia social groups may enable you and your family to meet others who understand what it is like to live with young onset dementia and engage in meaningful social outings and activities.

If you are a spouse/partner of someone diagnosed with young onset dementia

Think about your relationship with the person with young onset dementia and the relationships within your family. Young onset dementia brings many challenges. It is normal to feel scared, angry or frustrated, and to find your relationships feel strained. There are different interventions that may help you.

- Relationship counselling could help you maintain emotional intimacy with your spouse/partner.
- Individual counselling could help you with your own feelings.
- External support could help you take a break from caring.
- There are also interventions that could help you and your spouse/partner communicate better.
- Social activities with a group of people living with young onset dementia and family supporters, who understand your situation, may also be good for your spousal relationship.
- You might want to consider speaking with a professional who can help to signpost you to appropriate sources of support, so that you, your spouse/partner, and your family can feel like a cohesive team.

If you are a child of someone diagnosed with young onset dementia

Reflect upon your feelings and remember that you are not meant to face everything alone. Young onset dementia may instil a sense of loss of your parent as they used to be but you can still have a meaningful relationship with them and other members of your family. Sometimes putting distance from your family may feel like the best way to protect yourself from the changes you are experiencing. Although at times this may be true for a while, you might want to consider:

- Talking to a young onset dementia specialist about how you feel could help you better understand your emotions and how to cope with these and the changes brought about by the diagnosis. External support could also help you normalise dementia and eliminate any hidden feelings of fear or shame.
- You may be able to experience quality time with your parent with dementia while providing care to them or going to social outings with other families affected by dementia who understand the challenges you are going through.
- There are also interventions that could help you communicate better with your parent living with dementia.

If you are a professional working with families affected by young onset dementia

Reflect upon how each family and individual are unique and how best you can approach families affected by young onset dementia with an empathetic listening ear. Active listening is essential to help you understand their emerging individual and collective relational needs, family dynamics and circumstances, and the support required across their experience with dementia, including the period of formal care for the person with young onset dementia.

You might want to consider how you can develop a sense of connectedness with the whole family and each member individually, so that you can become a member of their 'extended family' that oversees and assesses their relational needs regularly and signposts or provides the support they need.

If you are a service manager or commissioner who provides or wants to provide services that support togetherness in families affected by young onset dementia

Reflect upon how you can enable each family to develop a sustainable alliance with a multi-specialist young onset dementia team that will enable them to confront dementia together and to have a say in their present and future care. Practical, emotional and relational support for all family members is essential, particularly during the period of diagnosis and challenging transitions, to maintain the family's sense of togetherness.

References

Allen, J., Oyebode, J.R. and Allen, J. (2009) Having a father with young onset dementia: the impact on well-being of young people, *Dementia*, 8 (4): 455–80.

Aslett, H.J., Huws, J.C., Woods, R.T., et al. (2019) 'This is killing me inside': the impact of having a parent with young-onset dementia, *Dementia*, 18 (3): 1089–1107.

Baldwin, C. and Capstick, A. (2007) *Tom Kitwood on Dementia. A Reader and Critical Commentary.* Maidenhead: Open University Press.

Bannon, S.M., Grunberg, V.A., Reichman, M., et al. (2021) Thematic analysis of dyadic coping in couples with young-onset dementia, *JAMA Network Open*, 4 (4): e216111. Available at: https://doi.org/10.1001/jamanetworkopen.2021.6111.

Bannon, S.M., Wang, K.E., Grunberg, V.A., et al. (2022) Couples' experiences managing young-onset dementia early in the COVID-19 pandemic, *The Gerontologist*, 62 (8): 1173–84.

Barca, M.L., Thorsen, K., Engedal, K., et al. (2014) Nobody asked me how I felt: experiences of adult children of persons with young-onset dementia, *International Psychogeriatrics*, 26 (12): 1935–44.

Bellass, S. (2016) *Intergenerational experiences of young onset dementia: A qualitative longitudinal study*, DPhil thesis, University of Salford.

Bergman, M., Graff, C., Eriksdotter, M., et al. (2016) The meaning of living close to a person with Alzheimer disease, *Medical Health Care Philosophy*, 19 (3): 341–49.

Brooker, D., Evans, S.B. and Dröes, R.M. (2017) Framing outcomes of post-diagnostic psychosocial interventions in dementia. *Working with Older People*, 21 (1): 13–21.

Brooker, D., Evans, S.C., Evans, S.B., et al. (2018) Evaluation of the implementation of the Meeting Centres Support Programme in Italy, Poland and UK: exploration of the effects on people with dementia, *International Journal of Geriatric Psychiatry*, 33 (7): 883–92.

Bruinsma, J., Peetoom, K., Millenaar, J., et al. (2020) The quality of the relationship perceived by spouses of people with young-onset dementia, *International Psychogeriatrics*. Available at: https://doi.org/10.1017/S1041610220000332.

Cabote, C. J., Bramble, M. and McCann, D. (2015) Family caregivers' experiences of caring for a relative with younger onset dementia: a qualitative systematic review, *Journal of Family Nursing*, 21 (3): 443–68.

Cartwright, A.V., Stoner, C.R., Pione, R.D., et al. (2021) The experiences of those affected by parental young onset dementia: a qualitative systematic literature review, *Dementia*, 20 (7): 2618–39.

Cheston, R. (2022) *Dementia and Psychotherapy Reconsidered.* London: Open University Press.

Chirico, I., Ottoboni, G., Linarello, S., et al. (2022) Family experience of young-onset dementia: the perspectives of spouses and children, *Aging and Mental Health*, 26 (11): 2243–51.

De Vugt, M.E., Stevens, F., Aalten, P., et al. (2003) Behavioural disturbances in dementia patients and quality of the marital relationship, *International Journal of Geriatric Psychiatry*, 18 (2): 149–54.

Draper, B. and Withall, A. (2016) Young onset dementia, *Internal Medicine Journal*, 46 (7): 779–86.

Flynn, R. and Mulcahy, H. (2013) Early-onset dementia: the impact on family care-givers, *British Journal of Community Nursing*, 18 (12): 598–606.

Gelman, C. and Rhames, K. (2020) 'I have to be both mother and father': the impact of young-onset dementia on the partner's parenting and the children's experience, *Dementia*, 19 (3): 676–90.

Groennestad, H. and Malmedal, W. (2022) Having a parent with early-onset dementia: a qualitative study of young adult children, *Nursing Research and Practice*, 2022: 7945773. Available at: https://doi.org/10.1155/2022/7945773.

Grunberg, V.A., Bannon, S.M., Reichman, M., et al. (2022) Psychosocial treatment preferences of persons living with young-onset dementia and their partners, *Dementia*, 21 (1): 41–60.

Grundberg, A., Sandberg, J. and Craftman, Å.G. (2023) Children's and young adults' perspectives of having a parent with dementia diagnosis: a scoping review, *Dementia*, 20 (8): 2933–56.

Hall, M. and Sikes, P. (2018) How do young people 'do' family where there is a diagnosis of dementia?, *Families, Relationships and Societies*, 7 (2): 207–25.

Harris, P. (2004) The perspective of younger people with dementia, *Social Work in Mental Health*, 2 (4): 17–36.

Hayo, H. (2015) Diagnosis and support for younger people with dementia, *Nursing Standard*, 29 (47): 36–40.

Holdsworth, K. and McCabe, M. (2018) The impact of younger-onset dementia on relationships, intimacy, and sexuality in midlife couples: a systematic review, *International Psychogeriatrics*, 30 (1): 15–29.

Johannessen, A., Engedal, K. and Thorsen, K. (2016) Coping efforts and resilience among adult children who grew up with a parent with young-onset dementia: a qualitative follow-up study, *International Journal of Qualitative Studies on Health and Well-being*, 11: 30535. Available at: https://doi.org/10.3402/qhw.v11.30535.

Kilty, C., Boland, P., Goodwin, J., et al. (2019) Caring for people with young onset dementia: an interpretative phenomenological analysis of family caregivers' experiences, *Journal of Psychosocial Nursing and Mental Health Services*, 57 (11): 37–44.

Lai, M., Jeon, Y.H., McKenzie, H., et al. (2023) Journey to diagnosis of young-onset dementia: a qualitative study of people with young-onset dementia and their family caregivers in Australia, *Dementia*, 22 (5): 1097–1114.

Lockeridge, S. and Simpson, J. (2013) The experience of caring for a partner with young onset dementia: how younger carers cope, *Dementia*, 12 (5): 635–51.

Massimo, L., Evans, L.K. and Benner, P. (2013) Caring for loved ones with frontotemporal degeneration: the lived experiences of spouses, *Geriatric Nursing*, 34 (4): 302–6.

Millenaar, J.K., Bakker, C., Koopmans, R.T., et al. (2016) The care needs and experiences with the use of services of people with young-onset dementia and their caregivers: a systematic review, *International Journal of Geriatric Psychiatry*, 31 (12): 1261–76.

O'Malley, M., Parkes, J., Campbell, J., et al. (2021) Receiving a diagnosis of young onset dementia: evidence-based statements to inform best practice, *Dementia*, 20 (5): 1745–71.

Poole, C. and Patterson, T.G. (2022) Experiences and needs of children who have a parent with young onset dementia: a meta-ethnographic review, *Clinical Gerontology*, 45 (4): 750–62.

Riedijk, S., Duivenvoorden, H., Rosso, S., et al. (2008) Frontotemporal dementia: change of familial caregiver burden and partner relation in a Dutch cohort of 63 patients, *Dementia and Geriatric Cognitive Disorders*, 26 (5): 398–406.

Roach, P. and Keady, J. (2008) Younger people with dementia: time for fair play, *British Journal of Nursing*, 17 (11): 690.

Roach, P., Keady, J., Bee, P., et al. (2014) 'We can't keep going on like this': identifying family storylines in young onset dementia, *Ageing and Society*, 34 (8): 1397–1426.

Stamou, V., Fontaine, J., O'Malley, M., et al. (2021) The nature of positive post-diagnostic support as experienced by people with young onset dementia, *Aging and Mental Health*, 25 (6): 1125–33.

Stamou, V., La Fontaine, J., O'Malley, M., et al. (2022) Helpful post-diagnostic services for young onset dementia: findings and recommendations from the Angela Project, *Health and Social Care in the Community*, 30 (1): 142–53.

Stamou, V., Oyebode, J., La Fontaine, J., et al. (2023) Good practice in needs-based post-diagnostic support for people with young onset dementia: findings from the Angela Project, *Ageing and Society*. Available at: https://doi.org/10.1017/S0144686X22001362.

Svanberg, E., Stott, J. and Spector, A. (2010) 'Just helping': children living with a parent with young onset dementia, *Aging and Mental Health*, 14 (6): 740–51.

Thorsen, K. and Johannessen, A. (2023) How gender matters in demanding caring for a spouse with young-onset dementia: a narrative study, *Journal of Women and Aging*, 35 (1): 81–97.

Van Rickstal, R., Vleminck, A., Engelborghs, S., et al. (2022) A qualitative study with people with young-onset dementia and their family caregivers on advance care planning: a holistic, flexible, and relational approach is recommended, *Palliative Medicine*, 36 (6): 964–75.

Wawrziczny, E., Antoine, P., Ducharme, F., et al. (2016) Couples' experiences with early-onset dementia: an interpretative phenomenological analysis of dyadic dynamics, *Dementia*, 15 (5): 1082–99.

Wiggins, M., McEwen, A. and Sexton, A. (2023) Young-onset dementia: a systematic review of the psychological and social impact on relatives, *Patient Education and Counselling*, 107: 107585. Available at: https://doi.org/10.1016/j.pec.2022.107585.

Zeleznikow, L. and Zeleznikow, J. (2015) Supporting blended families to remain intact: a case study, *Journal of Divorce and Remarriage*, 56 (4): 317–35.

16 The well-being and identity of children and young people who have or have had a parent with young onset dementia

Pat Sikes and Mel Hall

Overview

Research-based and anecdotal evidence suggests that having a parent with a young onset dementia seems to be a very different, and more challenging, experience than having a grandparent with dementia. The material in this chapter is drawn from narrative, auto/biographical research which explored 35 children and young people's perceptions and experiences of parental young onset dementia. Maintaining positivity can be difficult for several reasons, including how young onset dementia can disrupt cultural expectations and norms, social ignorance of young onset dementia, feelings of isolation, and limited support for children and young people. Recent years have seen growing awareness of young onset dementia amongst medics, social workers and the general public, which has helped to begin to address these issues. From the stories told to the authors, the following areas/themes were most likely to be mentioned in terms of positive consequences: family and personal relationships; educational and/or career choices; making memories and living one's best life; and finding a community.

Keywords

Parental young onset dementia, educational and career choices, familial relationships, biographical disruption, peer support.

Learning points

- Children, adolescents and young adults who have a parent with a young onset dementia often experience challenges to their emotional and mental well-being that can impact their personal lives and affect their educational and future careers.
- Parental young onset dementia does not necessarily adversely affect a person's entire life.
- Parental young onset dementia is, in most cases, very different from having a grandparent with a dementia, and therefore requires specific recognition and support.
- Young onset dementia services should ideally provide support for all family members.
- Educational institutions should be made aware when a young person is living with parental young onset dementia in order to be better able to offer support through educational milestones and career decisions.
- Peer support from others experiencing parental young onset dementia is extremely valuable and young onset dementia services and dementia support groups, often online, can help advertise and direct people towards them.

Introduction

When Jan Oyebode invited us to be involved in this book, she wrote:

> *As the leading researchers on the impact of young onset dementia for children and young people, you would be the obvious people to contribute a chapter on that area, so I am emailing to ask if you would consider writing one? The only thing that might be a challenge is that, as you can see in the attached summary info, I would like this to be a positive, solution-focused text – not meaning to deny the angst and difficulties but definitely to engender hope and solutions.*

Pat had initially been motivated to research the perceptions and experiences of children and young people who have/had a parent with young onset dementia when, in his early fifties, her husband, David, began to exhibit behaviours which were later diagnosed as being due to posterior cortical atrophy and vascular dementia. At this time their children were 13 and 15 and Pat found that where they lived, and indeed throughout the country, there were hardly any resources available to give advice and support to others who were also in this situation. That this was the case is undoubtedly due to the fact that, at that time, there had been very little research seeking to understand what experiencing parental young onset dementia was like.

Eighteen years on, and nearly 3 years after David's death, Pat read Jan's invitation to her daughter, Robyn, by now herself a child and adolescent psychiatrist, who said 'good luck with that one'. As Jan had intimated, parental young onset dementia does tend to be extremely painful for children, adolescents and young adults (as indeed it is for 'grown ups' experiencing their parents' old age dementia, albeit in some significantly different ways) and Robyn was questioning to what extent, or indeed whether, it is possible to be positive.

We certainly do not underestimate the challenge. However, having spent the last 11 or so years listening to the detailed and extensive stories of 35 people aged between 6 and 35, we believe that, alongside the difficulties and pain which appear to be characteristic of parental young onset dementia, there are some aspects which others could find supportive and/or inspirational. Obviously, whilst individual family circumstances and relationships, and individual personalities and dispositions vary, we are of the view that parental young onset dementia does not necessarily negatively impact a person's entire life. Young onset dementia will, for many, and in different ways, be a defining and shaping experience, but it will also be part of the whole and needs to be considered in the context of the other things that happen to someone throughout their life course (see Nielsen et al., 2024).

What we have to say is grounded in two research projects. The first was a UK-based study funded by the Alzheimer's Society, '*The perceptions and experiences of children and young people who have a parent with dementia*' (Grant R1388585). Mel was appointed as the research officer, hence beginning our productive collaboration. The study took a narrative, auto/biographical approach to collect the stories of 24 people aged 6–31 years over a period of 18 months, with most participants being seen two or three times, providing a longitudinal element that helped illustrate how the progressive nature of parental dementia is experienced. Participants were simply asked to 'tell me your story'. The study received ethical clearance from the University of Sheffield and has, so far, resulted in 10 publications in peer-reviewed journals and one book chapter. The second, currently ongoing, project involves Pat, Mel and Professor Caroline Gelman and Lea Wolf from the Silberman School of Social Work, Hunter College, City University of New York (which granted ethical approval) and looks at how people aged from 18 to their thirties, who are at risk of rare inherited dementias, make decisions about genetic counselling and testing. This work also takes a narrative, autobiographical approach and, to date, we have spoken with 11 people from the USA and UK. All participants in both studies were self-selecting, taking the initiative to respond to calls we put out on social media, university websites and dementia organisations. The youngest children were referred by their parents, although they took the final decision to take part themselves.

In terms of making sense of what we were told we, both individually and collaboratively, engaged in a process of reading, re-reading and identifying salient themes. We did not impose an analytical framework but were led by the participants' words. For us, the following headings reflect the areas/themes that were most likely to be mentioned in terms of positive, constructive and hopeful consequences. This is not intended as a definitive, exclusive or hierarchical list:

- Family and personal relationships.
- Educational and/or career choices.
- Making memories and living one's best life.
- Finding a community.

We will now consider each of these in turn.

Family and personal relationships

When a family member develops and then is diagnosed with a dementia, the disease and diagnosis occur in the context of pre-existing relationships (Keady and Nolan, 2003; Hall and Sikes, 2018). How these relationships move forward can vary, as is the case with all relationships, regardless of health and well-being. This is simply because people and the circumstances in which they live tend to change over time. That such change is an inherent characteristic of children growing to adulthood is, in the case of parental dementia we argue, particularly pertinent, given that communication with the parent will, eventually, probably become difficult, if not impossible. In this way, dementias differ from many other illnesses, including most cancers.

On a more general level, it does seem important to point out the 'normality' of change over a lifetime because we discern a tendency in some responses and strategies to deal with dementia, to try to recapture and reproduce a person as they were before they became unwell and received a diagnosis. Sometimes this is a valuable strategy, giving pleasure to all involved – as illustrated by various musical or art therapy interventions designed to tap into areas of the brain in order to resurrect memories of music and art a person enjoyed in the past. However, such approaches can also be seen to deny that personal change in interests, motivations, tastes, relationships, and so on, is not unusual. Do you, for instance, still like, to the same degree, all the people, foods, music, books that you favoured in your teens, or have your passions and dislikes altered?

This aside, the ways in which – and extent to which – dementia may alter someone's behaviours, personality and capabilities can be challenging, making it hard for family members to continue to relate to them as they previously did. It's worth reiterating here that it is common for relationships between children and parents to change as children mature and forge their own identities, with adolescence and early adulthood often being particularly difficult. The child with a parent with dementia is unlikely to have the opportunity to 'make things right' when they emerge from adolescence into adulthood, which a number of people we spoke with regretted. And then there are the cases where relationships were already not good or may even have deteriorated, sometimes as a result of behaviours later diagnosed as due to dementia. Gelman and Greer (2011) and Gelman and Rhames (2016) describe situations in cultural groups where familial dementia care is the expectation, when girls who had been sexually abused by a father have had to look after his intimate needs. Love is not a *sine qua non* of family relationships and assuming that parents (or partners) are 'loved ones' can add to the guilt that is often experienced when there is little or no love lost.

It is worth noting here that receiving a diagnosis can be significant for family dynamics in that it can offer an explanation for out-of-character and unpleasant behaviours by the parent with young onset dementia. Some of our participants said that it helped when they understood that, as a result of the dementia, their parent 'couldn't necessarily help' what they did and said. However, they all commented to the effect that the words and the behaviours were still hurtful and had negatively impacted the relationship, at least to some degree.

> *I know he 'couldn't help it' but that makes no difference to how I felt when he said those appalling things to me. I was devastated, hurt beyond telling and it was never the same again.* (Harriet, age 23)

Those who are lucky enough to have/had a loving relationship will likely mourn what has gone:

> *It's like there's two Mums in your head … but you're constantly grieving for the old Mum because she's sort of there but not … People who have a parent who dies when they are in their teens or twenties … it's awful but then you're allowed to grieve … whereas people don't see that with this, they just think actually you should be grateful that your Mum is still here and she's not dead and it's like, 'Well, it's really not that simple', but I think admitting that to anyone is really hard because people don't expect you to think that, I don't think.* (Elizabeth, age 28)

Some will try to maintain normal family practices:

> *I still try and keep presents and things nice and I did buy a present from him to Mum and it wasn't half funny because it was a necklace with two hearts intertwined and I gave it to Dad and I said, 'You give it to Joanne' – because if I say Mum, it kind of confuses him.* (Evie, age 17)

Relationships between children and the parent with dementia often, if not usually, become less reciprocal, with the child assuming the role of the active partner in terms of, for example, visiting and initiating activities which they, at least, find enjoyable, and which also may help them cope with their pain.

> *When I visit I take him a cake from what was his favourite bakery and feed it to him – I probably shouldn't 'cos he could aspirate – but it's the only thing I can do now that I know he enjoys and I like seeing that.* (Henri, age 23)

Sometimes facing dementia together strengthens relationships between children and 'well' parents and siblings and other family members:

> *It has brought me and my Mum closer together, I mean, we are super close now, that is a good thing.* (Evie, age 17)

In families facing the possibility of inheriting dementias, relationships can be affected by decisions around whether to seek genetic testing and the consequences of the choices made. Disclosing that there is dementia within a family, let alone that it is inherited, can be difficult for a variety of reasons, and particularly when potential marriage and children become considerations. Those who spoke with us as part of the inherited dementias study talked of how supportive their partners had been.

> Researcher: *Did you worry about your relationship* [with your boyfriend] *when you realised you had a 50/50 chance of getting dementia?*
>
> Cat: *It kind of did the opposite. Because it made it a lot stronger because where you go from just dating and he'd moved in with me ... he moved in at the same time as I moved back into my family home. And, and so we put up with so much from my family because it was such a nightmare, that that really brought us a lot closer. And then during that time I was going through the genetic counselling process, and it did make me realise how committed he was to me because of a fear that someone, you know, you might end up looking after. So I think we did have a lot of these discussions like, 'What if it's positive? Are you just gonna look after me then?' and I guess, and he was like, 'Well, yeah, I'm not gonna break up with you just, just because this will happen, we'll work around it.' So actually, it made us a lot closer and probably a lot quicker, you know, I noticed how my relationship compared to my friends of the same age has moved a lot quicker than theirs did ... I was lucky to have him. I don't know what I would have done otherwise. And I think that can be an issue where if you have got unstable family relationships, and you don't have someone to lean on.* (Cat, age 33)

Sisters who at the time we spoke to them had chosen not to have genetic testing, also took strength from the shared experience:

> *Me and my sister talk about like, oh, well if we both get it we're both gonna end up in the same care home and we're gonna have adjoining rooms, so we'll be together. Like, that's important. Like, that's what we want. And both of our partners know that, and we do joke about what that will be like, we'll be the crazy sisters like ram-raiding the door to try and get out, but, you know, we must have adjoining rooms next to each other like we must be together if we both get it, we have to be together. That's what we see.* (Martha, age 32)

Educational and/or career choices

The majority of people we spoke with were in school, further or higher education (at both undergraduate and postgraduate level), although a few had started their working lives. With regard to higher education, some had made decisions about which institutions to attend or courses to follow because they wanted to remain physically close to their parents. There were those who had chosen to live at home who would have gone away had their parent not had dementia.

> *One of the reasons I'd applied to do a Master's in London was to move closer to them and I was looking forward to going home every weekend and seeing them and actually that kind of turned out not to be the case [both parents died] but I'm really enjoying it anyway.* (Erin, age 24)

> *Looking after her was killing me. I was doing so much, was trying to do my uni work as well. I had one last term. I was working part time and trying to look after her, my Dad was working full time as well … So I've given it up now, left uni officially … I hope to go back one day. It's something that I've really enjoyed and I'd hate to waste it.* (Hannah, age 25)

It is not unusual for educational and or career interests to come out of personal experiences – indeed, Pat would never have become involved in dementia-related research had her husband not received his diagnosis. Thus, parental dementia led to three participants undertaking doctoral studies in neurology and then going into further research in the field. For instance:

> *Mum's diagnosis had come through – it probably was the fact that I started to get interested in neuroscience … When you relate to stuff like that you pick up a bit more in lectures rather than fall asleep at the back … I don't think I'd be doing the PhD I'm doing if it wasn't for that.* (Blair, age 21)

And, indeed, Blair's decision to opt for genetic testing came out of her research knowledge. Sally worked for a dementia charity, again as a direct result of her father's dementia.

Making memories and living one's best life

Few of us know exactly when we are going to die. Given a terminal diagnosis it seems a not uncommon response to take the attitude that there are significant benefits to knowing that time is limited because it means that active plans to 'live one's best life' and /or to make memories that involve the parent with dementia can be worked out and put in train. Rachel, for example, was hoping 'to get married quite soon because I want mum to be there and to *be there*'.

Others talked about having children earlier than they would otherwise have done in order to provide a grandparental experience for the family. Travel often featured in this sort of thinking. For instance:

> *We spent all our money on going to Florida, Disneyland Paris, Lego Land. (Rowena, age 6 and Mary, age 7)*

> *I feel like I'm just gonna live out – we can set goals knowing what we have in mind. So for us, we're in a very privileged place … where we can travel a lot with our kids, and so we prioritise doing that and doing it now. And you know, making the life for our kids, with both of us, as rich as it can be, so that their memories with their dad are really good. And hopefully, that'll last for a really, really long time … So that's for us we've been able to set how we approach life based on this information. (Simon)*

> *I know I try and live my life to the full because you just don't know. We had some family over from Canada and Dad was like, I really want to go and I just think let's do it. Dad said we'd have to go for a month. Yesterday we had a family day in Cambridge and Dad was just like I'm not going (to Cambridge), horrible to Mum about it, but he came … and Mum said she'd struggle to get him to an airport to go to Spain, let alone Canada for a month. It's so much money but I just think we just need to book the flights, get out there. Why not? We all work so hard for retirement, for what, we don't know what's going to happen tomorrow. And like tonight, my friend texted me for dinner and part of me is shattered, and got loads to do but I'm just doing it. I do believe there are positives. (Sally)*

Finding a community

Even though recent work has raised important questions around the under-diagnosis of young onset dementia (Carter et al., 2022), it is relatively rare when compared with the number of people who are diagnosed with a dementia after the age of 65. Inherited, familial dementias (usually detected in people under 65) are even rarer. This means that those living with young onset dementia, either as a person with the condition or as a family member, can be relatively isolated. Children, adolescents and young adults with a parent with young onset dementia may never have met anyone else in their situation. Indeed, we continue to receive emails from adults across the world who have come across our papers or references to our work, and who tell us that they thought they were the only child/young person to have had this experience. Although, and as this book demonstrates, there is a growing number of young onset dementia groups, in person and online, these are primarily aimed at people with a diagnosis and/or their partners making it a lonely business for children and young people.

In 2021, Lorenzo's House (https://lorenzoshouse.org), a Chicago-based but nationally and globally minded organisation, was founded and has established an online community that gives young people a chance to meet others like them. To date, the form Lorenzo's House takes is unique and user reviews suggest it offers considerable support. A Dutch initiative offers a different unique combination of an online platform combined with Summer camps for children who have a parent with young onset dementia (see Chapter 12).

The World Health Organisation offers iSupport for dementia carers (WHO, 2019; Masterson-Algar et al., 2023) and a version aimed at children and young people is now available (https://www.youtube.com/watch?v=ielR5YD1680). Within the UK, Admiral Nurses also have expertise in helping young family members (Harrison, 2024).

For those at risk of familial Alzheimer's disease, the Dominantly Inherited Alzheimer's Network (DIAN; https://dian.wustl.edu/for-families/) and the associated Youngtimers (https://www.youngtimers.org) provide communities for those who wish to participate in research and those who do get involved can find it a lifeline:

> *Thank God for the DIAN study … we chat, I chat with all of them every now and when I'm having a really bummed out day, or have a question that I can't seem to ask anyone or no one knows the answer. But without their support, without their knowledge and without their optimism. You know, 'It's gonna be okay, things are gonna be fine, and if they're not, we're all here to support you'. That's fantastic. (JC)*

Conclusion and implications for practitioners and those supporting children and young people with a parent with young onset dementia

Illnesses of any kind, and particularly terminal conditions, can disrupt the biographies of family members as well as that of the person who is unwell (Hall and Sikes, 2019, 2020: Nielsen et al., 2024). Children and young people who have a parent with a young onset dementia are particularly brought up against this as their mother or father loses abilities and capacities that are expected of parents. Maintaining positivity can be very hard, especially as research (Gelman and Greer, 2011) suggests children and young people may keep their fears and concerns to themselves for fear of further worrying their parents and as the disease progresses, the 'well' parent in particular.

As we have noted, and as scoping reviews of the extant literature show (e.g. Chirico et al., 2021; Kates et al., 2023; Kokorelias et al., 2024), there has been relatively little research focused directly on children and young people's accounts/ stories of their perceptions and experiences of parental young onset dementia, although this does seem to be changing, not least as qualitative research gains greater acceptability and young people's voices are also given greater credence than they were in the past. There needs to be more research since the more we know about how things are for those directly affected, the better able we will be to address their needs, ameliorate the negative consequences and accentuate the positives (Kokorelias et al., 2024).

Since we started our study in October 2014, young onset dementia has achieved a far higher profile as more people in the public eye, including actors, musicians, politicians, journalists and sportspeople, have 'come out' and shared their young onset dementia diagnosis and its impact on their families. There are also films like *Still Alice* (https://en.wikipedia.org/wiki/Still_Alice#Cast) and *Supernova* (https://www.dementiauk.org/supernova-film/) that have focused on young onset dementia and whilst these have, to some extent, taken a romanticised view, they have raised awareness. And then 'human interest' stories in popular newspapers about families affected by young onset dementia, whilst often taking a sensationalist view, emphasising the youth of the person with the condition, have also become more common. It seems fair to say that it is now more generally known that dementia is not just a condition of older people.

For our participants at least, this sort of general awareness could have been helpful. With regard to the medical and social services dealing with young onset dementia, it would seem that there is also a greater degree of recognition that children, adolescents and young adults who have a parent with a young onset dementia often experience significant challenges to their emotional and mental well-being that can impact their personal lives and affect their educational and future careers. But there is considerable room for improvement and for an end to the postcode lottery whereby many families experiencing young onset dementia in the UK do not have access to specialist Admiral dementia nurses.

In this chapter, we have touched on certain of the difficulties – as well as highlighting some positive outcomes – experienced by children and young people in young onset dementia families. This leads us to say that all those with professional responsibility for these young people (including educators in all sectors, those working in young onset dementia social, medical and psychological services, and general practitioners) need to make themselves aware, or be made aware through information programmes and initial and in-service education, of their potential needs and of the support that is available. At the time of writing, such support is mainly through the voluntary and charitable sectors or 'user groups' affected by young onset dementia. This is regrettable when the consequences can have wide-ranging and 'expensive' personal and social implications.

Dementia organisations such as DEEP, the UK Network of Dementia Voices (https://www.dementiavoices.org.uk), Dementia UK (https://www.dementiauk.org) and the Young Dementia Network (https://youngdementianetwork.org/) play an important role in publicising what is available. It seems a big ask – although it is the current state of affairs in the UK at least – to expect those who are experiencing young onset dementia, whether as a person with a condition or their family members, to do the hard work of researching what support is out there. In our view, the biggest *so what?* is that if professionals in the relevant areas fail to hear and to address what people have to say about what they need, *or* do not critically consider the findings of research of various kinds (be that reported in traditional academic papers, surveys undertaken by and personal accounts reported by dementia organisations), the negative consequences on the lives and futures of young people experiencing parental young onset dementia will far outweigh the positives.

Acknowledgement

We would like to thank all those who have spoken to us about their perceptions and experiences of having a parent with young onset dementia.

References

Carter, J., Jackson, M. and Gleisner, Z. (2022) Prevalence of all cause young onset dementia and time lived with dementia: analysis of primary care health records, *Journal of Dementia Care*, 3 (3): 1–5.

Chirico, I., Ottoboni, G., Valente, M., et al. (2021) Children and young people's experiences of parental dementia: a systematic review, *Dementia*, 36 (7): 975–92.

Gelman, C. and Greer, C. (2011) Young children in early-onset Alzheimer's disease families: research gaps and emerging service needs, *American Journal of Alzheimer's Disease and Other Dementias*, 26 (1): 29–35.

Gelman, C. and Rhames, K. (2016) In their own words: the experiences and needs of children in younger-onset Alzheimer's disease and other dementias families, *Dementia*, 17 (3): 337–58.

Hall, M. and Sikes, P. (2018) How do young people 'do' family when there is a diagnosis of dementia?, *Families, Relationships and Societies*, 7 (2): 207–25.

Hall, M. and Sikes, P. (2019) 'It's just limbo land': parental dementia and young people's life courses, *The Sociological Review*, 68 (1): 242–59.

Hall, M. and Sikes, P. (2020) The biographies of children and young people who have a parent with dementia, in A.C. Sparkes (ed.) *Auto/Biography Yearbook/Review 2019*. London: BSA.

Harrison, L. (2024) *Navigating the pressures of being a young carer*, Dementia UK. Available at: https://www.dementiauk.org/news/navigating-the-pressures-of-being-a-young-carer/.

Kates, J., Pogorzelska-Maziarz, M., Uppal, H., et al. (2023) The impact of dementia family caregiving on adolescent well-being: a scoping review, *Dementia*, 22 (4): 910–28.

Keady, J. and Nolan, M. (2003) The dynamics of dementia: working together, working separately or working alone?, in M. Nolan, U. Lundh, G. Grant and J. Keady (eds.) *Partnerships in Family Care: Understanding the Caregiving Career*. Maidenhead: Open University Press.

Kokorelias, K., Nadesar, N., Bak, K., et al. (2024) The impact on employment and education of caregiving for a family member with young onset dementia: a scoping review, *Dementia*, 23 (5): 850–81.

Masterson-Algar, P., Egan, K., Flynn, G., et al. (2023) iSupport for young carers: an adaptation of an e-health intervention for young dementia carers, *International Journal of Environmental and Public Health*, 20 (1): 127. Available at: https://doi.org/10.3390/ijerph20010127.

Nielsen, M.L., Björnskov, S., Gregersen, R., et al. (2024) Participation in everyday activities among young adult relatives of parents with dementia: a qualitative study, *Dementia*, 23 (6): 949–63.

World Health Organisation (WHO) (2019) *iSupport for dementia*. Available at: https://www.who.int/publications/i/item/9789241515863.

17 Peer support

Clare Mason

Overview

This chapter explores the role of peer support groups in supporting people diagnosed with young onset dementia and the unique challenges faced by them. Young onset dementia is characterised by symptoms which begin before the age of 65 or whilst the person is of working age. People with young onset dementia experience particular psychosocial and emotional complexities. The support they need should not only be tailored to their individual and group needs but also be age-appropriate, something that is lacking in much of the support provided both locally and nationally.

Keywords

Young onset dementia, peer support, peer support group, mutual support.

Learning points

- Peer support groups should have a clear structure. Although the structure can be loose and should be led by the members, it is best to have a format which includes introductions at each meeting. This supports those with cognitive impairment to be reminded of who is who and make connections. It also gives a platform for people to share their experiences and prompts discussion.
- Peer support groups need to be based on trust and friendship. Members trust one another and from that trust comes respect. Although each person's perspective is different, and people come from different educational and socioeconomic backgrounds, members need to respect these different views and in turn, they learn from them.
- Peer support groups need good facilitation. It is often necessary to 'move people on' during discussions or activities to ensure each person has the opportunity to be heard. It is also necessary so that people hear a wide range of views and opinions and benefit from a range of experiences. This can be a sensitive issue. Consideration needs to be given to those with communication difficulties, where some people may find it difficult to formulate sentences or make themselves understood.

- Groups should offer a range of means of communication. Some people are less able to participate during group discussion, so enabling people to communicate by text, email or social media after or between meetings can give a platform for anyone who has reflected on what has been covered in a meeting and give their input.
- Consider sharing a meal together. Although this has financial implications for the group as a whole and can take up a great deal of time during meetings, it can also provide a very relaxed social activity, where much 'low-level' support is shared between members. Environmental factors need to be considered, such as the colour and type of crockery, cutlery and utensils, and support for those with any disabilities to eat their meal in a relaxed, enjoyable way.

Introduction

Living with young onset dementia presents unique challenges for people living with dementia and their family and friends. Young onset dementia affects relationships, daily routines, employment, financial aspects and emotional well-being. This chapter explores the importance and benefits of peer support for people living with young onset dementia and their families. Although it summarises existing research evidence, much of the chapter draws from the experiences and insights of Pathways, a small charity based in Yorkshire, which runs regular face-to-face and online peer support groups, as well as an annual holiday. As well as highlighting the benefits of connecting with others in a similar situation, whether that be as a person living with young onset dementia or a family member, the chapter also provides some practical tips for running peer support groups, specifically for people living with young onset dementia and their family members.

Research evidence on the benefits of peer support groups for young onset dementia

There are widespread benefits from peer support for people living with dementia, including increased confidence and independence, and the sense of (re-) establishing a meaningful valued life and being socially included (Keyes et al., 2016). The benefits appear to stem from being able to identify with, and share lived experiences with, other group members.

However, there is very little research specific to young onset dementia. Peer support emerged as one of the forms of support viewed as positive by respondents to the Angela Project survey of what those living with young onset dementia and their family supporters found helpful in terms of support

(Stamou et al., 2021). The opportunity to share with others in an accepting environment seemed to be the most helpful aspect. A review of studies on peer support for people with young onset dementia and/or a rare dementia (Sullivan et al., 2022) found just three papers evaluating open-ended ongoing support groups or networks for those with young onset dementia, published over an 18-year period (Clare et al., 2008; Davies-Quarrell et al., 2010; Phinney et al., 2016). The evaluations found that groups/networks provided a forum for social connections, listening, sharing and mutual learning. From this scant research base, it would seem that being with others who have insider experience of living with young onset dementia provides a unique and helpful environment in which to share, learn and feel accepted.

There is also some ongoing work. A major study is evaluating the impact of multi-component support groups for those living with rare dementias, led by researchers at University College London with Rare Dementia Support. There is also a study in progress (Gerritzen et al., 2022) aiming to develop guidelines for establishing *online* peer support for people living with young onset dementia. The research team's initial work (Gerritzen et al., 2023) suggests that while online support can allow people to take part from home, there are also barriers to knowing about groups and many people are wary of talking to strangers online. So, while there is little rigorous research evidence on the value of peer support groups for those living with young onset dementia at the present time, more should be known in the near future.

Pathways peer support

Structure of peer support meetings

Pathways is a peer support group, formed by a group of people with young onset dementia, who felt they did not fit into the services provided for people with dementia. The services available at that time were in the elderly care sector. Pathways has been running for over 30 years and has evolved from a group that was embedded in a larger national dementia charity, to a small, self-funded organisation. Group members support one another, both those living with dementia and their partner-carers. Pathways holds monthly in-person meetings, online (Zoom) meetings, social activities and an annual supported holiday. All activities are chosen by the group. It also has a large social media-based group. Pathways is part of the DEEP Network (Dementia Engagement and Empowerment Project), which connects numerous groups across the country and provides a variety of dementia-related resources (see https://www.dementiavoices.org.uk/).

The lead facilitator of the Pathways group, who is also the chapter author, took on the facilitator role by default, after stepping in to help out when the previous facilitator was unwell. As an experienced facilitator and trainer, I am familiar with turn-taking, ensuring those less confident can speak, and managing time-keeping. All these are essential aspects of the role. Other group members take on different tasks, such as Sue, who organises trips and outings and Michael, who lives with dementia and is a trustee.

The Pathways peer support meetings, although informal, have a loose structure. This involves being greeted with drinks and an introduction by the lead facilitator who formally welcomes people. Each person at the meeting is then asked to introduce themselves, or 'pass' if they do not feel confident in speaking out or if communication is less fluent. This is done at each meeting to compensate for memory difficulties. Notices are then given, followed by the sharing of food. An activity usually follows which often includes a guest speaker, presentation or activity, such as photography, a quiz or discussion. These activities are chosen by group members, supported by volunteers. Meetings usually end with the sharing of upcoming events and information, thanks from the facilitator to those who have attended, and shared camaraderie whilst clearing away.

Functions of peer support meetings

Generational experiences related to young onset dementia

As noted throughout this book, there are many differences between the difficulties experienced by those living with young onset dementia and those who develop dementia at a later age. Often those living with dementia developed at a later age have already retired. Those living with young onset dementia are usually still in employment when difficulties develop but very few are able to continue working. Leaving employment has a huge impact on the income of the individual and their family, as well as on the identity that employment gives us, the sense of purpose, status in life and a reason to get out of bed each day. As people age and retire from working, many become less physically active but people with young onset dementia are generally still physically active. Those in the Pathways group often discuss the fact they still have dreams, plans and aspirations, something they can share with their peers.

Social contact

Young onset dementia also affects family dynamics and social relationships. Many people in the Pathways group, living with young onset dementia, experienced the loss of many friends who deserted them after hearing the news of their diagnosis. Sandra and Ian described their feelings about sharing news of Ian's diagnosis:

> *We haven't told our friends yet; we've only told a couple of close members of the family. We don't want people to start treating us any differently.* (Sandra)

> *I told one mate, and he hasn't been near since, not a word. It's put me off telling anybody else, so we just haven't. Now we don't know what to do for the best.* (Ian)

Another couple shared:

> *We thought we'd retire, get on a plane and go somewhere nice. It's put a stop to that. Everything's changed.*

In this situation, peer support groups can offer a valuable place for social contact.

Insights for partners

This also highlights that the diagnosis of one person in a relationship has a huge impact on the other and brings about a shift in the balance of power within that relationship.

The unique challenge posed by young onset dementia often creates a significant power imbalance in relationships where one person is affected. This imbalance can be confusing and emotionally draining for family carers who may struggle to keep up with the continuous change taking place. Peer support within the Pathways young onset dementia group provides family carers with valuable insights into dementia.

Benefits of peer support groups

A support group provides a space for shared experiences, strengthening understanding and empathy amongst members. Within group meetings and beyond, there is empathy amongst group members, and support for those struggling in similar circumstances; members exchange ideas, suggest coping strategies and provide emotional support. This collective knowledge not only serves as an educational resource, but also empowers members to navigate the complexities of dementia, with a sense of solidarity and resilience.

There are many known benefits of attending a peer support group for people diagnosed with young onset dementia. The following have been gathered from those who attend the Pathways group.

Emotional support

Peer support groups provide a platform for people living with young onset dementia and their families to share their experiences, thoughts, emotions and the many challenges experienced along the way, openly and honestly, without fear of judgement. Knowing others have intuitive understanding, through having gone through a similar situation, brings much comfort to people with dementia and family carers alike.

Connecting with others who are going through similar experiences can create a sense of belonging and validation; validation through being believed, with the acknowledgement of others who have experienced very similar situations. Peer support groups offer a safe space to express fears, frustrations and worries, without the anxiety of being judged. This can bring about a feeling of comfort, emotional well-being and resilience. The Pathways group is filled with joy and laughter. The group feel there is much humour in dementia, providing people are laughing together, laughing with one another and not at another person's expense. Michael who lives with young onset dementia said:

> *I only came in to ask for directions and I've been coming ever since!* (Michael)

Sandra and Ian, who were new members of the Pathways young onset dementia support group, said:

> *When we mentioned at our first meeting that we'd not told many people about Ian's diagnosis, it felt good to say it out loud, a few of them [members] said we did right not to tell anyone, but most of them said the sooner we tell people, the better, and our true friends would understand. We've since told a couple of close friends who we really trust and to be honest, they've been great, and we're glad we did.* (Sandra)

Longstanding members, both those with dementia and current and former carers and volunteers, welcome new members into the group. It can be a daunting experience to begin with, attending a peer support group for the first time and the emotion of sharing details of a recent diagnosis can be like 'shedding skin'.

Often, when new members share their story at their first meeting, emotions are raw and often spill out without warning. These emotions are felt by the group as a whole but are unchecked and allowed to flow. It is seen by many members as part of the 'healing process'. Group members often share experiences and feelings they would not – or have not – shared with anyone else, including close family, for fear of being judged or upsetting the other person. Peer support groups often provide the safe space that people feel they have been denied since diagnosis. The group feel that sharing experiences not only enables people to find solutions to current or potential problems, but to 'say it out loud' can help, particularly in the process of telling others such as family members, friends and neighbours. Michael, who lives with a rare form of young onset dementia, said:

> *I was originally sent to a day centre, but it was for older people. Even though I live on my own, I was locked in and not allowed out. I'd come on my own and went home on my own, but they still wouldn't let me out. It was full of old people, and we had to throw a ball to one another and say our name when we caught it. It was so childish, I hated it. When I first went to Pathways, I didn't know what to expect but we were all a similar age, most of us had had to stop working and a few of us had lost our driving licenses too, so we all understood how it felt. I didn't feel quite so alone after that.* (Michael)

Learning that others have very similar stories and have survived to live an active life can help people feel less afraid about the future.

Shared knowledge

Through mutual peer support, group members gain access to a wealth of collective, experiential knowledge. Members also learn new coping strategies from hearing the insights of others in a similar situation. Members often share practical tips on how to live life to the full, how to use technology or access information, and where to go for further support, advice and information. This new knowledge often provides hope and optimism for the future, something which is often lost when the diagnosis is first received. It is often only through meeting others who are living as well as they can with dementia that this realisation becomes a reality.

Members have shared information on gadgets and technology that makes life easier to live with dementia, such as using smart phones, smart watches and automated medication dispensers. Unlike many older people with dementia, most people with young onset dementia already use computers and smart phones. Information on useful apps, websites, easy-to-use phones, TV remote controls and kitchen equipment is regularly shared and valued by those living with a diagnosis (see Chapter 4 on technology to support people living with young onset dementia).

The group has close links with the Centre for Applied Dementia Studies at the University of Bradford. Students, researchers and educators often attend meetings, with a joint sharing of information and learning. Members can learn about research studies, and many have become Expert by Experience members, study participants and co-investigators, such as in the ongoing DYNAMIC study: DYNAMIC stands for Dementia at Younger Ages: Mapping Ideal Care. It is a study funded through the National Institute for Health and Care Research. The study is looking to improve current social care practice and resources for people living with young onset dementia. A person living with young onset dementia and a family supporter of a person with young onset dementia from Pathways have become members of the project management team for the study (see also Chapter 11, on being involved in research).

An example of using the pool of knowledge of Pathways members to a useful purpose is that one of the Pathways support group meetings was attended by a PhD student. James, the student, spoke to the group about his research proposal, looking at using artificial intelligence headsets linked to the memories of the wearer, with the purpose of triggering positive memories to improve well-being. The group were able to try the headset and give feedback what they thought of the project. As the individuals have gained confidence in speaking in front of one another, and feel most confident when together as a group, they felt able to give James open, honest feedback. The feedback not only gave James ideas of how to carry out his project, but also how to communicate with people with dementia in a way that enables them to understand and engage with the topic. The group also learned about new technologies and felt pride in being able to share their experiences and opinions with James and shape his research from the beginning.

The mutual sharing of knowledge not only provides a platform for learning but can break down barriers and stereotypes, often perceived about professionals or people with young onset dementia alike. For example, many group members have experienced difficulties with language and verbal communication and regularly seek advice from a speech and language therapist at the Centre. Members were also able to be involved in working with them to write national guidelines for the Royal College of Speech and Language Therapists. Julie Hayden, one of the members, writes:

> *The best groups are about fostering friendships between the members which can then be built upon to enable those people to create greater awareness and begin to influence others. Groups need effective facilitation, though this can be very difficult, as always there will be stronger voices who are more easily heard. Sometimes, due to shyness, or acquired problems with speech or word finding, people don't feel sufficiently confident to make their voices heard and accommodation needs to be made for those quieter voices to be a part of the group, as we all benefit from what they have to share. Everyone's experience is equally valid.* (Julie Hayden)

Reduced isolation and stigma

A key theme at Pathways young onset support group meetings is the stigma which surrounds dementia, particularly young onset dementia. People are often faced with comments such as 'you can't have dementia, you're not old enough' or 'you don't look like you've got dementia'. Worse than that are the jokes, such as 'I bet it's not so bad having dementia, you probably don't remember you've got it'. Similarly, the patronising tone taken by those without a diagnosis, a tone which is more commonly used towards children, can offend. This is also the case when a person talks to the person's spouse or partner, rather than the person with dementia. This all adds to the stigma and feelings of isolation. Being part of a peer support group can help reduce these feelings, as members meet others who look, sound and behave just like them. Their shared experiences with their many similarities bring them together, preventing them from feeling quite so alone.

The group has discussed how the fact that they still wear jeans, wear make-up, use a mobile phone or in some cases drive has been a cause for others to question their diagnosis. These doubts are felt to be rarely expressed to older people living with dementia. Members have spoken of feeling comforted by the knowledge that others in the group have experienced similar stigmatising comments, and they feel more able to 'shrug it off' through knowing they're not alone.

Being part of wider networks

Creating opportunities for mutual peer support requires establishing support networks. This can be done through partnerships with other local organisations and community groups, or online platforms. Ensuring that these opportunities are age-appropriate is important for those living with young onset dementia, so it is vital to seek the views and ideas of members to guide this.

As a group, Pathways has become part of a national network of peer support groups, run by the DEEP Network. Being part of the network has brought numerous benefits, including support for members and facilitators, sharing ideas and making connections nationally, as well as taking part in projects such as film-making: a project providing a new opportunity for many, a joint activity with lasting memories, and a way of educating others about young onset dementia and the benefits of joining a young onset dementia peer support group.

The use of Zoom for online meetings has also resulted in a wider spread network than was the case when Pathways only held face-to-face meetings. This came about during the COVID-19 pandemic and has since continued. This has enabled the group to connect with people living further afield and welcome them into their 'online peer support group'. The group also created an online peer support group on Facebook, the social media platform. Most posts are created by people living with young onset dementia and membership is worldwide, with over 650 members.

It is important to offer a variety of ways for people to obtain support, such as face-to-face or online meetings, telephone support, email support or support through social media. This not only enables people from a larger geographical area to access groups, but also meets the differing needs of a wide range of people.

Engaging professionals

At Pathways meetings, professionals from a variety of organisations attend each month. The group see the benefits as two-fold. It enables group members to learn about the work of different organisations and tap into the resources and services they provide. It also enables the group to have direct contact with professionals they wouldn't usually meet in such an informal setting, rather than at a diagnostic appointment, consultation or other appointments. It can often feel easier to ask a question at a group meeting, rather than on a one-to-one basis, which feels far more personal and direct. It also helps the group 'spread the word' about the needs of people with young onset dementia, demonstrating that people with young onset are very different from those who develop dementia at a later age, and that people with young onset dementia are human beings and can still contribute to life in a meaningful way, have dreams, aspirations, opinions and feelings.

Having professionals attend meetings regularly can not only offer valuable expertise and guidance to group members, but also offer continual learning opportunities for volunteers. For the Pathways groups, inviting professionals to attend meetings has led to some invaluable partnerships, such as that with the Admiral Nursing team in Bradford. At least two Admiral Nurses, who work with people with dementia and their carers, attend each meeting. This has enabled the team to learn about the needs of people living with young onset dementia first hand, and hear from their family members the difficulties and challenges they face as they develop their own work in this area.

Social activities

The activities of the group extend beyond the monthly online or in-person sessions, to social activities, outings and events. These events include the ordinary social activities people regularly enjoyed before receiving a diagnosis, which many now find challenging, due to the disabling nature of society. For example, many members discuss how a regular visit to the pub for a drink, food or to meet friends can become difficult due to the challenges of managing money, being able to easily communicate an order of drinks or food, being able to engage and follow conversation with friends, or locate and use the toilets, which are often difficult to find in dimly lit corridors with poor signage and confusing layouts. Many members have also experienced difficulties when attempting to attend social events with friends who do not live with dementia.

Members feel it is important to continue to carry out social activities and hobbies for as long as possible, where physical and cognitive abilities allow. However, often the activities on offer for people with dementia are felt to be inappropriate, patronising and childish for those with young onset dementia. Pathways group activities are chosen using a consensus approach; ideas are put forward by members, either during group meetings or by email, text or social media message, to allow those less confident at speaking out within the group a chance to have their views and ideas heard. A volunteer then investigates accessibility, price, distance, public transport and parking; he or she then feeds back to the group and a joint decision is made about event type, date and venue.

The group attend a local bowling alley and enjoy a game of ten-pin bowling, an activity people with dementia have been able to excel at and participate in with family carers and volunteers. Where older people may not be physically able to participate in such activities, most members of the Pathways group remain physically fit and enjoy the normality of outings such as these. The group also found that people with dementia, volunteers, and former and current family carers were able to participate equally in this activity. On each occasion, a person with dementia has won, with much celebration, adding to the enjoyment of the occasion and feelings of achievement for all.

Group holidays

The group also go on an annual holiday together. This came from a group discussion not long after Pathways had formed. Group members were asked what they missed doing since diagnosis. Many members mentioned holidays, and how these had become a thing of the past. Airports, ferry terminals and train stations are difficult at the best of times but when one member of the family has dementia, this can become tremendously difficult. Adding to the challenges is the fact that people living with young onset dementia, due to their young age and the fact that they usually don't 'look ill', are judged to be 'not doing their bit' in helping with things such as carrying luggage, supporting younger children, putting suitcases on baggage carousels or security desks. This can lead to comments or uncomfortable situations with other passengers, transport and holiday company staff. Similarly, hotels, particularly in foreign countries, can be very stressful places; they often have long corridors, painted white with numerous doors, all looking the same. It's very easy to get lost, or locked out of a hotel room, and it's then hard to explain any disorientation to another person or member of hotel staff, if they don't understand dementia and don't speak the same language.

Barry, a group member with dementia had an extremely frightening experience in France. Barry's wife Jenny explained:

> *We were on holiday in Paris, staying in a hotel. Barry got up to go to the toilet in the night. He thought he was going to the toilet door but instead of the toilet door, he went out of the hotel room door and of course it locked behind him. He found himself in the corridor, went the wrong way and got lost. Of course, all the corridors look the same, all the room doors look the same and he couldn't remember our room number. He used to speak fluent French but was starting to have difficulties with his language and couldn't make himself understood and the hotel staff couldn't understand him. It was very frightening and of course he didn't look like he had anything wrong with him. We soon realised we couldn't risk going abroad again, something we'd always both loved doing. (Jenny)*

Following these discussions, the group decided to hold an annual supported holiday, which has become a vital part of the support group's offer. Group members, including people with dementia, family carers and volunteers travel together to a hotel by coach. Volunteers liaise with the hotel long before the actual holiday takes place, ensuring that those with additional needs can be accommodated. Accessible bathrooms and bedrooms are provided for those with mobility needs. Sleeping arrangements are also considered and arranged. Many couples where one person has young onset dementia still wish to share a double bed, whilst others have ceased having intimate relationships or sleeping together for various reasons, maybe due to disability, continence issues or disrupted sleep-wake patterns. Walk-in showers, which are often in limited supply in older, more traditional hotels, are prioritised for those with mobility or visuospatial difficulties. Proximity to lifts is another consideration.

Prior to the holiday, the group put forward ideas for things they want to do during their stay, and vote on the most popular, after volunteers have researched prices, accessibility and suitability. A joint itinerary is planned, led by members' ideas and preferences, with group activities and free time planned in. Additional signage is put up inside the hotel to help members locate their rooms, toilets and facilities, and hotel staff are given information on group and individual needs. Entertainment is provided by the hotel and members can participate or 'do their own thing'.

The group has learned that the social activities, holidays, events and outings strengthen connections between members, providing opportunities for conversation away from the formality of meetings. The social activities also break the monotony of daily routines and create lasting memories for individuals, couples and the group as a whole. Julie Hayden, who attended the Pathways holidays in 2021 and 2022, writes:

Since my diagnosis of young onset, I have become increasingly involved in all aspects of activism. That means I am very busy the whole year round with little time for myself. However, for a few days each year the Pathways group gives me the opportunity to get away with a group of friends for a much-needed break. Assistance is available from the volunteers, but the beauty of the break is that we are allowed to just relax and be ourselves. Most supported holidays are very costly, yet the team at Pathways work very hard to greatly discount the price and so make it affordable. The health benefits are enormous to me as this represents my only chance to have a complete break from work. As I live alone, most of my meals are alone, but for the duration of the holiday I can enjoy socialising with my friends over the mealtimes. (Julie Hayden)

Karen, a family carer who has attended several Pathways holidays, wrote:

We were apprehensive before we went as we were going with people we didn't know, and with dementia it can be difficult to socialise with people not familiar with the illness, but with Pathways holiday this was not a problem. Everyone had different symptoms, but everyone was included in everything that was going on. Lots of things to do, but you don't have to take part if you want time to yourself or just to rest. Always felt included and could relax much more than on a holiday on our own. Got lots from talking to others, realising we are not alone. (Karen)

Financial considerations

Due to the disabilities young onset dementia presents and the fact that when symptoms begin many people are still working and must give up their jobs, finances become very restricted. The loss of a wage within the couple, family or for an individual is keenly felt, having a huge impact on paying energy and food bills, paying off debts such as mortgages, credit cards, loans, etc. (see Chapter 6 for more on financial issues). Often the family carer must also give up their own job or reduce their working hours to support the person with young onset. This can hugely restrict what a couple or person living alone can afford to do, such as travel to and from meetings, eat out, take part in social activities and hobbies, or go on holiday. Often, people with young onset dementia are not eligible for benefits and cannot access private pensions and finances.

Due to these financial difficulties, all Pathways activities are subsidised by the joint fundraising efforts of the group; they do not receive any government funding, so fundraising is vital. To avoid embarrassment, members are asked to let group volunteers know if they have difficulties paying for any activities and no judgements are made when funds are provided to pay for any individual to attend activities or events. Food is also provided at each meeting, and this is subsidised by group funds, with provision of food to be taken home at the end of meetings to enable members to have a meal the following day. Some members of the group previously reported having used local food banks due to financial difficulties, so the provision of food during meetings is welcomed by members. Due to the social aspect of eating together, this also provides a platform for relaxed interaction with one another, where lower level, informal peer support is gained, by people living with dementia and family carers alike.

Conclusions

In conclusion, young onset peer support groups can play a pivotal role in addressing the unique challenges faced by individuals diagnosed with young onset dementia. In this chapter, we have given detailed examples of the experiences of the Pathways charity young onset dementia group, based in Bradford. These show that through a blend of emotional support, shared experiences, knowledge sharing and inclusive activities, peer support groups can provide real support and hope for those navigating the complicated landscape of young onset dementia.

By providing a safe space where individuals can openly express their emotions, concerns and triumphs without judgement, peer support groups can foster a sense of belonging and validation that is vital for emotional well-being. Peer support groups can also provide a valuable link to others living with young onset dementia nationally, through membership of the DEEP Network and access to a wealth of resources available online.

Through sharing practical coping strategies and insights, peer support groups can empower their members to lead fulfilling lives and harness the resources available to them. Through the power of shared knowledge, individuals learn to overcome the obstacles presented by young onset dementia, guiding them towards a future filled with hope, resilience and optimism, something felt to be missing in many other services.

Support groups stand as a common strength against the isolation and stigma often associated with dementia. By bringing together individuals who share similar experiences and challenges, peer support groups unpick stereotypes and replace them with a sense of camaraderie and understanding. This collective effort not only reduces feelings of isolation but also paves the way for a more inclusive and empathetic society that sees the worth and potential of each person, regardless of their diagnosis.

A good way for peer support groups to continually learn and grow, is for them to collaborate with professionals from various fields. Through these interactions, both members and professionals can gain valuable insights and forge partnerships that contribute to improving the lives of those living with young onset dementia. These connections not only benefit the individuals directly involved but also have the potential to foster a broader understanding of the condition and its impact, as well as paving the way for a better life for those developing dementia in the future.

By extending their reach to encompass social activities, outings and holidays, peer support groups can create lasting memories and strengthen the bonds between their members. Dedication by those running peer support groups to providing financial support and ensuring accessibility ensures that all individuals, regardless of their financial circumstances, can benefit from these enriching experiences.

Health and care professionals and those living with young onset dementia and their families can benefit from the details given in this chapter, to consider what is offered locally for those in their area and can feel motivated and informed about how to set up peer support if it is currently lacking.

So what does this mean in practice?

If you are living with young onset dementia

The benefits described here may encourage you to attend a peer support group.

If you are a family member of someone with young onset dementia

This chapter may help motivate you to consider attending a peer support group either together with a partner with a diagnosis or separately.

If you are a professional supporting people with young onset dementia

This chapter will help you consider how you might facilitate dementia peer support groups, particularly those which also involve current and former family carers.

If you facilitate a peer support group

Considering that people have a range of communication needs, you can play a key role in ensuring people have enough time to process what has been said and formulate what they are going to say and say this out loud to the group. You can play a key role in ensuring the voice of people with young onset dementia is heard in group discussions, including those less confident in speaking in large groups. You play a vital role in ensuring a range of different views can be heard, in a non-judgemental, trusting environment, supporting a balance of seriousness and fun.

References

Clare, L., Rowlands, J.M. and Quin, R. (2008) Collective strength: the impact of developing a shared social identity in early-stage dementia, *Dementia*, 7 (1): 9–30.

Davies-Quarrell, V., Higgins, A., Higgins, J., et al. (2010) The ACE approach: promoting well-being and peer support for younger people with dementia, *Journal of Mental Health Training, Education and Practice*, 5 (3): 41–50.

Gerritzen, E., McDermott, O. and Orrell, M. (2022) Development of best practice guidance on online peer support for people with young onset dementia: protocol for a mixed methods study, *JMIR Research Protocols*, 11 (7): e38379. Available at: https://doi.org/10.2196/38379.

Gerritzen, E.V., McDermott, O. and Orrell, M. (2023) Online peer support: views and experiences of people with young onset dementia, *Aging and Mental Health*, 27 (12): 2386–94.

Keyes, S.E., Clarke, C.L., Wilkinson, H., et al. (2016) 'We're all thrown in the same boat …': a qualitative analysis of peer support in dementia care, *Dementia*, 15 (4): 560–77.

Phinney, A., Kelson, E., Baumbusch, J., et al. (2016) Walking in the neighbourhood: performing social citizenship in dementia, *Dementia*, 15 (3): 381–94.

Stamou, V., La Fontaine, J., O'Malley, M., et al. (2021) The nature of positive post-diagnostic support as experienced by people with young onset dementia, *Aging and Mental Health*, 25 (6): 1125–33.

Sullivan, M.P., Williams, V., Grillo, A., et al. (2022) Peer support for people living with rare or young onset dementia: an integrative review, *Dementia*, 21 (8): 2700–26.

18 Concluding thoughts

George Rook

This book is about many of the challenging issues facing those who find themselves developing symptoms of dementia under the age of 65. The title includes solutions, and we hope that the numerous key learning points in each chapter speak for themselves.

In Part 1, the authors consider issues connected first and foremost with maintaining autonomy, having control over your life. Our authors have discussed diagnosis and post-diagnosis contact with healthcare professionals. The need for emotionally sensitive behaviours and attitudes at these difficult times is overpowering, but the reality for many is that such sensitivity and understanding are often absent. This needs to be addressed in training and performance reviews, and in the culture of services.

We have explained some of the rarer forms of dementia, to help those working in health and social care to understand them. The common stereotype of what dementia 'looks like' needs to be challenged and better understood. The term 'Memory Service' is in itself a misnomer and misleading, as memory loss is not the dominant symptom in many dementias. Losing keys, that commonly quoted rejoinder from GPs, is perhaps classic memory loss. But not finding words is a form of memory loss; forgetting how to use a knife and fork, again a form of memory loss. Unsteady gait, perceptual confusion, behavioural changes, sensory changes – these are the stuff of most people's dementia. Health and care professionals need to learn that this is especially the case in young onset dementia. Again, training needs to change. And perhaps service names should too.

Technology is ever changing, so of course any written document on what is available will soon be out of date. Nevertheless, our chapter on technology demonstrates that there are many ways in which using technology, simple or complex, can be really helpful in enabling continued well-being and independence. We may joke about Alexa or other voices, but they provide really useful practical reminders and information. Equally, technology can enable distant friends and family to keep an eye on a person so that help is sought when needed. One lesson from this is that everyone who is diagnosed should be supported to get, learn and use the technologies that are out there. My (George) personal hobbyhorse is that on diagnosis everyone should be given and trained in how to use a smart tablet of some sort. Communication, reminders, purchases, entertainment, factual information – all available with a few taps and clicks. Of course, many people diagnosed under 66 will already have these skills, but some do not. Equity demands that we enable these people, not ignore them.

The chapter on cognitive rehabilitation demonstrates an evidence-based approach that helps people with dementia to continue to do things that are important to them. It is a set of very specific techniques and is not available in many areas yet, as it requires specific training. However, foundation level training is available free within the UK and internationally. It can help a person to maximise their cognitive capacity and/or help them to get around problems caused by cognitive impairment, and enable them to continue to be socially active, which is so important in slowing down symptom development.

The legal and financial implications of young onset dementia are discussed in full. These often have an enormous impact on those diagnosed and their families. Where to get information? How to find out what you don't know? (the Donald Rumsfeld question). A booklet at diagnosis does not cut the mustard here. We hope our chapter will fill a gap, for professionals as well as for those affected by the dementia.

And a voice in planning services? Oh, yes please! Co-design or co-production should be a given. Nothing about us without us! Why would health professionals not want to provide what the people in their care need? As with the need for emotional intelligence at diagnosis, healthcare professionals need to see through the eyes of those with dementia and their carers. They need to walk in our shoes. Those who have personal experience of dementia often provide the most understanding and useful services. So work with those you serve. It's easy – just ask them. Sit down with them. Understand them. Listen. Professionals have professional knowledge; people with dementia and carers have personal knowledge. So work together to provide the best possible services.

In Part 2, our authors write about identity, that sense of self and purpose and agency that is essential to the human condition. The differences in cultural attitudes and of health and care experiences in minority social or cultural groups are often talked about but rarely effectively addressed. The lessons in the chapter on the Indigenous population in Canada can be applied anywhere and everywhere. To work with minority cultures, indeed any culture, you need to understand the culture – and the people. Equity of care is not about providing the same for everyone; it is about providing what each individual needs, and making it possible for them to get good care on their terms. This requires knowledge, understanding and a real commitment to help, rather than box-ticking. Once again we return to the need for emotional intelligence. 'Seek first to understand, then to be understood.'

Legal and cultural attitudes to employing people living with dementia, at any age, are at best questionable, and often negative. Employers usually see a person who cannot work efficiently for them, and that their first course of action must be to get rid of them. No doubt this varies from company to company, but instead of seeing people living with dementia as an asset that needs a little looking after, employers often see them as a liability. This needs to change, and clearly the law as it stands, at least in the UK, is rarely observed in practice. Often small adjustments enable people to continue to work, perhaps part-time or with reduced tasks. We hope that the chapter on employment provides the knowledge and confidence that people need when diagnosed to work with their employer and negotiate a way forward.

Identity is closely bound up with employment, especially for those with regular employment and financial responsibilities. Similarly, meaningful activity, whether paid or not, is important for retaining identity and purpose. It provides social contact and interaction, and a sense of doing something worthwhile, and is a major contributor to well-being. Once again, the label of dementia can often be seen as a label of incapacity, of being no use to anyone any longer, and in fact a burden. We hope that this book addresses the need to change this deep-seated societal view.

Involvement in research related to dementia can be a worthwhile activity and has the extra benefit of providing researchers with lived experience to inform their work. The recent Dementia Enquirers project has demonstrated that people with young (or older) onset dementia can carry out research for themselves or work with academic teams as co-researchers. Thus not just being subjects in research, though that can be interesting and is essential for researchers, but actually working on an equal footing with research teams. The awareness and advantages of this are spreading across academic institutions.

We have not forgotten the role of family and friend unpaid carers in this book. As is often said, carers need to maintain their own health and identity if they are to provide support over the long term in sometimes challenging circumstances. We know that carers in the UK often find it very difficult to access support due to the myriad patterns of red tape and rules that govern the system. We know of stories about the only way for carers to get help is to declare that they cannot go on; but this is an inhuman way to solve the problem, and results in unbearable guilt and pain. Society must find better ways (and more funding) to provide the support our carers need. They are, after all, people who have a right to their own lives and choices; we should not take advantage of their loving commitment to providing care.

In Part 3, we addressed the importance of being socially connected, within and without the family. Social connection is a human need. Interaction with others uses many areas of the brain and helps to keep skills intact.

It is worth noting here that in the UK, up to a third of people living with dementia live on their own. They may have neighbours or distant family members to look out for them, but day to day they may have different needs to remain independent. Nonetheless, in this section our chapter authors address the central place of family relationships. Dementia is commonly said to affect the whole family. Families are probably more affected by young onset dementia than by later onset. In young onset dementia, the family may include older parents, young people still at home and a couple of working age (the person diagnosed and a partner or spouse). Family-centred support can be important to sustain relationships and help families maintain that sense of togetherness in the face of the unwelcome visitor of dementia. In the UK, there is a growing realisation that there should be specialist young onset services to support people and families with these unique needs, and it is our hope that these will grow and spread.

Some families of people with young onset dementia still have children in education, perhaps very young, who witness their parent's illness during a formative time of life, often assisting with care and at the same experiencing instability and distress. Being positive and finding hope can be difficult but sometimes adversity draws families together or strengthens young people's relationships. Children of those with young onset dementia may in the long run make career choices that draw from their experiences to help others.

Social connection provides opportunities to validate a person as a worthwhile individual with agency to make decisions for themselves. People living with young onset dementia told us that peer groups provide the best form of support for them, because others with dementia 'get it'. There's no pussyfooting around the subject, or talking over them, and people find they just have fun or a good moan and find out most of the information they need at these groups. But there are way too few, so we need more. Everyone with young onset dementia should have the opportunity to join a peer group.

Finally, this book is intended to provide insight *and* solutions. While readers can of course deduce for themselves solutions to some of the problems outlined, we hope that our chapter authors' learning points will be useful and lead to improved recognition of young onset dementia and better support for all those affected.

Index